D0713826

Legal Issues Confronting Today's Nursing Faculty

A CASE STUDY APPROACH

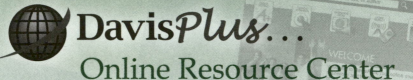

Davis*Plus*...
Online Resource Center

Davis*Plus* is your online source for a wealth of learning resources and teaching tools, as well as electronic and mobile versions of our products.

STUDENTS

Unlimited FREE access.
No password.
No registration.
No fee.

INSTRUCTORS

Upon Adoption.
Password-protected library of title-specific, online course content.

Visit http://davisplus.fadavis.com

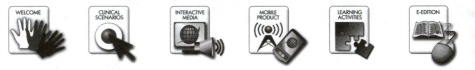

WELCOME · CLINICAL SCENARIOS · INTERACTIVE MEDIA · MOBILE PRODUCT · LEARNING ACTIVITIES · E-EDITION

Explore more online resources from F.A.Davis...

DAVIS'S DRUG GUIDE.com
powered by
Unbound Medicine®

www.drugguide.com

is Davis's Drug Guide Online, the complete Davis's Drug Guide for Nurses® database of over 1,100 monographs on the web.

Taber's Online
powered by
Unbound Medicine®

www.tabersonline.com

delivers the power of Taber's Cyclopedic Medical Dictionary on the web. Find more than 60,000 terms, 1,000 images, and more.

DAVIS'S Laboratory and Diagnostic Tests with Nursing Implications
powered by
Unbound Medicine®

www.LabDxTest.com

is the complete database for Davis's Comprehensive Handbook of Laboratory and Diagnostic Tests with Nursing Implications online. Access hundreds of detailed monographs.

www.FADavis.com

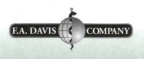

F.A. DAVIS COMPANY

Legal Issues Confronting Today's Nursing Faculty

A CASE STUDY APPROACH

Mary Ellen Smith Glasgow,
PhD, RN, ACNS–BC

H. Michael Dreher, PhD, RN

Carl Oxholm III, JD, MPP

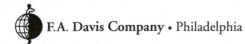
F.A. Davis Company • Philadelphia

F. A. Davis Company
1915 Arch Street
Philadelphia, PA 19103
www.fadavis.com

Copyright © 2012 by F. A. Davis Company

All rights reserved. This book is protected by copyright. No part of it may be reproduced, stored in a retrieval system, or transmitted in any form or by any means, electronic, mechanical, photocopying, recording, or otherwise, without written permission from the publisher.

Printed in the United States of America

Last digit indicates print number: 10 9 8 7 6 5 4 3 2 1

Publisher, Nursing: Joanne Patzek DaCunha, RN, MSN
Director of Content Development: Darlene D. Pedersen
Project Editor: Jamie M. Elfrank
Electronic Project Editor: Tyler Baber
Manager of Art & Design: Carolyn O'Brien

As new scientific information becomes available through basic and clinical research, recommended treatments and drug therapies undergo changes. The author(s) and publisher have done everything possible to make this book accurate, up to date, and in accord with accepted standards at the time of publication. The author(s), editors, and publisher are not responsible for errors or omissions or for consequences from application of the book, and make no warranty, expressed or implied, in regard to the contents of the book. Any practice described in this book should be applied by the reader in accordance with professional standards of care used in regard to the unique circumstances that may apply in each situation. The reader is advised always to check product information (package inserts) for changes and new information regarding dose and contraindications before administering any drug. Caution is especially urged when using new or infrequently ordered drugs.

Library of Congress Cataloging-in-Publication Data

Glasgow, Mary Ellen Smith.
  Legal issues confronting today's nursing faculty : a case study approach / Mary Ellen Smith Glasgow, H. Michael Dreher, Carl Oxholm III.
    p. ; cm.
  Includes bibliographical references.
  ISBN 978-0-8036-2489-4 (pbk. : alk. paper)
  I. Dreher, Heyward Michael. II. Oxholm, Carl. III. Title.
  [DNLM: 1. Education, Nursing—legislation & jurisprudence—United States. WY 33 AA1]
  LC-classification not assigned
  610.73—dc23   2011030987

Authorization to photocopy items for internal or personal use, or the internal or personal use of specific clients, is granted by F. A. Davis Company for users registered with the Copyright Clearance Center (CCC) Transactional Reporting Service, provided that the fee of $.25 per copy is paid directly to CCC, 222 Rosewood Drive, Danvers, MA 01923. For those organizations that have been granted a photocopy license by CCC, a separate system of payment has been arranged. The fee code for users of the Transactional Reporting Service is: 8036-2489-4/12 0 + $.25.

To my husband, Tom, whose love and support I cherish
MESG

To my brother Donald
and
to Drs. Townsend, Zaccardi, Baseman, Panzera, Montgomery, Kunaszuk, Lorenz, Clark, Kiefer, Weitz, Walker, Teixeira, Valle Ortiz, Byrne, Moore, Cotter, and Zwicker
17 courageous DrNP graduates who challenged conformity
for the advancement of nursing knowledge
HMD

To the Nurses, Administrators, and Assistants of the Eleventh Street Family Health Services
of Drexel University,
who demonstrate each and every day their passion and commitment to social justice and a vibrant, caring society.
CTO

"You'll be hearing from my lawyer!"

Unfortunately, this is a phrase that all too many of us get to hear in our lives. In many sectors, including academia, it has become the "trump card" in how students and faculty think they can get a dispute resolved their way: threaten to get "the lawyers" involved, and people cave.

If you practice the healing arts and teach others who will do the same, your objective is to care for patients and teach students to do so; but you will not always be able to help individuals as much as you (or they) will like, and sometimes there will be an adverse result. In academia, there will be disputes—about agreements allegedly made, quality of services rendered, costs incurred, attitudes expressed. With our society becoming increasingly diverse, the opportunities for misunderstanding—and causing offense—are expanding rapidly.

The law is the framework that allows each of us to deal with others in a predictable way.[1] For centuries, the courts have been where disputes were resolved. Our modern legal practices date back almost eight centuries to England in 1215 and the Magna Carta—a reform imposed upon the king by the populace, which, among many other things, guaranteed that disputes between the people would be decided by the people themselves in their own community, in public. This system of justice—trial by jury—remains the dominant feature of American law, but it is no longer the primary way that disputes are resolved. In most cases and for most people, lawyers and courts are too formal, too slow, and too expensive. But they are always there, waiting for when other methods fail.

The first chapter will discuss rights and claims, the different ways they get resolved, and the process that dispute resolution typically takes. The next chapters will provide a quick overview of the legal principles and specific laws that all nursing faculty need to know and will provide some instruction on how to read "a case." Then the role of university counsel is addressed. The remaining chapters will analyze academic nursing cases in order to provide the reader with legal background, prevention tips, and resources to navigate common and not-so-common legal issues in nursing education. Society has become increasingly litigious. This book will serve as a resource to nursing faculty and academic administrators on how to manage legal issues encountered in their daily professional lives.

---

[1]Everybody knows the famous quote from Shakespeare's *Hamlet:* "The first thing we do, we kill all the lawyers." While this is commonly thought to be a slam against attorneys, it is in fact an accolade. The persons discussing this strategy were intent on causing social chaos. They knew that, in the absence of law and those who "guarded" it, they could better achieve their ends.

The book, *Legal Issues Confronting Today's Nursing Faculty: A Case Study Approach* was conceptualized from a doctoral nursing course that bears a similar name. This text provides faculty and academic administrators with practical advice on how to deal with the vast array of legal issues that arise in nursing education. These issues are ***rarely addressed*** in the literature, and faculty often struggle with how to solve some of the legal issues they confront daily in the classroom and clinical environment. This book assists faculty in making real-life decisions about academic issues such as incivility, discrimination, academic dishonesty, and conflict of interest, with the legal bases in mind. The two nursing faculty authors, Drs. Mary Ellen Smith Glasgow and H. Michael Dreher, have an extensive background in academic nursing administration; management of large, complex nursing programs; and expertise in the faculty role. The university attorney author, Carl "Tobey" Oxholm, has served as Chief Legal Counsel at a large, private university. The authors offer their knowledgeable perspectives on how to address simple and complex nursing academic legal issues based on their collective experience.

Whether you are a new or seasoned nursing professor/academic, nursing administrator, or graduate student taking a master's or doctoral nursing program in legal issues in nursing education course, we believe this text can serve as an important guide for your career. The nursing education environment today is complex and challenging. Navigating the legal issues that every faculty member will at some point face (regardless of role) requires, at minimum, some familiarity with critical higher education legal issues and their management.

MESG

HMD

CTO

Mary Ellen Smith Glasgow, PhD, RN, ACNS-BC is a Tenured Professor and an Associate Dean for Nursing, Undergraduate Health Professions, and Continuing Nursing Education at Drexel University College of Nursing and Health Professions. In this role, she is responsible for all undergraduate health professions and nursing programs in the college, approximately 3,310 students, including curriculum, faculty development, institutional and accrediting body quality assessment, and fiscal planning. In her former position as Director of the Undergraduate Nursing Programs, she developed the Accelerated Career Entry, BSN Co-op, and RN-BSN Online programs. Her research interests include bone marrow donation in minorities and leadership development in nursing education and practice.

Dr. Glasgow received a Master of Science in Nursing degree from Villanova University and a PhD from Duquesne University, School of Nursing. She completed a postdoctoral fellowship at Bryn Mawr College and HERS, Mid-America Summer Institute for Women in Higher Education Administration. She is the recipient of the 2010 Villanova University College of Nursing Alumni Medallion for Distinguished Contribution to Nursing Education. She is certified as a Clinical Specialist in Adult Health Nursing by the ANCC and is on the Editorial Board for Holistic Nursing Practice and Oncology Nursing Forum. She also serves as the Associate Editor for Oncology Nursing Forum responsible for the Leadership and Professional Development Feature. Dr. Glasgow is also a Trustee of Princeton HealthCare System in Princeton, New Jersey. Dr. Glasgow was selected as a 2009 Robert Wood Johnson Foundation Executive Nurse Fellow. She recently coauthored a book, *Role Development for Doctoral Advanced Nursing Practice*, with Dr. H. Michael Dreher.

H. Michael Dreher, PhD, RN is Associate Professor with Tenure in the Advanced Nursing Role Department at Drexel University and was founding Chair of the Doctoral Nursing Department 2004–2010. His PhD is in Nursing Science from Widener University (2000), and his AS (1984), BSN (1988), and MN (1991) are from the University of South Carolina, Columbia. Dreher is a dynamic leader, innovator, and educator. He has taught in associate, baccalaureate, master's, and doctoral nursing programs and has been an academic nursing administrator in BSN, MSN, and DrNP degree programs. He has led Drexel to the forefront of practice doctoral nursing education and spearheaded the Drexel DNP Conferences on DNP Education in Annapolis, Maryland, in 2007 and Hilton Head Island, South Carolina, in 2009. In 2006 he established the first mandatory doctoral study abroad program in nursing, sending students to the United Kingdom (UK) and Ireland. His clinical nursing experience (1984–2000) has focused primarily on Adult Health/Coronary Care/Home Care of Cardiac Patients, and he has completed a postdoctoral fellowship in sleep and respiratory neurobiology at the University of Pennsylvania (2001–2003). He participated in the Harvard Macy Institute Program for Leading Innovation in Healthcare and Education (Harvard Business School/Medical School, 2007) and established the first MSN in Innovation (2007). Dr. Dreher has published more than 70 journal articles and has been principal investigator (PI) or co-PI on over 20 funded projects. His current scholarship focuses on professional/practice doctorate issues and in expanding his Model of Practice Knowledge Development. He presented at the Second International Conference on Professional Doctorates in Edinburgh (2011) and was the only non-UK contributor on a commissioned report (2011) *Professional Doctorates in the UK 2011* (Fell, Flint, & Haines, eds.). Dreher is coauthor with Dr. Michael Dahnke of *Philosophy of Science for Nursing Practice: Concepts and Application* (2011) and coauthor with Dr. Mary Ellen Smith Glasgow (2011) of *Role Development for Doctoral Advanced Nursing Practice*. He is currently Associate Editor and Column Editor for "Practice Evidence" in *Clinical Scholars Review: The Journal of Doctoral Nursing Practice*.

Carl Oxholm III received his Juris Doctor from Harvard Law School, cum laude, in 1979, and his Masters in Public Policy from the Kennedy School of Government. Thereafter followed a very successful 22-year career as a trial lawyer in Philadelphia in private practice and government service, including 5 years as a Chief Deputy City Solicitor, 5 more as a named partner in a mid-sized law firm, and over two decades in leadership of the city's public interest legal community, during which time he received several awards for exemplary public service, including being elected a Fellow of the University of Pennsylvania Law School. In 2001, he joined Drexel University as its General Counsel, Senior Vice President, and Secretary to the Board of Trustees. In the decade he has been with Drexel, he has played a leadership role in many of Drexel's most significant developments, including the academic merger with MCP Hahnemann University, including its colleges of Nursing, Public Health, and Medicine; development of Drexel University College of Medicine's medical malpractice mediation program, which received a Certificate of Appreciation from the Supreme Court of Pennsylvania Medical Malpractice Task Force in December 2005 and remains a national model; the creation of a captive insurance company that today insures Drexel's medical students, nurses, psychologists, and doctors from the Drexel University College of Medicine; creation of the Earl Macke School of Law, which today has a top-ranked concentration in health law; and creation of Drexel's Center for Graduate Studies in Sacramento, California, of which he served as Dean and Chief Executive Officer and General Counsel of Drexel University.

Oxholm has taught extensively in the field of litigation tactics and ethics as well as on mediation; has published a guide to health-care professionals caught up in litigation *So You've Been Sued: Medical Malpractice Litigation in the Court of Common Pleas of Philadelphia County* (Philadelphia Health & Education Corporation, 2003; third edition, 2007); and has coauthored a leading article on on-line and blended education titled "Re-examining and repositioning higher education: Twenty economic and demographic factors driving online and blended program enrollments," *Journal of Asynchronous Learning Networks* 9(1), published by The Sloan Consortium (2010).

Today he serves as President of Arcadia University.

Contributors

Stephen F. Gambescia, PhD, MEd, MBA
Assistant Dean of Academic and Student Affairs
Associate Professor
Drexel University College of Nursing & Health Professions
Philadelphia, Pennsylvania

Marcia R. Gardner, PhD, RN, CPNP, CPN
Associate Professor
College of Nursing
Seton Hall University
South Orange, New Jersey

Barbara Granger, PhD, CPRP, LLC
Granger Consultation Services
Philadelphia, Pennsylvania

Deborah R. Lorber
Assistant Vice President, Risk Management
Drexel University College of Medicine
Philadelphia, Pennsylvania
Chief Operating Officer
Schuylkill Crossing Reciprocal Risk Retention Group

Faye A. Meloy, PhD, RN, MSN, MBA
Assistant Clinical Professor
Assistant Dean for Pre-licensure BSN Programs
Chair, BSN Co-op Department
Drexel University College of Nursing & Health Professions
Philadelphia, Pennsylvania

Terry Jean Seligmann, J.D.
Arlin M. Adams Professor of Legal Writing
Director of the Legal Writing Program
Earle Mack School of Law
Drexel University
Philadelphia, Pennsylvania
Former President, Legal Writing Institute
Member, Board of Directors
Association of Legal Writing Directors

Mary-Anne Andrusyszyn, RN, BScN,
MScN, EdD
Arthur Labatt School of Nursing
The University of Western Ontario
London, Ontario, Canada

Toni O. Barnett, PhD, APRN, BC,
FNP-C, CNE
North Georgia College & State University
Dahlonega, Georgia

Cynthia Francis Bechtel, PhD, RN,
CNE, CEN, EMT-1
Framingham State University
Framingham, Massachusetts

Wanda Bonnel, PhD, GNP-BC, ANEF
University of Kansas
School of Nursing
Kansas City, Kansas

Patricia Bradley, MEd, PhD, RN, CNE
York University
Toronto, Ontario, Canada

Janis Browne, RN, MEd, DNSc
York University
Toronto, Ontario, Canada

Michelle M. Byrne, RN, PhD, CNE,
CNOR
North Georgia College & State University
Dahlonega, Georgia

Evelyn Cesarotti, PhD, FNP, GNP
Arizona State University
Phoenix, Arizona

Cynthia L. Dakin, RN, PhD
Elms College
Chicopee, Massachusetts

Marilyn L. Dollinger, DNS,
FNP-BC, RN
St. John Fisher College
Rochester, New York

Sally Doshier, EdD, RN, CNE
Northern Arizona University
School of Nursing
Flagstaff, Arizona

Frances R. Eason, EdD, MSN,
RN-BC,CNE, ANEF
College of Nursing
East Carolina University
Greenville, North Carolina

Pamela B. Edwards, EdD, MSN, BSN,
RN-BC, CNE, FABC
Duke University School of Nursing
Duke University Health System
Durham, North Carolina

Sally Elizabeth Erdel, MS, RN, CNE
Bethel College
Mishawaka, Indiana

Alayne Fitzpatrick, APRN, CS, BC,
EdD
Fairleigh Dickinson University
Teaneck New Jersey

Linda Grimsley, RN, DSN
Albany State University
Albany, Georgia

Neena Grissom, EdD(c), MSN, RN
College of Nursing
University of Arkansas for Medical
Sciences
Little Rock, Arkansas

Patricia Grust, MSN, RN, CLNC
State University of New York Institute of
  Technology
Utica, New York

Jamesetta Halley-Boyce, RN, PhD,
  FACHE
Seton Hall University
South Orange, New Jersey

Kathleen Geiger Hoover, PhD, RN, CNE
Neumann University
Aston, Pennsylvania

Joyce Young Johnson, RN, MN, PhD
Albany State University
Albany, Georgia

Elizabeth Kinion, EdD, MSN,
  APN-BC, FAAN
Montana State University
Bozeman, Montana

Norma Kiser-Larson, PhD, RN, CNE
North Dakota State University
Fargo, North Dakota

Vera G. Kling, DHSc, MSN, RN, BC
Charleston Southern University
Charleston, South Carolina

Ramona Browder Lazenby, EdD,
  MSN, RN, FNP-BC, CNE
Auburn Montgomery School of Nursing
Montgomery, Alabama

Karen S. March, PhD, RN
York College of Pennsylvania
York, Pennsylvania

Jane C. Norman, PhD, RN, CNE
Tennessee State University
Nashville, Tennessee

Lisa M. Ogawa, PhD, RN
University of Massachusetts, Worcester
Worcester, Massachusetts

MJ Petersen, EdD
College of Saint Mary
Omaha, Nebraska

Mary Carol G. Pomatto, EdD,
  ARNP-CNS
Pittsburg State University
Pittsburg, Kansas

Carla E. Randall, RN, PhD
University of Southern Maine
Lewiston, Maine

Priscilla L. Sagar, EdD, RN, ACNS-CS,
  CTN-A
Mount Saint Mary College
Newburgh, New York

Susan Parnell Scholtz, RN, PhD
St. Luke's School of Nursing at Moravian
  College
Bethlehem, Pennsylvania

Lynda Shand, RN BSN, MA, PhD,
  CNE, CHPN
The College of New Rochelle
New Rochelle, New York

Linda A. Streit, RN, DSN
Associate Dean for Graduate Programs
Georgia Baptist College of Nursing of
  Mercer University
Atlanta, Georgia

Lois Tschetter, RN, EdD, CNE
South Dakota State University
Brookings, South Dakota

Mary B. Williams, MS, RN
University of West Georgia School of
  Nursing
Carrollton, Georgia

Lynn Cathy Wimett, EdD, MS, APRN-C
Regis University
Denver, Colorado

The case studies in this book are drawn principally from the experiences of the two nurse educator coauthors of this book. The judgments about the facts, the conduct, and the better practices are theirs alone, not that of Drexel University nor of the lawyer coauthor, Carl Oxholm. He has participated in the editing of each chapter, and we thank him here for his contributions; but we hasten to note that, as in legal practice, the lawyer does not have to share his client's opinions, and "for the record," we do have our differences—but the clients get to decide. As Drexel's General Counsel (chief attorney) for 7 years, his experience and expertise are broad; quick to recognize when more in-depth legal knowledge is appropriate, he has called on several colleagues with whom he worked in Drexel's Office of the General Counsel to take the lead in editing. We wish to acknowledge and thank them here:

- **Laure Bachich Ergin, Esquire**—Ms. Ergin is currently Associate Vice President and Deputy Counsel at the University of Delaware. During the period 1997–2010, she was a member of Drexel's Office of the General Counsel, with many years' service as its Deputy General Counsel. In that capacity, she not only acquired expertise in student conduct issues but also updated and administered many of the policies we describe in this book. Her review and advice was particularly helpful to us in matters affecting disability, mental health, and conduct issues (Chapters 21, 22, 23, 24, and 35).

- **John R. Gyllenhammer, Esquire**—Mr. Gyllenhammer is currently Associate Vice President and Chief Counsel for the Drexel University College of Medicine. For close to a decade, he was charged with primary responsibility for counseling and representing the College of Nursing and Healthcare Professions, and he remains our "go-to" attorney whenever the College faces a "hot issue." He is the primary author on Chapter 2, "Legal Issues Commonly Encountered by Faculty and Academic Administrators," and he also reviewed the chapters dealing with civility and evaluating performance (Chapters 19, 20, 29, 31, and 32).

- **Timothy J. Raynor, Esquire**—Mr. Raynor is Associate General Counsel, Office of the General Counsel, Drexel University. He has served as the university's principal attorney involved with intellectual property issues, including commercialization and technology transfer. He reviewed our chapters on intellectual property and "intellectual theft" (Chapters 11 and 12).

Acknowledgments

I would like to acknowledge my parents, Nancy and Frank Smith, and my in-laws, Doris and Tom Glasgow, who are always there for me. Thank you for being such a huge blessing in my life. *MESG*

I want to acknowledge the patience and support of my partner Dr. Michael Dahnke, who did so many things I just could not do because I was writing intensively for the last 14 months. *HMD*

To Kimberly Ann, my *sine qua non* for 35 years and counting. *CTO*

List of Tables

List of Figures

Table of Contents

We have a combined 40 years of university nursing education experience and 27 years of university legal experience. The case studies utilized in this book are not "fact" but composites drawn from that experience as well as from the decided case law so that we can discuss the specific points at issue in the chapter. All the names of the characters in the case studies are fictional.

We have included copies of policies and procedures in use at Drexel University at the time this book was being written, which can be located online at http://davisplus.fadavis.com. We are happy to share these as examples, but they are only examples. Drexel University is a private university—in corporate form, a private not-for-profit corporation. It is governed by a charter, articles of incorporation, and bylaws. Its faculty members are not unionized, and there are no collective bargaining agreements with faculty. It has not adopted, officially or unofficially, the policies or procedures of the American Association of University Professors (AAUP), whose policies and procedures we have also referenced. Finally, Drexel is located in Philadelphia, Pennsylvania, which has a fairly well developed body of judicial case law applicable to higher education. As a result, the Drexel policies and procedures have been developed to fit Drexel's situation and should only be considered only as an example. And our lawyer-authors are quick to add that they are offered entirely without any warranties or representations. You really should check with your university counsel before using these examples at your institution.

As this book will make clear, "the law" is not a "one size fits all" menu, nor is it a list of rules and regulations that you can consult and get specific answers in every situation. Lawyers are famous for giving "two-handed advice"—"on the one hand, this; on the other, that"—for good reason: judges have issued opinions that are diametrically opposed in virtually identical situations, and legislators have not been comprehensive (or even thoughtful) when they add the "next" piece of legislation to an already complicated area.

What this means is that judgment on your part is always involved; and what the lawyer does is provide advice on how to increase the likelihood that one answer will be the final answer in a particular situation. What this also means is that this book provides examples, but not specific legal advice, on ways to address situations that we face regularly if not every day. How we interact with students is driven by the same legal principles that apply to how we interact with colleagues (employees), so there is overlap in the discussion; and you ought to read pairs of chapters (for students/for faculty) to more fully understand what is going on in the legal realm.

In many ways, the point of this book is to get you to the point of appreciating the legal framework that provides the structure of our business. Sometimes—even most of the time—the principles will be easy to apply, and the way to resolve a situation will be clear. The higher the "price" of a wrong decision, the more the bottom line becomes clear: consult your own university counsel.

The Legal Process: A Primer

CHAPTER 1

An Introduction to the Legal Process: A Primer

The Origin of Rights

"You cannot do this to me. I know my rights!"

In fact, virtually none of us knows our rights. What we have is a sense of entitlement that results from living in one of the world's richest countries, having the privilege of attending a college or university, and enjoying the luxury of reading and thinking. Add to this situation an excess of lawyer advertising[1] and the publicity given to some seemingly outrageous jury awards.[2]

In a legal sense, rights come from a number of sources that can be identified and consulted.[3] These include the following:

- Contracts: agreements both oral and written in which one party obligates itself to do something for another
- Common law: rules and principles arising from the judgments of juries and judges and the way that they articulate the bases for their decisions
- Statutory law: rules that legislatures of all levels have enacted
- Administrative law: rules and procedures that have been developed by government agencies, charged with the interpretation and enforcement of statutes
- Constitutional law: pronouncements made in a federal or state government's highest charter
- International law: treaties among nations and the laws of other nations

---

[1] It is virtually impossible to complete a round-trip to campus from home without seeing or hearing an advertisement for a lawyer, making it clear that a (bad) situation is someone else's fault, and that the lawyer will fight "to the death" to vindicate your rights. They have toll-free numbers and promise that there will not be a fee "unless we win for you." What's not to like?

[2] How many tens of millions of dollars did that woman win from McDonald's, after she sued because the fresh cup of coffee she had purchased from the drive-through and placed between her legs spilled and scalded her?

[3] This is to distinguish the discussion of rights as lawyers and judges argue about them, from the kinds of inherent rights that flow from religious or political philosophies. The latter typically inform the former, but only the former can be cited to a court or a judge as justification for a particular position.

A variety of rights can be involved in a particular event. For example, it is a crime to hit someone. That means the conduct violates a written law that is part of the criminal code (perhaps of both the state and federal government). It is also a violation of the common law (battery), because that law protects the "right to bodily integrity" even if the state had not also stepped in. These rules have different consequences if they are broken. Break a criminal statute, and one can be put in jail and made to pay a fine, which goes to the state; violate the common law, and one will pay money (damages or restitution) to the victim.

There are also two systems of justice at work: state and federal. In most cases, it is only the law of the state in which the dispute arose that will matter. In some instances, however, there is an overlay of federal rights and obligations stemming from the Constitution of the United States, the laws enacted by Congress and the president, and the rules and regulations promulgated by federal agencies. When a federal contract or right is involved in a dispute, federal law is triggered, and the federal courts can become involved. If the person one has punched has rights that are protected by federal law (e.g., the right to be free of discrimination on the basis of age, sex, race, disability, or national origin), one's conduct may be subject to investigation in two proceedings at the same time.

In academia, rights under the law can acquire new and added dimensions. It is likely, for example, that a faculty member's university prohibits him from punching a colleague or a student—it's far enough removed from academic freedom to be punishable as a violation of the university's code of conduct. One could be suspended or even lose a job. That's a matter of contract law: when that faculty member took the job (or when the student accepted the offer of admission), he agreed to live by the rules of the university. Not knowing that was a possible consequence of his actions is not a defense.[4]

Another example worth considering is academic dishonesty. Suppose a junior member of the faculty, intent on tenure, is "creative" in the research she does, borrowing data from another source and claiming it as her own, and entirely making up other data. The original author had her work stolen, so there is a violation of the common law. The university has its most fundamental precept of integrity dashed, so the employment contract was broken. The researcher may also have violated the terms of a grant that was funding the research, threatening adverse consequences to the university (possibly disqualification from future grants, not

---

[4] This is where the phrase "ignorance of the law is no excuse" comes from. Because the law is what sets the boundaries of behavior, all of us have the right to expect that those boundaries will be observed—whatever they are. If one crosses a line unknowingly, this violates someone else's rights; and the fact that it was not intended, and the offender didn't realize it, does not reduce that other person's right. Where ignorance does come into play is often in considering the remedy for the misconduct: intentional bad acts get punished far more severely than do innocent ones. In most instances, the amount of the punishment is left to the discretion of the decision-maker (judge, juror, arbitrator, or other decider).

to mention damage to its reputation). It may have violated federal or state regulatory requirements, for which there might be fines or penalties. And what about those who read of the fraudulent results and relied on them—perhaps using a therapy that really was not proved and that ended up causing them harm? All of a sudden, satisfying tenure requirements seems inconsequential.

Deciding Who's Right

We all decide dozens of disputes every day—conflicts in our calendars, disagreements in an approach to a problem, competition for a parking spot, and confrontations with aggressive drivers. We don't spend much time or effort on them because they are so small. The bigger the issue—the more important to our future, our family, or our wallet—the more time and effort we'll spend. And when it's really important, that's when most of us head for a lawyer.

Because of the way that our country was founded, we strive to make our courts open to those who have complaints. Not only are the filing fees relatively low, but in the United States, plaintiffs can engage their attorneys on a contingency fee basis, meaning that the attorney will be paid only out of money won for the plaintiff; and the attorney is even allowed to pay the out-of-pocket costs for the plaintiff on the same basis.

Going to court can be incredibly expensive for defendants—costs can easily rise to six figures to defend hotly disputed claims such as employment discrimination or medical malpractice. Oftentimes the defendant won't get the opportunity to testify or to defend herself at trial because she signed away that right to her insurance company in the policy she bought: for the insurance company, it's only money, and it is not obligated to worry about her reputation. Insurance companies also know that juries (and judges) make mistakes, and sure-win claims can be lost. Even a "win" at trial won't mean it's over (or that the meter has stopped running), because decisions can be easily taken to an appellate court.

The expense, the time, and the publicity involved in litigation are all reasons that people have decided to take their disputes to other places to have them resolved. "Alternative dispute resolution" is a phrase that encompasses many different methods, each of which one may experience as a member of a college or university faculty.

Ombudsman

Often a university has a standing position called the *ombudsman*. This is not a process but a person who is available to help resolve certain kinds of complaints or issues. This person has no power, cannot order anyone to do anything, and cannot punish anyone for not participating. The university cannot force anyone to use him. He doesn't decide anything. All he can do is ask questions, make suggestions, and help the disputants work through their issues. Typically, the ombudsman is someone whom everyone respects and holds in high regard; typically, the ombudsman is sworn to secrecy, keeps no notes, and cannot be forced to divulge what anyone said to him. But "typically" means not always: the role of the ombudsman is defined by university policy or procedure, which must be read carefully.

Mediation

Like the ombudsman, a *mediator* helps disputants reach an agreed-on solution, but the mediator's role is more formal than that of the ombudsman, there is a process to be followed, and the expectations for each are better defined. The disputants often get to choose the person who will serve as the mediator. The mediator is subject to a code of ethics. The mediation process is typically described in a written document to which the disputants are required to agree, but in all respects it is a voluntary process that requires agreement of both sides every step along the way.[5]

Before actually tackling the problem at hand, the mediator will typically require the different sides to discuss and agree on the way the mediation will be handled, dates, what issues will be discussed, whether they will submit written materials (e.g., their statements of claims and defenses), ground rules for behavior (complete confidentiality being the most important), and when and how the process might end. The role of the mediator then becomes that of "shuttle diplomat," operating in the zone between the two sides and working to bring them closer together.[6] Sometimes mediation will resolve the whole dispute, sometimes just part; it can clear away collateral issues and forge agreements on how the remaining parts of the dispute can be handled. It is important that it ends with an agreement between the parties—an enforceable contract—if it results in anything at all.

Administrative Hearings

Codes of conduct, student and faculty handbooks, and collective bargaining agreements routinely specify ways of resolving certain kinds of disputes in a way that is more formal than mediation but less formal than going to court.

---

[5] Drexel University College of Medicine has developed a process for resolving health-care disputes between its doctors and their patients. It begins with an agreement that the patient signs when seeing the doctor for the first time, and is described in a pamphlet that covers virtually all the steps along the way. The process uses two lawyers as mediators—one who usually represents patients/plaintiffs and the other who usually represents doctors/defendants—who are both chosen from a list of experts who have been specially trained in mediation. Before the mediation begins, the parties and their lawyers sign a mediation agreement that specifies the rights and obligations of everyone involved, including the fact that everything that happens during the process must be kept entirely confidential. Mediations that succeed (and they do succeed more than 90% of the time) result in written agreements signed by the parties. The courts in Philadelphia have regularly ratified this process, dismissing lawsuits filed by patients who did not first take their claims to mediation and otherwise enforcing the terms of the agreement.

[6] The word mediate comes from the Latin word for "middle," *medias*. The mediator is the one in the middle.

Objections about how a member of the faculty has been treated (grievances) or behaved (disciplinary problems) are typically required by the university to be submitted to this kind of process. Universities do this because the courts will enforce that kind of requirement and not allow lawsuits to be filed until the process is over.

The governing document (code, handbook, policy, or contract) will specify both what the process is and who will sit as the hearing officer(s); the disputants typically are given very little say in either matter. The hearing officers are members of the university community—faculty, staff, or students as appropriate given the nature of the panel and dispute. They are given certain stated powers—for example, they can require university employees to appear and give evidence. They also have certain specified duties, including performing their duties in fairness to all and rendering a decision within a set period of time. Lawyers may or may not be allowed to participate. The time for presenting each side may be limited. Witnesses may or may not be allowed to be called to testify. The decision-makers may be allowed to render only certain kinds of decisions or dispense only certain kinds of remedies. All of these issues are typically specified in the governing documents, but never with enough specificity to answer every question; in those cases, the panel members make the decisions.

The disputants may or may not have rights to appeal the decision to another university official (e.g., dean of students in the case of student disciplinary matters, provost in the case of faculty grievances, president in case of tenure denial), but the "scope of review" (what issues can be considered) is typically very small. Once this step is over (or if no appeal is taken), the decision is called final and it must then be implemented. Sometimes one side or the other will take a further appeal to the courts, but the appeal will not postpone (or stay) the duty to comply with the decision. The law strictly limits the issues that a judge can consider. On the merits of the dispute, the law requires judges to defer to the expertise of the university in certain key areas, promotion and tenure being prime examples, unless there is a clear and convincing reason that the university is wrong. In the end, it is only in the rarest of circumstances that the law gives judges the authority to undo a decision made during a grievance or disciplinary proceeding, either about who should win or what the remedy should be.[7] In virtually no case is one party or another ever given the chance to start over.[8]

---

[7] Appeals from administrative hearings are typically limited to claims that there was a fundamental problem with the hearing (it did not follow the process that the handbook or agreement specified) or with a hearing officer (he had a fundamental conflict of interest that was not disclosed). Under some states' laws, decisions of administrative panels can be modified if the judge finds that there was "capricious disregard of the evidence" or "gross abuse of discretion" but as the words themselves show, the bar is set very high for these kinds of rulings.

[8] A de novo hearing is one that starts "from the beginning." It is awarded extremely rarely, as when a judge determines that one side or another was completely deprived of a fair hearing the first time.

Arbitrations

Arbitrations are like administrative proceedings, but have broader applicability. The parties to a contract may have agreed (at the start of the contract) that they would submit to arbitration all disagreements arising out of or relating to the contract. They can agree to arbitration after a contract is in place and a dispute has arisen. A judge can force them to take their claims to arbitration before they go to trial before a jury.

There are several ways that the arbitrators can be selected: they can be assigned by a judge, chosen from a list of qualified individuals from which unacceptable candidates have been "stricken" by the parties, or selected by agreement. Once selected, the process that is followed will either be set by the document signed by the parties or governed by court rules.

In general terms, arbitrations may follow court procedures but will be less formal. There will be lawyers, and the lawyers will give opening statements. Witnesses will be called, examined, and cross-examined. Documents will be formally marked as exhibits and offered to the arbitrator. Legal memoranda will be submitted. The arbitrator will then issue a decision, rendering an award to one side or the other and specifying the remedy to be provided. In most cases, the award is for damages—money—but where the rules or agreement allows, the arbitrator can specify equitable relief—orders that certain actions must be done (e.g., return to work) or must stop and not happen again (called *injunctions*; e.g., ending a policy).

Whether there can be appeals from arbitration awards depends on the agreement or the rules under which it was conducted. Arbitrations can be binding—that is, the decision rendered by the arbitrator(s) can be final like those in an administrative hearing—or not.[9]

Trials

Disputes can go to trial and be resolved by jury verdicts or judicial awards. That happens in a very small percentage of the disputes that find their way to court. There are many reasons for this: trials are very expensive (costs plus time that people must spend preparing for them and sitting through them), it takes a long

---

[9] Because so many lawsuits are filed each year and there is only a set number of judges, courts in most jurisdictions have adopted rules of procedure that require disputes of a certain kind and amount to be tried in arbitration before they are allowed to be listed for a trial before a judge or jury. The parties to the dispute have no choice about this—it is a rule—but although the process is mandatory, the decision of the arbitrator(s) is not final. The loser has the right to appeal and receives a de novo hearing. Although this may seem a waste of time, the vast majority of cases referred to arbitration are resolved either by the arbitrators or shortly after an appeal is filed. The principal reasons for this are that the lawyers use the arbitrators to get a fair evaluation of the case and the filing of an appeal is often used as a last step to provoke a negotiated settlement rather than incur the substantial costs associated with formal trials. Judges receiving cases on appeal from arbitrations also see them as ripe for settlement, and use their power to encourage the parties to settle.

time to get to trial (during which time emotions tend to lessen and financial reasons tend to dominate), the process reveals information that makes right and wrong less clear (making settlements possible), and judges regularly use their power to force settlements. Few people actually make it through the entire process, and only a small subset of them think the experience was worth it.

The following section outlines the process that leads from the filing of a complaint to the issuance of a decision ending the case. Virtually every lawsuit will go through each of these steps (unless it is earlier settled).

Parties

The person who believes she has been wronged and who starts the lawsuit is called the plaintiff. The plaintiff chooses who must respond to her charges of misconduct, and those are called defendants because the law obligates them to defend themselves (if they don't, a judgment by default will be entered against them almost automatically). Being named a defendant, and being served with legal papers, often catches people by complete surprise. Sometimes the plaintiff names people who had nothing to do with the claim; more often, the people had something to do with the events that had something to do with the claim. The defendant(s) and the plaintiff(s) are together termed the parties.[10]

Lawsuits are begun when the facts are least clear; the facts get clearer as the lawsuit progresses, and that often allows innocent defendants to get out of the case before it goes to trial. But at the beginning, an attorney representing a plaintiff will err on the side of including as a defendant anyone who may have played a role in causing the injury to his client. This is because the law puts a very hard deadline on when people can file lawsuits (or, in administrative setting, assert claims). These limiting rules are called statutes of limitation because they are usually enacted by the legislature (statute) and limit access to the court. If a lawyer learns after the time period has expired that someone else really did have something to do with causing the injury, even the guiltiest person can escape liability. Therefore, it is often out of an abundance of caution that people who are not really responsible—including nurses and nursing students—can find themselves named in medical malpractice cases.

Individuals can be served with legal process by anyone anywhere at any time—at home, in the office, even in the middle of teaching a class.[11] Written in

---

[10] The term comes from contract law, as in "the party of the first part" and "the party of the second part" who are on opposite sides of the transaction, as they are in court. Like the word "brief" used to describe a lawyer's long memorandum of law, it is no party being involved in litigation.

[11] Many universities have policies that require all legal processes addressed to any employee to be served on a specific administrator. This includes lawsuits that have nothing to do with the university, suits in divorce being an easy example. This is not to pry, but to avoid disruption to the class and embarrassment to the faculty member. The process server is not required by law to obey the policy. Process servers are not required to be considerate; they are hired to get the job done.

rather stilted English, presented in numbered paragraphs, and referring to long-ago events in which one has no real or current interest, a legal document from the court is exactly the kind of thing that one will be inclined to put to one side to read later. Don't. Process servers and the piece of paper they are delivering are the modern-day equivalent of a person being physically arrested by a sheriff and there are penalties (which can include arrest) if the instructions contained in the paper are not followed within the (usually short) period of time allowed. If the claim has anything whatsoever to do with a faculty member's or administrator's service to the university, it is in her best interest (and probably required by university policy) to deliver that paper to a university administrator immediately.

Pleadings

A long time ago, those who were aggrieved submitted pleas to the judiciary to help them. Today, the pleadings are the written statement of what the claims and defenses are. In some jurisdictions (including many state courts) the claim must be stated with specificity, providing a detailed account of what happened and why the grievant (called a *plaintiff*, who starts the process by filing a com*plaint*) should be given some help (called relief): money damages, return of his property, orders forcing the other party to do something, and so on. In other jurisdictions (such as the federal courts), all the plaintiff needs to do is give a short-form notice that he has a complaint of a certain type against the defendant.

The defendant then has a short amount of time to respond, and is given a choice: she can file a motion that challenges the legal sufficiency of the complaint, or file an answer to it. In most cases, a motion is filed because the defendant's lawyer thinks it might actually succeed in removing some of the claims, or will get the judge involved in the case faster, or just buys time. Few cases are actually dismissed at this point because even if the defendant is right, judges will usually allow the plaintiff a second (and often a third) time to plead a claim properly.

Once the motions practice is concluded and the judge has issued any preliminary orders, the defendant has to file his answer to all of the claims that remain—a response that not only challenges the facts (and defendants are often required to state their own contrary view of what happened, so the court knows where the factual disputes actually lie) but also asserts legal principles that either excuse the conduct or prove that the conduct was not wrong in the first place (defenses). The plaintiff then has the opportunity to test the legal sufficiency of the defenses through motions practice.

Discovery

When the motions practice has ended and the pleadings are closed, the parties engage in what is called *discovery*. This is the period of time in which each party gets the chance to ask questions to discover the truth. They can ask questions of any of the other parties, of independent witnesses,[12] and of experts who have been hired to testify in the trial; the questions can be about the facts, the claims, the defenses, the opinions of the experts and the reasons for them, and anything else that might be important—including the mental abilities and capacities of the people who are witnesses. Great care must be taken in answering questions, because false answers suggest that someone is not a truth teller, and that opens up the questioning to other instances and events in which the person may not have told the truth. But everyone who has ever been involved with litigation will say that the questions are endless, require enormous effort to answer, and are terribly intrusive.

The manner in which the questions get asked are up to the attorneys. They can be in the form of written questions (interrogatories), oral questions (depositions), and requests to produce anything tangible for their inspection and copying. Virtually everything arising out of or relating in any way to the facts that are at issue is fair game for the questioning. The law also permits the attorneys to review any document (graphic, electronic, or other form of recording) and all files—even those marked personal, because they get to prove for themselves that one of the parties has been accurate in filing the information away and is not hiding something.

Electronic records are the greatest source of dispute because of how much we use e-mail and e-documents. Once served with legal process, one's personal obligation is to provide access to every device that might have been used to store or communicate information relevant to the dispute.[13] In addition, there are also federal and state laws that require that any and all records that might be related to a case be preserved, and the lawyers are allowed to check the parties' hard drives (and everyone else's, it seems) for deleted items. Discovery that one has destroyed documents or other kinds of evidence not only leads to the inference that it would have proved bad things against that party, but it can, under certain laws, subject one to criminal penalties, such as fines and even jail.[14]

For everyone involved, discovery represents the largest investment of time and the biggest intrusion into privacy, and the right of the parties (and their

---

[12] If one is not a party to the lawsuit, she will receive these questions by way of a subpoena commanding her presence at a deposition and requiring her to bring various documents with her. The word subpoena comes from the Latin words for "under punishment," and the document is as powerful as a complaint in terms of the force of the law that stands ready to enforce it. As with a complaint, this document should also be taken to a university administrator as quickly as possible.

[13] If the parties cannot agree, it's the judge who ultimately decides what is relevant, but the party asking will ask for as much as possible and the party responding will try to limit the request as much as possible.

[14] Federal law, for example, prohibits the alteration or destruction of documents, or interference with witnesses, in any matter that is the subject of an investigation or could become so. For that reason, complaints about sexual harassment or misconduct, or wage and hour violations, or safety in the workplace, all of which involved federal laws, all involve the potential federal penalties.

lawyers) to look almost everywhere explains why universities have policies that state nothing on an employee's office computer, laptop, or cell phone is exempt from inspection review by the university, at least in certain situations. Collecting and imaging hard drives not only costs quite a lot of money but substantially interferes with everyone's work; and because the law imposes a continuing obligation to disclose, collecting information may have to occur more than once. For those who have undergone this process, it is easy to understand why the university (typically in the role of the defendant) settles cases more often, or more quickly, than the merits of the cases suggest it should: as a purely economic matter, it is often far less expensive to pay early to get out fast.

Motions Practice and Pretrial Proceedings

For those subject to it, the process of discovery seems endless, but a date does arrive when the questioning is required to end. At that point, the parties and their lawyers spend enormous amounts of time organizing all of the evidence, presenting it in motions to the court, arguing about the legal sufficiency of the claims and defenses, and getting ready for the actual trial. This can take months. It is also during this period that the parties—by their own decision, or directed by the judge—may try to settle the case through mediation, or agree to have it resolved by arbitration instead of trial.

Trials

Real-life trials are nothing like those on television crime dramas. They can span weeks at a time. The lawyers often meet with the judge behind closed doors, while everyone else sits in the courtroom, waiting without explanation. One is not allowed to have cell phones on in the courtroom or to talk above a whisper. If one has been subpoenaed to testify, he may even be required to sit out in the hallway (so he doesn't hear what other witnesses are saying), and he will have to remain there until the judge releases him. If one is a party, the university will most likely require him to be in court every day, from the moment the jury is picked to the minute the judge gavels that the proceeding has ended. Depending on legal rulings made by the judge and tactical decisions made by the lawyers, he might not even testify. It is a huge imposition on everyone's time and the university's funds.

Almost no one finds the experience satisfying. Witnesses are not allowed to give their stories; instead, they are confined to answering the lawyers' questions, even if that means the full story is not given. The lawyers interrupt each other and the witnesses with objections that are very distracting (and sometimes intended to be). The lawyers will know the facts even better than the witnesses (that's their job), and they will be ready to impeach anyone's testimony with facts they have learned during the discovery process. Their objective is to prove that their client's side of the story is the right one, the one that the judge and jury should believe, and that anyone who speaks against that version is wrong, or lying about it. It may not even seem fair—but it is, in the larger sense that everyone is playing by the same rules.

After all of the evidence has been presented, the lawyers will give their closing arguments in which they marshal all of the facts they have brought out in the trial into the story that they want the jury to accept, and argue why the other party's story is inconsistent with the facts and not worthy of belief. The judge then charges the jury on what the law is and the jury's obligation to interpret those laws to the facts of the case and decide who is right. This charge is not written: as in the rest of the trial, the members of the jury must try to remember what they have to been told, as they are not allowed even to take notes in most jurisdictions. They retire to the jury room to discuss the facts and make their decision, and are allowed to be finished only when they have reached and announced their verdict in open court. Unlike criminal cases, the jury does not need to be unanimous: each jurisdiction decides for itself the number of juror votes required to make the decision.

Post-trial Proceedings and Appeals

After a verdict has been entered, the parties will try to persuade the trial judge that the jury was wrong, and the judge does have the ability to reject the whole of the jury's verdict or to modify it. When the judge is finished with that process, the parties have the right to appeal whatever part of the decision they don't like to a higher court called a court of appeals. At that level, the judges (typically a panel of them) will hear the argument and make what is in most instances the final decisions in the case.[15]

It is in this posttrial process that the law changes from oral (the jury's decisions) to written form. Before the decisions are submitted to an appeals court, the trial court is required to confirm the reasons for its decisions in a written opinion. The appellate court, in turn, reviews that decision and issues its own, which is also written. These are public, recorded in the courthouse, published, and, at the appellate level, reported in both hard copy and electronic journals. It is these decisions to which the lawyers and judges look for guidance in presenting and arguing their next cases, and where most of the law is found.

---

[15] These courts are called intermediate appellate courts because there is usually one higher court, called (in most states and in the federal system) the supreme court. In most cases, however, the supreme court gets to decide whether it will hear the appeal, and the vast majority of requests are denied.

CHAPTER 2

Legal Issues Commonly Encountered by Faculty and Academic Administrators

As noted in Chapter 1, the law comes from a wide variety of sources, including the interpretations of hundreds of thousands of judges. There is nothing close to unanimity or consistency across all of their decisions, the main reason lawyers can find precedent (a judge's decision) to support virtually any argument and claim. Therefore, it can be difficult at times to know what the law is or what your rights are.[1]

This chapter provides a broad overview of the law in areas that faculty administrators commonly encounter. The decisions that are most important to faculty administrators are those that have been rendered by judges in the state where they work, because those decisions are binding on the judges who will hear the claims in which they are involved. (The decisions rendered by judges in other states or system are "advisory only" and do not have to be followed.) Familiarity with major legal causes of action that arise in the educational setting can help the faculty administrator to avoid stepping on legal landmines while running a program or department.

Breach of Contract

Whether one works at a state or private institution of higher education, the most common legal claim raised in a lawsuit is a breach of contract claim. It is often alleged in the plaintiff's complaint that the institution breached its contract, meaning that it failed to abide by or violated some provision of the contract. A contract can be oral, written, or a combination of both; it can be created formally (e.g., in a legal-looking document with signatures at the bottom) or informally (e.g.,

---

[1] This is also why "it depends" is the answer your questions will most likely receive from a lawyer.

through a letter or a telephone call); and it can be formed by action and conduct as well as by words. Both state and private institutions can be held liable for breach of contract to a student, faculty member or employee because each of these relationships is of a contractual nature. Courts have upheld breach of contract claims under both express and implied theories.

Express Theory

Under the express theory of liability, the court finds that the school has violated the terms of a written agreement or document, such as an employment, housing, dining or scholarship agreement which the student or faculty member has signed. The court may rely on some other institutional document to establish the terms of the contract, such as an appointment letter, a handbook, a catalog, a brochure, or a course-offering bulletin. As the intermediate appeal court in Pennsylvania held:

> [T]he relationship between a private educational institution and an enrolled student is contractual in nature; therefore, a student can bring a cause of action against said institution for breach of contract where the institution ignores or violates the portions of a written contract. . . . The contract between a private institution and a student is comprised of the written guidelines, policies and procedures as contained in the written materials distributed to students over the course of their enrollment in the institution. (Swartley v. Hoffner, 734 A.2d 915, 919 [Pa. Super. Ct. 1999])

Therefore, in order to succeed in a breach of an express contractual provision, the plaintiff must be able to point to some provision in the written contract that the institution has not followed. This is frequently difficult for a plaintiff to do. In many cases, the judge dismisses the breach of contract claim because the plaintiff cannot point to a commitment specific enough to hold the institution liable.

Implied Theory

Because courts have been reluctant to rigidly apply commercial contractual principles on the student–college relationship, several state courts have also recognized an implied contractual relationship between students and their school. The exact terms of this contract are more nebulous and not as easy to find. The implied theory has its modern origin in a 1962 decision of New York's highest appellate court, the New York Court of Appeals, which wrote:

> When a student is duly admitted by a private university, secular or religious, there is an implied contract between the student and the university that, if he complies with the terms prescribed by the university, he will obtain the degree sought. (Carr v. St. John's University of New York, 187 N.E.2d 18 [N.Y. 1962])

Under either theory, the prudent faculty administrator will always consult the applicable policies, procedures, regulations, and other institutional documents and seek to apply them in a consistent manner. Institutional counsel should be consulted before deviating from established policies, or in situations where such policies are vague, ambiguous, inconsistent, or nonexistent.

Discrimination, Harassment, or Retaliation Claims

Federal, state, and local laws prohibit discrimination on the basis of race, national origin, sex, disability or handicap, religion, and age. Some state or local statutes also prohibit discrimination based on other protected categories such as sexual orientation. Academic institutions will also have established policies and procedures on this subject matter that the faculty administrator should become familiar with. It is very common for educational institutions to designate a specific office, department, or officer to ensure institutional compliance. This designated official will often have responsibility for the internal investigation and resolution of complaints. To protect the institution, the faculty administrator who becomes aware of discrimination or harassment allegations should immediately consult with the institution's designated official.

Race and National Origin

Discrimination on the grounds of race, color, or national origin is prohibited under Title VI of the Civil Rights Act of 1964 (42 U.S.C. § 2000d) for an institution that receives federal funds. The statute simply says the following:

> No person in the United States shall, on the grounds of race, color, or national origin be excluded from participation in, be denied the benefits of, or be subject to discrimination in any program receiving Federal Financial assistance.

And in the context of employment, discrimination on the basis of race, color, or national origin discrimination in any employment decisions is illegal under Title VII of the Civil Rights Act of 1964 (Title VII) (42 U.S.C. § 2000e et seq.). This includes employment decisions concerning hiring; firing; promotions; demotions; discipline; compensation; and any other terms, conditions, or privileges of employment.

Sex or Gender

Discrimination on the basis of sex is prohibited under Title IX of the Education Amendments of 1972 (Title IX) (20 U.S.C. § 1681 et seq.) for those institutions receiving federal funds and, in the employment context, is also prohibited under Title VII.

In situations in which a student claims sexual harassment by a teacher, in order for an institution to be held liable under Title IX the student-plaintiff must prove that an appropriate person at the educational institution had actual knowledge of the alleged discrimination and responded with deliberate indifference to the allegation. Actual notice must be given to a person at the institution who has authority to address the alleged discrimination and implement corrective actions. In order to establish institutional liability for student-on-student sexual harassment, the plaintiff must also prove that the offending behavior is so severe, pervasive, and objectively offensive that it denies its victims the equal access to education that Title IX is designed to protect.

Courts recognize two types of sexual harassment claims under Title VII. The first, quid pro quo, occurs when a supervisor requires a subordinate to submit or perform sexual favors or advances as a condition of receiving some tangible job benefit. The second, hostile environment, involves unwelcome, offensive conduct that becomes sufficiently severe and pervasive that it alters the victim's conditions of employment. A hostile environment can be created by a supervisor or non-supervisors such as other employees or third parties. The employer will be held strictly liable if the harassment resulted in some type of tangible or adverse employment action. If there is no tangible or adverse employment action, the employer will not be held liable if it shows (1) that it exercised reasonable care to prevent and promptly correct any harassing behavior; and (2) that the employee unreasonably failed to take advantage of any preventive or corrective opportunities provided by the employer.

One of the key disputes in many discrimination and retaliation cases is whether the plaintiff experienced an adverse employment action. It is clear that courts will consider major actions such as a termination, reduction in pay, demotion, failure to promote, suspension, reassignment, removal, or diminishment of duties and responsibilities to be tangible or adverse. Other minor types of action may not rise to the legal standard of tangible or adverse action. In situations in which an employee or student has raised allegations of discrimination or harassment, is it always a good idea to consult with institutional legal or human resource offices before any type of negative or adverse action is taken.

Federal regulations implementing both Title IX (34 C.F.R. § 106.40) and the Pregnancy Discrimination Act of 1978 (29 C.F.R. § 1604.10) prohibit discrimination on the basis of pregnancy, childbirth, or related illnesses. These laws need to be considered when a nursing program wishes to impose limitations on pregnant students and employees out of concerns that during their work or educational program they could be exposed to substances or diseases that might cause birth defects.

Disability Discrimination and Reasonable Accommodations

State and private schools are prohibited from discriminating against individuals (including employees and students) with disabilities. Although both federal and state laws address disability discrimination, the two leading federal statutes on this subject matter are section 504 of the Rehabilitation Act of 1973 (29 U.S.C. § 794) and the Americans With Disabilities Act of 1990 (ADA) (42 U.S.C. § 12101 et seq.). In most jurisdictions, courts analyzing claims under state disability discrimination law will follow or adopt decisions interpreting the ADA and section 504 federal laws.

The ADA protects qualified individuals with a disability. Under the law, a person is considered disabled if he or she (1) has a physical or mental impairment that substantially limits one or more major life activities, (2) has a record of such impairment, or (3) is regarded as having such an impairment. Temporary impairments of short duration, such as a broken leg, will usually not be considered a protected disability absent long-term or permanent complications. The individual must also be "otherwise qualified," meaning she or he must meet the education, experience, expertise, or other qualifications for a program or position. Courts typically defer to an educational institution's determination of its own qualification standards for applicants, students, and academic programs. The deference is far greater when the university has specified the essential functions of the position through a job description or established technical standards stating the key requirements for admission to, participation in, and graduation from the academic program.

The law imposes a duty to provide reasonable accommodations. This duty arises once a disabled individual indicates that she or he has a disability and needs accommodations. The law does not require that the employee or student use any specific words to invoke the law's protection. There is also no duty if the institution is not aware of the disability and the need for an accommodation. Most colleges and universities will have policies that designate a specific office or administrator to handle all aspects of accommodation requests, from evaluating whether the impairment meets the legal definition of disability to considering and approving specific reasonable accommodations. One of the most important roles that the faculty administrator has is recognizing when a student or employee is making a request for accommodations and then referring the individual to the appropriate office for consideration of the accommodation request.

Once the institution becomes aware that there is a disability and a need for accommodation for an individual, the law requires an interactive process to occur between the institution and that person to determine what reasonable accommodations should be provided. Both sides are required to participate in this interactive process. The institution need not provide the specific accommodations requested by the individual. Reasonable accommodations can include almost anything. However, the institution does not need to make an accommodation that would cause it undue hardship. Courts have found an undue hardship occurs when an accommodation would substantially modify the academic program or if there is a direct threat to the health and safety of the disabled individual or to others.

In response to U.S. Supreme Court cases interpreting the ADA, Congress passed amendments to the ADA in 2008 (Pub. L. No. 110-325, 125 Stat. 3553). The amendments changed the ADA and section 504 to overrule several Supreme Court decisions that limited the number of persons covered by the law. Among the most significant changes to the ADA made by the amendments were those (1) eliminating consideration of mitigating measures when making disability assessments, and (2) expanding the definition of "major life activities" to include major bodily functions and impairments that are episodic in nature or in remission. Many legal commentators believe these amendments will make it easier for plaintiffs to succeed with their disability discrimination claims. It remains to be seen whether subsequent court decisions interpreting the 2008 amendment will bear out these predictions. Because the law will be rapidly evolving in this area, faculty administrators dealing with student or employee accommodation requests should consult institutional counsel or the disability services office to make sure they are handling disability issues in compliance with the most current interpretation of the law.

Religious Discrimination and Accommodations

Title VII also prohibits employers from discriminating against or harassing employees and applicants because of their religious beliefs. It also requires employers to provide employees with reasonable accommodations based on religious beliefs unless the accommodation would cause an undue hardship to the employer. Although the accommodation request process is similar to that followed in disability accommodations, the undue hardship standard is easier for the employer to meet in religious accommodation cases in that they need to show that the accommodation would incur more than a *de minimum* cost.

Age Discrimination

It is illegal for any employer, public or private, to discriminate against persons who are forty (40) years or older under the Age Discrimination in Employment Act (ADEA) (29 U.S.C. § 621 et seq.).

Retaliation Claims

Most federal and state law prohibiting illegal discrimination and harassment also contains provisions that prohibit retaliation by the institution against individuals who bring complaints or participate in the investigation of such allegations. It is not unusual in employment or student discrimination litigation for the institution to prevail on the underlying discrimination complaint but have the court find it liable for retaliating against the plaintiff. In order to state a claim for retaliation, the plaintiff will need to show that she or he engaged in a protected activity and suffered an adverse employment or academic action, and that there is a causal connection between the protected activity and the adverse action. Many faculty administrators find managing a student or employee who has previously raised an allegation of discrimination or harassment to be particularly challenging.

Sarbanes-Oxley Protections

The Sarbanes-Oxley Act of 2002 (15 U.S.C. § 7201) is commonly understood as applying only to publicly traded corporations. In fact, it has two parts that apply to all entities. The first, the Corporate and Criminal Fraud Accountability Act of 2002 (Title VIII), which makes it a crime to "knowingly" alter documents "in relation to or contemplation of" the investigation of "any matter within the jurisdiction of any department or agency" and establishes penalties for retaliating against whistle-blowers. The Corporate Fraud Accountability Act of 2002 (Title XI) makes it a violation of the criminal laws to "tamper" with documents involved in, or "otherwise impede," an "official proceeding." The law imposes both civil and criminal penalties for violations.

There are any number of federal laws that apply to universities that go beyond employment and access to education: research, financial aid, housing, occupational and workplace safety, and environmental, just to name a few obvious ones. Any violation of these laws leads to the possibility (or possibility of contemplation) of a federal investigation; the involvement by the U.S. Equal Employment Opportunity Commission (EEOC) in a claim of employment discrimination is almost commonplace at many large universities. What Sarbanes-Oxley does is add a level of prohibitions to what can be said and done once there is the possibility or existence of an official proceeding; and the charge of retaliation or destruction of evidence is often easier to allege and prove than the underlying misconduct.

Judicial Deference to Academic Decisions

Be it a student challenging an academic dismissal or a faculty member challenging a decision to deny tenure, both federal and state courts will defer to legitimate academic decisions of the faculty and institution. There are many reasons courts give this deference. The two seminal U.S. Supreme Court cases on this question, *Board of Curators of the University of Missouri v. Horowitz* (435 U.S. 78, 98 S.Ct. 948) (1978) and *Regents of the University of Michigan v. Ewing* (474 U.S. 214, 106 S.Ct. 507) (1985), involved the dismissal of two medical students. The principles enunciated in these two decisions establish the broad deference granted by courts in academic decision-making and are frequently cited by subordinate federal and state courts.

The Supreme Court's 1978 decision in the *Horowitz* case involved a student's dismissal from medical school. During Horowitz's first year of clinical rotations, faculty noted dissatisfaction with her clinical performance, attendance at clinical sessions, and personal hygiene. Although the student was advanced to the next year on probation, faculty dissatisfaction with Horowitz's clinical performance continued and, when her performance was again reviewed by a faculty committee, it was recommended that she not be permitted to graduate at the end of the year and that she be dismissed unless she showed "radical improvement." Horowitz was permitted to appeal the decision by taking a set of oral and practical examinations given by seven practicing physicians who were to recommend whether Horowitz should be dropped immediately or remain in the program on probation. Two of the evaluating physicians recommended graduation, two of the evaluating physicians recommended immediate dismissal, and three recommended delaying graduation and continuing probation. After receiving the physician evaluations, the committee reconfirmed its decision to withhold graduation, and after receiving poor evaluations in two more clinical rotations, the committee unanimously voted to dismiss Horowitz from medical school. Students were not typically allowed to appear before either of the evaluating committees when the student's academic performance was being reviewed.

In her lawsuit against the medical school, Horowitz claimed that she had not been given procedural due process prior to her dismissal. Assuming that Horowitz had a constitutionally protected interest requiring procedural due process, the Supreme Court held that during her dismissal, Horowitz had been provided with as much due process as the Fourteenth Amendment required:

> The school fully informed respondent of the faculty's dissatisfaction with her clinical progress and the danger that this posed to timely graduation and continued enrollment. The ultimate decision to dismiss respondent was careful and deliberate. (474 U.S. at 85, 98 S.Ct. at 953)

In its opinion, the Court distinguished between decisions to suspend or dismiss a student for academic versus disciplinary reasons:

> Academic evaluations of a student, in contrast to disciplinary determinations, bear little resemblance to the judicial and administrative fact-finding proceedings to which we have traditionally attached a full-hearing requirement. . . . The decision to dismiss [Horowitz], by comparison, rested on the academic judgment of school officials that she did not have the necessary clinical ability to perform adequately as a medical doctor and was making insufficient progress towards that goal. Such a judgment is by its nature more substantive and evaluative than the typical factual questions presented in the average disciplinary decision. Like the decision of an individual professor as to the proper grade for a student in his course, the determination whether to dismiss a student for academic reasons requires an expert evaluation of cumulative information and is not readily adapted to the procedural tools of judicial or administrative decisionmaking. (435 U.S. at 89–90; 98 S.Ct. at 955)

The Court found that the committee's consideration of Horowitz's clinical attendance and personal hygiene did not convert the dismissal into one for disciplinary reasons. The Court noted that personal hygiene and timeliness may be factors that are as important in a school's determination of whether a student will make a good medical doctor as is the student's ability to take a case history or diagnose an illness.

After finding that Horowitz had no procedural due process right to a formal hearing prior to her dismissal on academic performance grounds, the Supreme Court considered whether the dismissal had violated her rights to substantive due process. On this question, the majority opinion stated,

Courts are particularly ill-equipped to evaluate academic performance. University faculties must have the widest range of discretion in making judgments as to the academic performance of students and their entitlement to promotion or graduation. (435 US 78, 96, n. 6., 98 S.Ct. 948, 958, n. 6)

The U.S. Supreme Court provided additional guidance on the substantive due process requirements in its 1985 decision in *Ewing.* In the fall of 1975, Ewing had enrolled in a 6-year program at the University of Michigan, known as the Inteflex program, which offered both an undergraduate and medical degree upon completion of the program. Although encountering academic difficulties, including marginal passing grades, a number of incompletes, and makeup examinations while on a reduced course load, Ewing had by the spring of 1981 completed all of the courses required for the first 4 years of the Inteflex program. One of the requirements of the Inteflex program was for a student to pass the National Board of Medical Examiners (NBME) Part I examination. In his first attempt at the Part I examination, Ewing failed with the lowest score ever received by an Inteflex student in the program.

The school's Promotion and Review Board reviewed the status of several Inteflex program students, including Ewing, and voted to drop him from the program. At Ewing's written request, the board met a week later to reconsider its decision. Ewing personally appeared before the board to explain why he believed his score did not reflect his academic progress or potential. However, the Promotion and Review Board members unanimously reaffirmed their decision to drop him from the program. He then appealed the board's decision to the Executive Committee of the medical school. After giving Ewing an opportunity to be heard in person, the Executive Committee denied his appeal for a leave of absence and another attempt at the Part I examination.

After exhausting internal appeals within the school, Ewing sued the university, claiming that the school's refusal to allow him to retake the examination was an arbitrary departure from the school's past practice. He claimed the other medical students at the school who had failed the NBME Part I examination had routinely been allowed to take the test a second time.

Ewing pointed to the fact that all 32 medical students who had previously failed the NBME Part I had been permitted to retake the test. He also pointed to a promotional pamphlet issued by the school that stated that a student who failed the examination would be provided an opportunity to retake it. After losing at the trial level, Ewing succeeded before the court of appeals, which held that the failure to permit him to retake the test although all other students who failed had been allowed to do so resulted in Ewing being deprived of his Fourteenth Amendment property right to continued enrollment in the state's medical school program free from arbitrary state action. The Supreme Court reversed, holding that the court of appeals had misapplied the doctrine of "substantive due process." Writing for a unanimous court, Justice Stevens characterized Ewing's claim to be that the university misjudged the student's fitness to remain in the medical school program. Justice Stevens's opinion strongly counsels judges from second-guessing the judgment of faculty:

> *The record unmistakably demonstrates, however, that the faculty's decision was made conscientiously and with careful deliberation, based on an evaluation of the entirety of Ewing's academic career. When judges are asked to review the substance of a genuinely academic decision, such as this one, they should show great respect for the faculty's professional judgment. Plainly, they may not override it unless it is such a substantial departure from accepted academic norms as to demonstrate that the person or committee did not actually exercise professional judgment. (474 U.S. at 225; 106 S.Ct. at 513)*

The *Ewing* Court believed that restrained judicial review of the substance of academic decisions is appropriate because of the lack of standards to guide judicial review, a reluctance to interfere in the prerogatives of state and local educational institutions, and the school's right under the First Amendment to academic freedom and institutional autonomy (474 U.S. at 225–226; 106 S.Ct. at 513–514).

The rationale for judicial deference articulated in these the *Horowitz* and *Ewing* opinions are frequently cited by lower federal and state courts. It provides powerful arguments that a nursing program can rely on to defend itself in litigation and makes it extremely difficult for a student to successfully challenge an adverse academic decision in a court of law.

Distinction Between Academic and Disciplinary Matters

As noted above, courts distinguish between academic dismissals and disciplinary dismissals. They require more due process in disciplinary matters than in academic ones. Although the line is not always clear, it is important to properly classify whether the issue at question is an academic or a disciplinary one. Courts have found the following matters to be academic in nature:

- Matters of personal hygiene, interpersonal skills, and attendance
- Inability to handle stress, make sound judgments, and set priorities
- Repeated failure to produce thesis data when requested
- Incompetent clinical performance because of absence from class and unethical conduct by missing patient appointments
- Sleeping in class, turning in assignments late, and exhibiting behavior that causes concerns about students' commitment to a profession
- Failure to follow supervising faculty's directions or the delivery of unsupervised health care

In contrast, courts have required that institutions provide more due process in situations involving academic misconduct or academic dishonesty issues such as cheating or plagiarism. Generally, courts require that the accused student be given adequate notice of the charges and opportunity for a hearing appropriate to the nature of the case.

The University–Faculty Relationship

In addition to teaching and supervising students, the nursing administrator may also have responsibility for the management and supervision of faculty members within the department, program, or, as is becoming more common in nursing programs, the delivery of a single course taught by a team of faculty members.

Much of the university–faculty relationship will be governed by the provisions of the individual employment contract or faculty appointment letter as supplemented by any written faculty handbook and applicable policies, rules, regulations, and procedures (hereafter referred to as "institutional policies" of the institution, the nursing college or school, and the faculty member's department or program). Such matters can also be governed by unwritten practices that have been routinely applied or followed in the past to address the same type of matter.

It is critical for the nursing administrator to be familiar with these institutional documents and common conduct because they will govern critical faculty matters such as promotion, nonreappointment, dismissal, tenure, discipline, ownership of intellectual property created or invented by the faculty member, assignment of duties and responsibilities, performance evaluation, and grievance rights, to name just a few. Failure to follow or to consistently apply institutional policies can expose the institution to liability on breach of contract or discrimination grounds.

Of course, it is inevitable that situations will arise in which no written institutional policy or unwritten practice exists to guide decision-making. In those circumstances, consultation with the nursing administrator's supervisors is advisable before any action is taken.

At those educational institutions where faculty are part of a union or collective bargaining unit, the terms of the collective bargaining agreement between the institution and the union will also govern the relationship.

Academic Freedom Issues

As an administrator, you will encounter faculty members who may claim an institutional policy or a decision you have made violates the faculty member's right to academic freedom. Despite its importance as a fundamental principle in academia, it is a bit strange to learn that there is no real consensus about the precise meaning of academic freedom and that as a legal principle guiding courts it remains "poorly understood and ill-defined" (Lawrence White, Fifty Years of Academic Freedom, 36 Journal of College and University Law 791 [2010]). Your response to this assertion of academic freedom will depend, in part, on whether you work at a state or governmental institution (i.e., public) or at a private one.

Faculty members employed by a public college or university are protected by the First Amendment of the U.S. Constitution. Therefore, they can sue for violation of their constitutional rights when their employer improperly punishes them for engaging in protected speech or expression. A public institution cannot limit or punish faculty members for speech expressed on a matter of public concern or in his or her role as a private citizen, as opposed to being a public employee. However, this does not mean the faculty member can do or say whatever he or she wants in the classroom. The faculty member can be subject to discipline if his or her speech or conduct in the classroom is unrelated to the course or at variance with the established curriculum. Therefore, he or she will not be protected by the courts under either First Amendment or academic freedom principles.

First Amendment constitutional claims cannot be brought against a private institution. However, a private institution (as well as a state institution) may promise academic freedom to faculty members through the faculty contract or an institutional policy. For example, many private and public institutions of higher education have adopted the American Association of University Professors (AAUP) 1940 Statement of Principles on Academic Freedom and Tenure. The AAUP statement defines academic freedoms as including the "full freedom in research and in the publication of the results," "freedom in the class room in discussing their subject" and freedom from institutional censorship or discipline when the faculty member speaks or writes as a citizen. At institutions that have adopted the AAUP statement or some other definition of academic freedom, a faculty member may assert that this is part of the employment contract.

Tort Claims

Negligence

Institutions and individuals can be held liable for deaths or injuries to person or property that are caused by the negligent acts or omission of the school, its employees, or agents. Although negligence is determined by state law, in general, liability can occur if (1) the institution owes a legal duty of care toward the injured party; (2) the institution has failed to meet the requisite standard of care; and (3) the institution's breach of duty was a proximate cause of the plaintiff's injury. However, liability may not be imposed if the defendant can show that the plaintiff was contributorily negligent or assumed the risk. State institutions may have additional defenses or immunity depending on the state's tort claims act. Consultation with your institution's risk management department or legal office is recommended.

Medical Malpractice

Medical malpractice (professional negligence) liability is usually based on tort law. Malpractice occurs when the health-care provider breaches his or her duty to exercise reasonable skill and care in the treatment of the patient.

Malpractice claims may be brought against both nursing faculty and students who are involved in patient care activities because of educational and training requirements of the nursing school program. The operation of the clinical training program will usually be governed by the terms of the contract (often referred to as an affiliation agreement) between the nursing school or program and the hospital or health-care facility where the clinical training occurs. These contracts almost always contain requirements that the faculty and students assigned to the clinical site have appropriate levels of professional liability and other types of insurance coverage. Usually this insurance coverage is provided for both the employed faculty and students by the school under its own insurance policies. However, in some instances, schools do not provide this insurance coverage for their students and require that the students purchase their own personal, professional liability policy. In either event, it is important for the nursing administrator responsible for the affiliation agreement to make sure that all participants have the required coverage or the institution may be in breach of its contract with the training site, as well as exposed to uninsured financial loss.

Defamation

A claim of defamation can be brought in instances in which the faculty administrator communicates negative information about a student or employee to a third party. This could occur in any number of contexts, such as providing a reference for a student or employee, giving an assessment of a tenure candidate, or responding to a questionnaire from a state board or health-care facility. A defamatory statement is a written or verbal publication of a statement or information that is false and has a tendency to injure a person's reputation. Because defamation is a matter of state law, the elements of a defamatory claim can vary slightly from state to state. In general, to succeed in a defamation case, the plaintiff must prove that a false statement of fact was made that is defamatory in nature and was published to a third party who is not the defendant or plaintiff. Although truth is always a defense to a defamation claim, it may not be easy to prove in court. Because the defamatory statement must be one of fact, an opinion will not be actionable. Another defense to a claim of defamation is that the defamatory statement is protected by an absolute or a qualified privilege. Absolute privileges are available when the plaintiff gives consent or in a legal proceeding. A qualified privilege can be raised when there is a shared legitimate common right, duty, or interest between the defendant publishing the information and the third party receiving it.

Educational Malpractice

Courts have generally not recognized claims of educational malpractice, whether framed in terms of tort or breach of contract, made by students or third parties where the allegation is simply that the educational institution failed to provide a quality education or its pedagogical methods were questionable. Courts are reluctant to recognize educational malpractice as a cause of action because of the difficulty in determining an appropriate standard of care to measure a teacher's conduct, the uncertainty in determining if poor teaching is the reason for the student's failure to learn, the potential burden that permitting such claims might impose on schools and courts, and recognition that courts are not equipped to oversee the daily operations of an educational institution. The Iowa Supreme Court in *Moore v. Vanderloo* (386 N.W.2d 108) (Iowa 1986) relied on these reasons in rejecting an educational malpractice claim brought by a patient against a school, alleging that the patient's injuries were caused by the school's inadequate training of the chiropractor who treated him.

Summary

This chapter provides only a very basic and introductory explanation of the more common types of legal issues that the faculty administrator is likely to encounter in his or her job. Later chapters in this book build on this summary of basic legal issues with more specific situational examples and discussion.

Our objective here is to help you "spot the legal issues" so you can be sensitive to the fact that there are legal ramifications that can form relationships, breach obligations, and expose your institution (and even yourself) to potential financial liability. When you *start* feeling you are out of your depth, *that* is the time you should go to your supervisor and consider contacting university counsel.

CHAPTER 3

How to Read a Judicial Decision

Thanks to Lexis, Westlaw, and other commercial companies, it is easy to research the law and find decisions that have been reported.[1] One has to know what she is reading, though, before she can decide it is meaningful. This chapter explains how judicial decisions are written and reported, to give a sense about how to read and use them.

Cases are always referred to by their citations, an example of which follows:

Wilson v. El-Daief, 600 Pa. 161, 964 A.2d 354 (2009)

What this tells the reader is that those involved in the lawsuit was a person named Wilson, and he was opposed by a person named El-Daief. Their dispute was so seriously contested that they took it all the way to the Supreme Court of Pennsylvania (Pa.), which decided the case in 2009. The court's opinion can be found in two different books (Pa. and A.2d), but it can also be found in LEXIS, Westlaw (WL), and even through Google (go ahead and try it).

Readers will see that the opinion is divided into the parts described below.

Caption

At the very top of the decision will be the names of the people or entities that were having the dispute. The title of the case is called its *caption*. At the trial level, the person or organization (called a *party*) who started the lawsuit is called the *plaintiff* (sometimes the *petitioner*). Their names come first. The person who was sued is called the *defendant* (or the *respondent*). At higher levels (i.e., once the case goes up on appeal), the first-named party is typically the one who lost and who is called the *appellant* (the one who is calling on the appellate court for justice). The party that won is called the *appellee*. The v. that separates the plaintiff/appellant from the defendant/appellee stands for *versus*. The abbreviation *et al.* is sometimes included on one or both sides of the v., which stands for et alia, meaning "and others."

---

[1] Whether one uses LEXIS or Westlaw is really just a matter of personal preference. Each offers different ways of researching the law. Both are excellent.

Court

The next segment of the judicial decision will indicate the name of the court from which the decision was reported, and the name of the judge(s) who wrote it. In the federal system, the trial court is called the United States District Court, the appellate court is called the United States Circuit Court of Appeals, and the highest appellate court is the United States Supreme Court. The states have named their courts in inconsistent ways, so be careful. New York State's supreme court is actually its lowest-level court, and its appeals courts have divisions. The *Bluebook* has a list for each state of the state courts from the highest down to the lowest trial court.[2]

Key Numbers

The commercial companies that publish legal decisions have done their best to break down every decision into the specific points that the judge(s) made. They have then organized all of those legal issues into an outline of the law that is astonishing in its scope and complexity (because of how interrelated the law is). The company has assigned each small legal issue its own place in the outline by giving it a unique identifying code (library and number). By doing so, they are collecting in the same location every decision rendered by any judge in any jurisdiction (trial or appellate, state or federal) in any decision that the company has reported. It's a service the company offers, but is neither foolproof nor official.

This organization of the law does not make any effort to distinguish between the actual holding in the case (the bottom line of the decision) and the legal principles that were specifically required to reach that decision, and the more general discussion about the law that the judges typically employ to frame the issues or describe the process they used to get to their decision. This latter is called *dictum* and, although interesting, instructive, or even persuasive, it is not of precedential value, authoritative, or binding in any way.

Summary and Holding

In a short paragraph, the company then summarizes the parties, claims, and disposition. This is provided as a service by the company; it is not official but usually very instructive concerning the larger points.

---

[2] The *Bluebook* began in 1926 as *A Uniform System of Citation: Abbreviations and Form of Citations*. In 1939, the paperback was published with blue covers. It formally took the name the *Bluebook* in 1991. As it accurately says of itself, it is "the definitive style guide for legal citation in the United States. For generations, law students, lawyers, scholars, judges, and other legal professionals have relied on *The Bluebook*'s unique system of citation" (http://www.legalbluebook.com). It is the legal profession's equivalent to Strunk and White's *Elements of Style* or APA style for scholarly papers.

The Court's Opinion

The court's opinion is actually the text of the judge's decision. It is typically written in parts: (1) who the parties are, (2) at what point in the process the decision is being rendered, (3) the questions to be addressed in the opinion, (4) the answers the judge gives to them, and, often, (5) what happens next. The commercial reporters typically reproduce the full text of the decisions.

Judges are empowered to make their own decisions, but they are required to follow the law. Some decisions are binding on them, namely, decisions rendered by the appellate courts that are higher than theirs in the same system and decisions made in courts that have primary jurisdiction over the issues. This means, for example, that federal courts have primary jurisdiction over federal laws and the U.S. Constitution, and the courts in Pennsylvania have primary jurisdiction over disputes in Pennsylvania.

To show that they are following the law, judges will specifically refer to other decisions that have been rendered on the point they are discussing. These are called *precedents,* and the opinion will therefore cite the decision by the names of the parties (all underlined) and give the address in the libraries of the commercial reporters where those decisions can be found.

Reporters and Citations

When a decision is first issued by the court, it is a separate opinion, by itself, not yet collected for publication with others. At this stage, it is called a *slip opinion.* Most written decisions by judges are then collected and published in sets of books called *reporters* that can be either official or unofficial.[3] There will often be two different publishing companies that have taken the official opinions and reproduced them, in hard volumes and/or over the Internet, adding additions to them that they hope will make people want to buy and use their specific services. The text of the decisions should not be different, but the ways of searching for useful or applicable decisions will be.

Each decision (called a *case*) has its own unique identifier, called a *citation*— usually the name of the reporter, the volume, and the page number on which the case begins. Reporters are generally organized by the kind of court and its location. For state court decisions, the official reporter will usually have a state abbreviation as its name, such as *Pennsylvania Reports* (abbreviated as Pa.). The major commercial publisher has grouped the states into regions and publishes regional reporters containing decisions from that group of state courts. Pennsylvania cases

---

[3] Official reporters are those the state or federal court designates as its own. There are also unofficial reporters containing the same decisions that are published in print by commercial publishers. The same written decisions can also be retrieved on the Internet from commercial databases such as Westlaw and LEXIS, or on other sites, including sites the particular court runs. For example, the Supreme Court of the United States posts its decisions on its Web site as they are issued each term.

are published in the Atlantic regional reporter (abbreviated as A.), which covers the mid-Atlantic states (Delaware, Maryland, New Jersey, and Pennsylvania). There are so many decisions that there will be a second, third, fourth, and fifth series of the reporters (abbreviated as 2d, 3d, etc.).

When a decision is published in more than one place, the citations are called *parallel citations,* usually referencing the official journal as well as the commercial one (or two) where it can be found. Recall the example from the beginning of this chapter:

Wilson v. El-Daief, 600 Pa. 161, 964 A.2d 354 (2009)

In this example, the same written decision of the Pennsylvania Supreme Court can be found in volume 600 of the *Pennsylvania Reports* (Pa.) beginning on page 161, and also in volume 964 of the *Atlantic Reporter, Second Series* (A.2d), beginning on page 354. One could retrieve the decision either by using books in a law library or by typing one of the citations into a commercial database.

The following are examples of citations of federal court cases:

Miranda v. Arizona, 384 U.S. 436, 16 L.Ed. 2d 694, 86 S.Ct. 1602 (1966)

This Supreme Court decision would be found in volume 384 of the *United States Reports* beginning on page 436. That is the official reporter. The decision is also published in two other unofficial reporters: the *Lawyers Edition* (L.Ed.), and the *Supreme Court Reporter* (S.Ct.). They are parallel citations.

Enron Oil Corp. v. Diakuhara, 10 F.3d 90 (2d Cir. 1993)

This decision from the Second Circuit Court of Appeals, which is an intermediate federal appellate court, would be found in volume 10 of the *Federal Reporter, Third Series,* beginning on page 90.

When there is a published reporter that contains an opinion, the proper citation is to cite the reporter. Before reporter citation is available, cases may be cited in a more complicated way, typically at Westlaw or LEXIS, that identifies the case by name and the commercial database identifier:

Ji v. Bose Corp., 2010 WL 4722276 (1st Cir. 2010)

Once the case receives a citation to the *Federal Reporter* (it will be included in the F.3d series), that would become its proper citation. There are also some opinions that are never officially published, often because the court has made the judgment that the case does not add to the law and is not significant to persons other than the parties involved. Because a court's decisions are public, the commercial databases will often obtain these opinions from the clerk and publish them anyway. There are rules set by each court about using their so-called unpublished opinions, so caution is needed before relying on one of these.

Remember, just because a case has a citation, don't assume that it is good law or even law at all. The citation just tells someone where to find it. What's inside the decision is what lawyers get paid to fight about!

CHAPTER 4

The Role of the University Attorney: When the Academic Nursing Administrator Comes Calling

Society has become very litigious. Everyone seems to want to fight for their rights instead of compromising to find some mutual accord. That's one of the reasons that the law fills so many volumes, is so complicated, and hardly ever provides one definitive, single answer to a question. Academia might once have been protected from these pressures, but the day of the ivory tower is long gone. Today, the law is a constant visitor to the campus. It audits every class and faculty meeting and personal interaction. Its millions of pages are accessible over cell phones to those who believe they have been wronged, and a carefully worded search will produce a decision right on point to support their positions.

A multitude of legal issues confronts the contemporary nursing faculty members in the classroom, in clinical settings, and in their professional role as members of the faculty. Academic nursing administrators not only see these issues directly but also must help guide others through them and manage them as business matters, adding new dimensions (and new exposures to liability) to situations that are already complicated. But although all this may appear overwhelming and poised to swamp the academic enterprise at every possible turn, the fact is that the world is largely no different on campus than it is off. The major difference is that everyone on campus is accustomed to inquiry and argument, and to being rewarded for persistence.

This book was written to help nursing faculty and administrators identify, address, and resolve some of the legal issues that you are likely confront in the classroom and clinical environment during your tenure as a faculty member and/or academic administrator. It should help you in making real-life decisions with legal and ethical bases in mind about academic issues that range from interpersonal incivility to unconstitutional discrimination. But it cannot address every issue you will face, nor provide the specific guidance that you might need in any particular instance. That's why universities have lawyers.

When to Call

The old medical saying "An ounce of prevention is worth a pound of cure" also rings true in the legal setting. When you become aware of an issue that could have legal implications, or can see a situation that might get out of control, you should get someone else involved in helping you think it through—a more senior member of the faculty, your department head, or your dean. In the majority of universities and colleges across the country, that's about as far as you will be able to go, because there is no one else to consult.[1] But more and more universities are hiring attorneys as part of the staff, and larger universities may have several in the Office of General Counsel. As its name suggests, it is there to provide advice and counsel on a wide variety of matters to members of the university. It is also the gateway to attorneys who specialize in particular fields such as intellectual property, tax, employment discrimination, federal regulations, and litigation.

If a university has one or more attorneys on staff, be sure that they are busy helping the university's administrators conduct university business: reviewing and negotiating contracts, helping the director of human relations with specific employment-based issues, dealing with insurance companies and municipal authorities, and assisting the president and chief financial officer. Although all these tasks are important and will fill any attorney's day, if you are served with legal process and the time to respond is running out, then dealing with your problem takes precedence over them all. If and when you receive a summons, complaint, or lawyer's letter, do not put it aside: call the university counsel and deliver that document to her immediately.

The best time to involve the university counsel, however, is before that lawyer comes looking for you, or when you have to seek your own lawyer. At the core, the university attorney's role is managing risks. In almost every context, her objective is to be predictive about all of the things that might go wrong, and build into the situation steps that will reduce the university's exposure to disruption and loss. In contracts, these are the written terms of the deal being negotiated; in ongoing relationships, this is practical advice that will help her clients avoid issues or solve them before they grow much larger.

---

[1] But do not give up if legal counsel is not directly available to you. Other institutional resources may be available at your college or university to help you manage matters that have legal issues associated with them such as the human resources department, risk management, student and employee disability services office, campus security or police department, campus counseling center, or an equality/equity office. Each of these offices will be staffed by administrators who, although not attorneys, have a wealth of professional experience and training.

The Rules of Engagement

When you call university counsel, you are making an official call, from one university employee/official to another. Under the legal profession's Code of Ethics, lawyers owe the duty of undivided loyalty to their clients. That means that everything a lawyer does must be done in her client's best interests (or at least, what she thinks them to be). In conducting her client's affairs with others, the lawyer must conduct herself with honesty and integrity as well as be a zealous advocate for her client, using her best efforts at all times. The lawyer must keep her client well advised about what she is doing and about any developments that are material to the client's interests. Finally, a lawyer is duty bound to keep confidential everything that her client tells her in confidence. Therefore, clients may be totally honest and in return receive the best possible legal advice, based on the circumstances having been presented factually.

These ground rules may seem pretty straightforward, and when the client is an individual, they are. But what happens when the client is a corporation, as is a university? To whom is the duty of undivided loyalty owed? The president? The dean? The board of trustees? Whose lawyer is she really? If you tell her something, from whom must it be held in confidence? When the issue is a lawsuit filed against you, alleging that you caused harm to a student or a third party, the answers to these questions are clear: your interests are the same as the university's, and you want everyone to know what is going on because you are all working together. But what happens if your dispute is with your department head or dean? Does it matter if your interest is personal (you think you have been unfairly treated) or organizational (you think your superior is breaking university policy)?

These are some of the toughest issues that university counsel have to decide, and they are the topics of regular continuing legal education for them. But they are the attorney's issue, not yours. When you seek the advice of university counsel, begin by telling them the nature of the issue and the dispute and ask them if they will keep in confidence what you are about to tell them. They should respond by telling you that they will do so until such time as they recognize a conflict of interest. At that time, they should tell you that they can no longer help you on a confidential basis and you will have to decide whether to proceed further. Until then, though, you have been the attorney's client and they must not tell anyone else what you have told them unless you give them authorization (consent) to do so.[2]

---

[2] There are exceptions to this general rule, but they are extreme. For example, a lawyer may disclose to others a client's intention to break the law or to do someone else bodily harm. You can be sure that university counsel would quickly do so.

University Counsel as Advisor

From the discussion of the law in Chapter 2, you can tell that there is a wide variety of laws that apply to universities that are, in many respects, like small cities. No lawyer can claim to be a master of all legal issues, and it is unlikely that university counsel will be a specialist in any. Instead, university counsel are typically generalists, equipped to handle most matters presenting themselves in the university context because they can do the legal research that is required to produce a reasonably reliable result. In most circumstances, that is enough.

Although it may be the first time that you have ever faced the issue that is troubling you, it is likely that the university's legal counsel has faced it before—you may just not have heard of it because it was handled confidentially. When you call the attorney, you may get the answer right then; however, it is more likely your question will itself be met with lots of questions. You won't find this frustrating after reading the preceding chapters, because you will recognize at once what is going on: the attorney knows the outline of the law and is using her questions to discover the facts to discover and learn where the issue best fits in that outline, so she can give you the most precise answer to your question.

That answer may not be what you expected or wanted. Instead of being a final decision, the answer may be a recommendation that you perform some action or take some step. This is because lawyers know that most disputes are actually resolved not on the merits of a decision, but through procedures that lead to agreements. The advice may include suggestions about things to say as well as steps to take, and will almost always include documenting and making a record of what you are doing. Thinking down the line, the lawyer knows that juries feel more confident in finding the facts if there is a document that was created at the time that proves what the facts were. Take, for example, employment disputes: saying that you met with someone who reported to you and discussed the problems you had with her performance several times before you terminated her is far more credible if you kept notes from those meetings at the time and placed them in her personnel file. When the attorney receives a copy of her client's file (as she quickly will) and sees your notes, the employee's attorney will feel very differently about whether to take the case and how zealously she can advocate for her client than if those notes were not there.

A major benefit of university counsel is their ability to help you think of alternatives.[3] If she does her job well, she will be more broadly versed in the university as a whole, and be able to identify resources within the university community unknown to you that may help resolve the situation. You will know more about the

---

[3] This is not a skill that all attorneys have. Unfortunately there are counsel who view their role as simply that of being able to reject requests. The more experienced and valuable counsel are those who say, "You cannot do it the way you propose, but there are other ways to reach the same objective."

subject matter and context in which the problem arises. Working together, you have a better opportunity to figure it out.

The other major role of university counsel is to advise you regarding the obligations you owe—and the rights you have—as a representative of the university. This may be in interpreting the regulations of a government agency or the terms of a grant you have been awarded; analyzing the conflicting duties you may owe to funder, patient, or student; or defining what *due process* means in the context of a grievance hearing or what *academic freedom* means in the context of classroom behavior or academic research. What you think is fair really is not important (or material, as a lawyer would say), and the answers to your questions will not always (or even predictably) be rational. The best course of action is to ask. You won't be faulted if you followed the advice of university counsel or were not provided it when you asked for it.

University Counsel as Mediator

Because the primary role of university counsel is that of risk manager, she will be ever on guard to reduce the likelihood that disputes within the university community will rise to the level of formal complaints requiring adjudication by grievance officers or courts. The university has many levels of employees and officers, from the most recently hired secretary to the chairperson of the board of trustees, all of whom form the client. On a day-to-day basis, they may have the same interests, or they may not. Because everyone is different, perceives things differently, and communicates imperfectly, conflict can easily arise within the group. In an era of economic shortage and increasing demands, opportunities abound for personnel issues to arise.

In the formal construct, an attorney must choose her client and take a side. In fact, university counsel often acts more as a mediator than an attorney. This can take two different forms: shuttling between disputing colleagues and being an active participant in helping them work out a problem, or advising both sides behind the scenes on how each might approach the other. In this case, the lawyer owes the same obligations to each side. He can only reveal confidential facts to the extent permitted by the one who gave the facts to him, which requires him to create an internal barrier to separate the confidences and instructions of one from another. He cannot help one more than the other. If the dispute is not resolved, he cannot represent either and must recuse (remove) himself from further involvement.

These are the ground rules that the lawyer should explain to the university employee whenever advice regarding an intrauniversity issue is sought. You need to know that the university attorney is providing this service to you because her client is the university and, in performance of the ethical and professional obligations the attorney owes to that client, she is going to do her very best to resolve the issue at the lowest possible level, thereby reducing the risks and costs to her client. There is a conflict of interest in performing these two very different roles at the same time. You waive that conflict when you seek the attorney's advice on the personal matter because you accept the fact that she is trying to do her best for the university. If you are out for your own purposes, then you need to hire (and pay for) your own attorney.

University Counsel as Advocate

In dealings with third parties, university counsel has an undivided loyalty to zealously advocate for the university. Within the university, the university counsel's job is to enforce the university's rules and procedures and advance its (corporate) interests. In both realms, there is a hierarchy of authority that begins at the top, above the university president, with the chairperson of the board, and is constrained by published university bylaws, codes, policies, and procedures.

In these circumstances, there is a right answer, and the university counsel can be relied on to give it and enforce it. If you have been sued because of something you did within the scope of your duties for the university, you can be confident that university counsel will advocate zealously in your defense—subject to the university making the final decisions about whether to defend the claim and when to settle it.[4]

The role of advocate is different from that of decision-maker. A lawyer does not make substantive decisions. He can advise you about the consequences of certain actions, but the client always has the right to decide which action to take, even if the lawyer thinks it is a bad idea and recommends against it. If the lawyer believes the course of conduct you have decided on is not in the university's best interests, she will tell you that you (and she) cannot proceed with it without getting the approval of someone at a higher level of authority.

There is one part of the university that university counsel does not represent, and that is the student. University counsel will always defend and advocate for the university and any of its employees against a student. The duty that the attorney owes the student derives solely from the promises the university has made to the student, and even here the duty is indirect: the lawyer will advocate to university personnel on behalf of students, but once an issue is decided, the lawyer's duty to

---

[4] Indeed, virtually every university will carry a variety of insurance policies (such as general liability, errors and omissions, professional liability, etc.) that cover employees and agents when they are alleged to be legally responsible (liable) for actions committed while acting within the scope of the employee's or agent's scope of duties for the university. Often these universities will have an institutional policy that describes the circumstances and conditions under which their employee or agent will be eligible for indemnification and defense from the institution; and that policy will also indicate, directly or by inference, when the university will not protect the employee. Many universities require their employees to disclose potential conflicts of interest. One of the reasons that it is important for the employee to do so thoroughly is to make sure that the university knows what he or she is doing, so that there won't be any question about whether the insurance later covers the employee in case a claim is asserted.

the university takes over, and she will advocate to the student whatever that decision is.

University Counsel and You

University counsel adds an important dimension and can play a valuable role in the academic community. You will find that attorneys will ask you questions (because of their training) that will help you get a clearer picture of the situation you are confronting. If the matter involves something inside the university, the help you get may be more practical than truly legal in nature, because (as every lawyer will tell you) the facts are key. Change the facts just a bit, and the legal implications can be substantial. That's why it is smarter to involve the university counsel earlier in the process rather than later, so that she can help you create and develop options for resolution. It will also give you confidence that you are doing the best you can and that you will be defended by the university if the issue cannot be resolved and develops into a claim.

Legal Cases With Nursing Students and Nursing Faculty

CHAPTER 5

The Role of the Ombudsman for the Student

CASE STUDY

A Student Files a Complaint With the University Ombudsman

Your role: You are Dr. Fairchild, the Associate Dean for Graduate Nursing Programs.

Davinia Morris, CNM, is an experienced certified nurse-midwife who first earned her certificate in nurse midwifery in 1990—years before master's preparation for nurse midwives became the standard. Ms. Morris (who has a BA degree in psychology) decided to enter an MS completion program in midwifery that would allow her to obtain the MS degree but not repeat most of her previous midwifery clinical courses. Ms. Morris looked for a program that would take the least amount of time and have the lowest cost. A fellow nurse-midwife friend told Ms. Morris that she should contact a nearby university, the University of Alcoa, which all her nurse-midwife friends had attended for their MS completion degrees, indicating she could earn it quickly there. Ms. Morris made an e-mail inquiry to the nurse midwifery program director, Ms. Anna Strauss, and Ms. Strauss informed her by e-mail that she would need to take only 15 credits to receive her MS degree. Ms. Morris was thrilled because, although this program was not online, it required the fewest credits of any she investigated and was within easy commuting distance. Ms. Morris subsequently proceeded to take her five courses over the next 2 years.

At this same time, the College of Nursing (where this degree program resides) migrated from a paper-and-file student record system (with centralized filing in respective departments) to an online system in which paperless/electronic files are now maintained in the registrar's office. Upon completing her five courses (15 credits), Ms. Morris applied for graduation, but to her horror she was informed that a minimum of 30, not 15, credits must be taken *at the University of Alcoa* for any graduate student who seeks a master's degree. Ms. Morris immediately notified the program director about this issue, and Ms. Strauss declared there must be some mistake, stating that "we have always awarded the MS Completion for Nurse Midwifery after 15 credits." Ms. Strauss called the registrar and attempted to bully her into awarding the student the MS degree. When the registrar would not award the degree, she (the registrar) decided to do some historical checking and found out that at least 12 other nurse-midwife students had been awarded the completion MS degrees in the past with only 15 credits. When the registrar notified Ms. Strauss of this violation of policy, Ms. Strauss denied knowing of the policy, but blamed the registrar for her lack of oversight stating, "Don't blame me, you yourself signed off on all these degrees!" Trying to prevent widespread exposure of this violation of policy and procedure by both the midwifery department and the registrar's office, Ms. Strauss stated it wouldn't happen again, told the registrar she would work something out with the student, and said that there was no need to do anything else.

Ms. Strauss subsequently attempted to strike a deal with the student, but Ms. Morris refused to take any additional credits. Furious, Ms. Morris (and without going through any further channels) immediately notified the university ombudsman and copied you, the Associate Dean for Graduate Nursing Programs. She was emphatic that she had a credit agreement "in writing" (the e-mail) from the program director, and she demanded that the university own up to its commitment to her and award her the MS degree.

Questions

- As associate dean, how would you first proceed?
- Who should take the lead in solving this issue: the ombudsman or the associate dean who was copied on the complaint?
- Independent of the student's issue with the ombudsman, what should your course of action as associate dean be toward the program director who reports to you?
- What is the role of the registrar's office in this incident?

Student Use of a University Ombudsman: Legal Principles and Review of the Literature

The use of some type of ombudsman is prevalent in academia and is one of the roles in the field of *alternative dispute resolution* (ADR) (Gadlin, 2000). *Merriam-Webster's Online Dictionary* (2010) defines *ombudsman* as "one that investigates, reports on, and helps settle complaints" (p. 1). The first use of the role of the ombudsman was in the early 1800s, when Sweden used the ombudsman post to hear grievances against the government, parliament, and administrative offices (Levin, 2009). There are, however, many different models of *ombudsmanship*.

The first type of ombudsman is the *classical ombudsman*, which "emphasizes statutory independence from governmental control, the power to investigate complaints, and the authority to publish findings and recommendations" (Gadlin, 2000, p. 38). The classical ombudsman's role and function are established by statute. There are some instances in which this type of ombudsman is prevalent in the university setting, discussed later in the chapter. Gottehrer and Hostina (1998), in *Essential Characteristics of a Classical Ombudsman*, indicate the classical ombudsman role must have the four following characteristics: independence; impartiality and fairness; credibility of the review process; and confidentiality.

The second type of ombudsman is the *organizational ombudsman,* whose roles are similar to those of the classical ombudsman. However, the position or role has not been established by statute; rather, it was established by organizational forces such as a vote of a faculty senate or student body (Gadlin, 2000). Some universities also have ombudsmen that operate more organizationally than they do classically. However, both types are represented in the International Ombudsman Association (IOA) (formed in 2005 with the merger of the University and College Ombudsman Association [UCOA] and The Ombudsman Association [TOA]). According to the IOA Web site, "IOA is the largest international association of professional organizational ombudsman practitioners in the world, representing over 500 members from the United States and across the globe" (2007, p.1)

The IOA publishes three documents that are critical to the implementation and function of the ombudsman role:

1. *IOA Code of Ethics* (posted January 2007)
2. *IOA Standards of Practice* (posted October 2009)
3. *IOA Best Practices* (posted October 2009)

These documents are all open source and available from the IOA's Standards & Practice Web site (http://www.ombudsassociation.org/standards/). The *IOA Code of Ethics* is briefly summarized here and the *Standards of Practice* and *Best Practices* documents are discussed in Chapter Six.

IOA Code of Ethics

There are four ethical principles—independence, neutrality and impartiality, confidentiality, and informality. First, "The Ombudsman is *independent*[1] in structure, function, and appearance to the highest degree possible within the organization" (International Ombudsman Association [IOA], *Code of Ethics,* 2007, p. 1). According to Shelton, "It is intended that this independence be protected, as much as possible within the institution, by placing the appointment at the highest level of authority" (2000, p. 84). In other words, petitioning students cannot perceive the university ombudsman as inherently favoring faculty or university officials but as an independent agent who will review a grievance independently of the other, often more powerful individuals in the organization.

Second, the ombudsman must show *neutrality* and *impartiality.* The IOA states, "The Ombudsman, as a designated neutral, remains unaligned and impartial. The Ombudsman does not engage in any situation which could create a conflict of interest" (2007, p. 1). Neutrality is essential, particularly if the ombudsman is going to have credibility among various different agents within the university. It is

---

[1] Emphasis added.

obvious to both undergraduate and graduate students that individuals in the university, especially faculty with a PhD, for instance, or a department chair or associate dean have both personal status and power. The ability of the ombudsman to evaluate each side equally, no matter the status or position, is indeed one of the particular skills of an adept ombudsman. The definition of neutrality expressed in the ombudsman policy at Albany State University (Albany, Ga.) states "[neutrality] enables the Ombudsman to see and appreciate both sides of the problem and places him or her in the best possible position to promote solutions that will be accepted by all parties involved"(p. 1, n.d.). Impartiality is a slightly different concept than neutrality. Bauer favors the term *ombudsperson* (the more gender-neutral title) used at the University of Western Ontario, in London, Ontario, Canada, and indicates that impartiality "speaks to the way I behave towards different constituents within the university" (p. 61). She further elaborates, "I like the fact that impartiality is the way I behave, rather than the way I think or feel. It is clearer than neutrality, which the dictionary associates with war and adversarial conflicts" (p. 61).

The third principle is *confidentiality*. Again the IOA defines it as meaning that "the Ombudsman holds all communications with those seeking assistance in strict confidence, and does not disclose confidential communications unless given permission to do so. The only exception to this privilege of confidentiality is where there appears to be imminent risk of serious harm." It should be elaborated, however, that "if the complainant wishes only to talk, that will be respected. But if action is desired for a specific problem, total confidentiality becomes impossible" (Stieber, 2000, p. 53).

A differentiation should further be made between the concept of *anonymity* versus *confidentiality*. Absolute anonymity, although desired by the student complainant or any other complainant, may not be feasible or practical, especially if competing parties ultimately want some form of mediation or compromise. The Houston Community College Web site indicates that "the Office of the Ombudsman will not provide specific information with the *reasonable hope of preserving the anonymity*[2] of the person alleging the claim" (Young, 2008, p. 5).

The last IOM principle is the concept *informality* (2007). Here, "the Ombudsman, as an informal resource, does not participate in any formal adjudicative or administrative procedure related to concerns brought to his/her attention" (p. 1). The ombudsman will attempt to resolve conflicts or disputes through mediation and recommendation, whereas going to human resources to file a complaint for a violation of university policy, using any available ethics hotline to report a wide range of unethical behaviors, or perhaps contacting the campus-based Equal Employment Opportunity Commission (EEOC) authority

---

[2] Emphasis added.

(e.g., for charges of discrimination) are all alternative but *formal* dispositional ways of resolving issues.

Some university ombudsman positions may be structured so that they see appeals made by students only, whereas some universities may have a separate faculty ombudsman position that is aimed at protecting faculty interests, such as is the case at Ohio State University (2010). It is important for students to ask to which ombudsman (if there is more than one type) they should direct their complaints.

Discussion of Case

In the Case Study for this chapter, the first question is, As associate dean, how would you first proceed? Dr. Fairchild was flabbergasted by this incident and wondered what was really going on. The midwifery program had been independently placed in the organizational structure for a long time and had only recently been moved to Dr. Fairchild's portfolio of departments and programs for which she had administrative responsibility. She really was unaware that there was a post-master's option in midwifery because no one ever talked about it. Therefore, she was a little more suspicious than usual about what was going on.

The second question is, Who should take the lead in solving this issue: the ombudsman or the associate dean who was copied on the complaint? In this case, Dr. Fairchild communicated with the ombudsman that he should first rule on the case of the student complaint before any further discussion took place about how to evaluate the actions of the program director.

The third question is, independent of the student's issue with the ombudsman, what should your course of action as the associate dean be toward the program director who reports to you? Once she had initiated communication with the ombudsman, Dr. Fairchild immediately notified Ms. Strauss that all communication between the student and herself (Ms. Strauss) must cease until the issue is resolved. Further, although not discussed with the ombudsman, Dr. Fairchild also wondered to what degree the office of the registrar had been either complicit or negligent with the awarding of previous master's degrees in this program in violation of the university policy. Dr. Fairchild did notify the dean of the college about the pending case and brought her up to date with the facts.

Findings and Disposition

The university ombudsman concluded that indeed there was evidence that the student was informed by the program director that she would receive her completion master's degree after accruing 15 semester credits or five courses. The ombudsman ruled that this type of communication was incorrect and was not in line with standard university policy at the time of the student's matriculation. Further, although the ombudsman was sympathetic with the student's complaint and her request to be awarded the degree because she had completed her requirements in good faith, the ombudsman did not agree that the e-mail communication should be upheld. Instead a compromise was made and the student was allowed to apply for graduation when she completed 27 credits, not 30. In other words, the student was given a one-course reduction because of the miscommunication on the part of the program director. Again, although sympathetic to the student complaint, the ombudsman ruled that it would be improper and a violation of higher education standards, including those of Alcoa University, that anyone would be awarded a master's degree after taking only 15 credit hours. The ombudsman did not rule on any actions toward the program director, Ms. Strauss. However, upon disposition of the student complaint, the associate dean subsequently wrote up Ms. Strauss for her violation of the university policy and indicated that any further deviation from university policy, with regard to graduation requirements or *any other standard university policy* would result in Ms. Strauss being terminated.

The last question is, What was the role of the registrar's office in this incident? Dr. Fairchild, in consultation with the dean, opted not to pursue any action against the registrar mainly because in this case the registrar did rebel and refuse to award the degree. Although the associate dean and dean agreed there was obviously some sloppiness in the registrar's office, they opted to give the registrar the benefit of the doubt. They considered that only with the introduction of electronic files was it possible to ensure that all credits toward individual degrees could be absolutely accounted for. Ms. Morris accepted the ombudsman ruling as she thought it fruitless to appeal to the president of the university. Ms. Strauss accepted her punishment, although she was angry that it would likely appear in her annual evaluation and affect her annual merit raise. The registrar contacted the dean and assured her that their electronic systems would certainly prevent this from ever happening again.

Relevant Legal Case

Student Files Personal Injury Lawsuit in Federal Court Over Final Grade of "C" After Negative Ruling by University Ombudsperson

Brian C. Marquis v. University of Massachusetts at Amherst, No. 07-30015 (D. Mass. Jan. 31, 2007).

In the fall of 2006, the plaintiff, Brian Marquis, enrolled in an undergraduate course in philosophy, Philosophy 161: Problems in Social Thought, at the University of Massachusetts–Amherst. Mr. Marquis was a 51-year-old paralegal seeking a double major in legal studies and sociology. The course was taught by a teaching assistant, Jeremy Cushing. On the first day of class, Mr. Cushing passed out a syllabus in which he indicated there would be three examinations each worth 25%

of the final grade (75%); four response papers each worth 5% each (20%); and the remaining 5% for class participation. According to the lawsuit filed in the district court of Massachusetts, the syllabus read as follows: "Each paper will receive a number grade (from 0–5) in .5 point increments" (2007, p. 4).When the semester concluded, the plaintiff had the following grades: 23, 22.5, and 19.5 (out of a possible 25%); response paper grades of 5, 4, 4, 4.5 (out of 5s); and a 5% class participation grade that appears to be unknown, but the plaintiff calculated in the full 5%. The plaintiff therefore calculated his grade to be 92.5% and thus an A–. Upon receiving his grade report, however, he was given a final grade of 84 and thus awarded a C. After the plaintiff first appealed to the teaching assistant, Mr. Cushing claimed that "to make the grades more representative of student performances, I set a curve (or, more accurately, I drew up a new grade scale)" (Complaint, 2007, p. 5). It should be noted that a curve grading scale was not mentioned on the syllabus (Elder, 2010). As written about in the *Boston Globe*: "Cushing wrote back that he graded the students more stringently on the third exam because they had a full semester to learn how to write for a philosophy class....But the students' scores struck Cushing as too high, so he graded everyone on a curve before assigning letter grades" (Saltzman, 2007, p. 2).

Subsequently, Mr. Marquis appealed to the department chair, Phillip Bricker, who denied the appeal and who later stated, "I think suing over a grade is somewhat absurd....It ended up just wasting a lot of people's time and money"(Saltzman, p. 2). An appeal was then made to the ombudsperson, Catherine Porter, who also denied the appeal, writing, "I would urge you to accept this grade and continue with your course work as these are no grounds for an academic grievance" (Complaint, 2007, p. 5). Porter also stated that in 30 years at the university she had never had never heard of a grade appeal like this one. With all appeals denied, the student's attorney filed a 15-count lawsuit in federal court claiming violation of the First, Fifth, and Fourteenth Amendments; six violations of the U.S.C. (U.S. Code); violation of Massachusetts General Law; Promissory Estoppel[3]; Breach of the Special Relationship; Breach of Contract; Intentional Infliction of Emotional Distress; and Tortuous Interference with Economic Advantage. The attorney emphasized that Marquis had suffered personal injury, because a grade of C on his transcript would hurt his chances of being admitted to law school (Complaint, 2007).

After a brief hearing with the plaintiff and an attorney for the university, who asked, "Does the court really want to put itself in the business of reviewing, under

---

[3] *Promissory Estoppel*—"when a person makes a false statement to another and the listener relies on what was told to him/her in good faith and to his/her disadvantage. To see that justice is done a court will treat the statement as a promise, and in a trial the judge will preclude the maker of the statement from denying it" (TheFreeDictionary.com, 2010, p. 1).

some constitutional or federal statutory doctrine, the propriety of the grades which a student has received?" (Elder, 2010, p. 2). District Court Judge Michael A. Posnor dismissed the lawsuit against the university. What do you think? Do you think the judge ruled properly in this case? At our own university there is no official university grading scale (however, individual colleges or departments may adopt a grading scale, and the nursing division in our college does have one) for either undergraduate or graduate grades—our grading scale is very similar to the undergraduate scale at this university, whereas A– equals 3.700 points, B equals 3.00 points, and so on. Therefore, unless the individual professor prints a corresponding grading scale on the course syllabus (e.g., A– = 90–92, B = 84–87), the student may actually may not know exactly what a final grade will be if all assignments are graded with a letter grade, or in this case on a 0–5 scale. Indeed, as the ombudsman in this case indicated, "faculty have their own grading scales and . . . one professor might view an 84 as an A minus, while another might view it as a C"(Saltzman, 2007, p. 2). Our point is that where there is no corresponding grading scale to an assigned letter grade, there is lots of room for very divergent grade calculations and in this case even the teaching assistant appeared to have instituted a grading curve (based on a review of final grades) that was not disclosed on the syllabus. What do you think about the comments of the department chair? Might you inquire as to what kind of teaching pedagogy skills the graduate teaching assistant has been given?

Although there is no indication this was the first time Mr. Cushing had taught, the decision to institute a grading scale at the end of the course without due process explanation to the students, at least in our view, seems awfully arbitrary. And most important, how do you view the decision and comments of the ombudsperson, Ms. Porter? Did you get the sense that she was ruling with the IOA's *Code of Ethics* in mind with due attention to independence, neutrality and impartiality, confidentiality, and informality? Our concluding viewpoint is that in a climate of intense litigation in the United States and with more accountability required in higher education, an individual faculty member is perhaps more protected from charges of bias in grading if the syllabus is more precise in both grading criteria and grading scales for respective grades awarded.

Summary

Although in the preceding case, the student did not have a positive outcome from use of the university ombudsperson, at least it is notable that the student did pursue his appeal with the university ombudsperson once there was a denial by the department chair. And although litigation in state and federal courts is almost always a legitimate possibility for most claims, courts are often wary of interfering in university activities that are in the domain of the faculty, particularly with regard to grading (Roth et al., 2009). Nevertheless, the role of the ombudsman or ombudsperson is an important addition to higher education, and any student who has a legitimate claim must consider whether to consider a formal complaint to the official offices listed earlier in this chapter, or more informally to the office of an ombudsman, where mediation, recommendation, and hopefully equitable resolutions can be sought and delivered.

CRITICAL ELEMENTS TO CONSIDER

As was shown in the legal case but not in the nursing case presented in this chapter, students are almost always advised to follow the chain of command in an organization to pursue a complaint. If the complaint occurs within a course, then normally the student should first appeal to the course professor, then perhaps the department chair, and there may be additional levels to whom to appeal, including associate/assistant dean and even dean.

If you are a student and you believe you have a legitimate claim, you must decide to either pursue either a formal complaint to the appropriate university official (e.g., human resources, confidential ethics line, office of equality officer) or an *informal* complaint if at all possible.

If there is no satisfactory resolution within the respective college or school, then identifying the office of the ombudsman is a proper next step. Again, because some ombudsmen represent faculty only, make sure you have an ombudsman who hears student complaints.

Put your complaint in writing and be very specific.

Try to refrain from using any derogatory terms or inflammatory language, and present your case in a precise but professional way.

Try to avoid gossip or indiscreet discussion of your issue to wide numbers of parties. Speak confidentially only to individuals you trust who you also believe will be discreet and offer professional, unbiased advice.

If you are called to the ombudsman's office to evaluate your complaint, dress professionally, present yourself in the most professional way and communicate whether you are seeking to be completely anonymous or merely confidential. You should understand that in some cases, for an ombudsman to rule specifically on your case, you may have to reveal your identity. In these cases you should seek reassurance that the defendant whom you are bringing a complaint against cannot harass you or seek reprisal. Inquire if there are any specific university policies that might protect you in these cases.

Continued

CRITICAL ELEMENTS TO CONSIDER—cont'd

Document all conversations you have with university officials at all levels. Include dates, times, and exactly what each party said.

Go to your university or college ombudsman Web site for more information, but do not be surprised if it is not highly visible. Our own ombudsman Web site is not as visible as we would like, and there isn't much detail there about the role of the ombudsman.

If you have any questions that you may want answered prior to contacting any department in an official capacity, you may be able to contact your undergraduate or graduate student government association for peer advice.

HELPFUL RESOURCES

- Department of Education Student Loan Ombudsman
  http://www.studentloaninfo.org/blog/student-loan-ombudsman
- Student Press Law Center
  http://www.splc.org/knowyourrights/legalresearch.asp?id=2
- University of Michigan Student Mediation Services
  http://www.umich.edu/~sdrp/
- Indiana University Code of Student Rights, Responsibilities, & Conduct
  http://www.indiana.edu/~code/

References

Albany State University. (n.d.). The ASU ombuds office. Retrieved September 16, 2010, from http://www.potentialrealized.org/admin/student-activities/ombuds.dot

Bauer, F. (2000). The practice of one ombudsman. *Negotiation Journal, 16*(1), 59–79.

Gadlin, H. (2000). The ombudsman: What's in a name? *Negotiation Journal, 16*(1), 37–48.

Gottehrer, D. M., & Hostina, M. (1998). *Essential characteristics of a classical ombudsman.* Retrieved September 16, 2010, from http://www.usombudsman.org/documents/PDF/References/Essential.PDF

Elder, G. (2010). Final grade of a "C" prompts personal injury lawsuit. Totallawyers.com. Retrieved September 19, 2010, from http://www.totallawyers.com/legal-articles-grade-lawsuit.asp

International Ombudsman Association. (2007). *Boards & committees.* Retrieved September 16, 2010, from http://www.ombudsassociation.org/about/

International Ombudsman Association. (2007). *Code of ethics.* Retrieved September 19, 2010, from http://www.ombudsassociation.org/standards/Code_Ethics_1

International Ombudsman Association. (2009). *Best practices.* Retrieved September 19, 2010, from http://www.ombudsassociation.org/standards/IOA_Best_Practices_Version3_101309.pdf

International Ombudsman Association. (2009). *Standards of practice.* Retrieved September 19, 2010, from http://www.ombudsassociation.org/standards/IOA_Standards_of_Practice_Oct09.pdf

Levin, P. T. (2009). The Swedish model of public administration: Separation of powers—the Swedish style. *Journal of Administration and Governance, 4*(1). Retrieved September 14, 2010, from http://www.joaag.com/uploads/4-_4_1___LevinFinal.pdf

Marquis v. University of Massachusetts at Amherst, No. 07-30015 (D. Mass Jan. 31, 2007), Retrieved September 19, 2010, from http://kevinunderhill.typepad.com/Documents/Pleadings/Marquis_v_UMass.pdf

Merriam-Webster.com. (2010). Definition of *ombudsman.* Retrieved September 15, 2010, from http://www.merriam-webster.com/dictionary/ombudsman?show=0&t=1284575547

Ohio State University. (2010). Faculty ombudsman. Retrieved September 19, 2010, from http://ombudsman.osu.edu/

Roth, J. A., McEllistrem, S., D'Agostino, T., & Brown, C. J. (2009). *Higher education law in America* (10th ed.). Malvern, PA: Center for Education & Employment Law.

Saltzman, J. (2007, October 4). Student takes his C to federal court. *The Boston Globe.* Retrieved September 19, 2010, from http://www.boston.com/news/local/articles/2007/10/04/student_takes_his_c_to_federal_court/

Shelton, R. L. (2000). The institutional ombudsman: A university case study. *Negotiation Journal, 16*(1), 81–98.

Stieber, C. (2000). 57 varieties: Has the ombudsman concept become diluted? *Negotiation Journal, 16*(1), 49–57.

TheFreeDictionary. (2010). Estoppel. Retrieved March 24, 2011, from http://ncyclopedia.thefreedictionary.com/Promissory+estoppel

Young, R. J. (2008). *Houston Community College Office of the Ombudsman quarterly report, January 1, 2008 through March 31, 2008 and April 1, 2008 through June 30, 2008.* Retrieved September, 19, 2010, http://www.hccs.edu/hcc/System%20Home/Departments/Ombudsman/SYS4313_OmbudsmanReport_Web.pdf

The Role of the Ombudsman for the Faculty

CASE STUDY

A Faculty Member Files a Complaint With the University Ombudsman[1]

Your role: You are the department chair.

Dr. Monica Solheim makes an appointment to see you. Although she does not report directly to you, she does teach 50% of her load in the BSN programs that you oversee. You have heard that the pediatric nursing faculty members are upset about a suddenly announced resignation of one of their own members. You have also heard rumors about their fury that they were not involved in choosing her replacement. As the department chair, you are in a serious predicament; the faculty member who resigned was the senior coordinator of the pediatric clinical nursing course, and she had a course reduction for these administrative responsibilities. She resigned just 2 weeks before the fall term was to begin. Given that time span and with large sections of pediatric courses about to commence, there was no time for a search committee to be appointed. You know you need to make a replacement quickly, and in fact you already have. Before doing so, you consulted with the associate dean for your division (who will be voting on Dr. Solheim's possible promotion in the fall) and shared your judgment that none of the undergraduate faculty in this specialty really has the leadership skills (and perhaps the work ethic, as this is a very time-consuming endeavor) to undertake such a large responsibility. You considered appointing a highly qualified graduate nursing faculty member (a proven and experienced leader), but she is nearing retirement and likely does not want this huge responsibility (although you did not ask her). The associate dean informed you there is a brand-new doctor of nursing practice (DNP) graduate who is very experienced, has teaching experience, and has exhibited strong leadership qualities—something this nursing organization lacks depth in, despite its large number of full-time faculty. You jointly decide to inquire if she would be interested in this position. Learning that she was, you quickly interviewed her and, very impressed, offered her

---

[1] Note: At the beginning of Chapter 4, which deals with a student's use of the ombudsman, is a note about the dissatisfaction with the term ombuds*man*. It is used here for the reasons indicated there.

the position and she accepted. She is currently in the process of becoming a new employee. Somehow, word got out before you were able to manage the announcement, and word spread like wildfire.

When Dr. Solheim meets you, she expresses her personal outrage, and that of her faculty colleagues, that there was no search committee and no real search at all. You had already heard she is upset that one of her best friends on the undergraduate faculty was not offered the position. In your meeting, you indicate that the resignation was sudden and close to the beginning of the term and that a formal search was not possible. You inform her that you are well aware of all the pediatric faculty's credentials and that the new hire was best positioned to undertake this new role. You further tell Dr. Solheim that this DNP graduate was known to be a "work horse" and at the top of her graduating class. Once you raised the issue of merit, Dr. Solheim begins to advocate vigorously for her friend, but you interject noting that her friend had never expressed any interest in the position, nor had Dr. Solheim recommended her, even though she knew the position was vacant. You civilly inform Dr. Solheim that her advocacy, although perhaps well meaning, is nonetheless inappropriate, and you reinforce that the position has been filled. The meeting ends, but not well.

The next day you receive notification from the university ombudsman that Dr. Solheim has filed a complaint against you for not following due process in hiring a member of the faculty and giving her senior administrative duties.

Questions

- How would you first proceed?
- Have you followed the university policy on hiring or violated a required faculty hiring protocol?
- When you either meet with the ombudsman or provide your side of the case in writing, what will you say or write?

Faculty Use of a University Ombudsman: Legal Principles and Review of the Literature

Chapter 5 presented a common definition of an ombudsman and identified two primary types: classical and organizational, with the former instituted by statute and the latter instituted by other agents or bodies. The International Ombudsman Association (IOA) is the leading international organization for establishing common global standards and best practices, and these are discussed in this chapter, as they emanated from the IOA's first developed *Code of Ethics* (2007). According to Alcover (2009), "University and academia are, due to its nature, its structure and its inside relationships, a perfect breeding ground for the conflicts, disputes, problems, and grievances. In these settings, mediation is one of the dispute resolution mechanisms most used by University" (p. 275).

Whereas Chapter 5 discussed the ombudsman or the ombudsperson who works with university students, staff, *and* faculty (in other words, the full university community), this chapter will focus on the role of the ombudsman who is specifically

assigned to work with faculty and who is perhaps exceptionally skilled (or has specialized) in faculty ombudsmanship issues (Dunn, 2010).[2,3] The IOA's *Standards of
Practice* (2009) were developed from the aforementioned *Code of Ethics*. According
to the *Standards of Practice* preamble, "Each Ombudsman office should have an
organizational Charter or Terms of Reference, approved by senior management,
articulating the principles of the Ombudsman function in that organization and
their consistency with the IOA Standards of Practice" (p. 1). In many ways, the
Standards of Practice are extensions of the *Code of Ethics* and provide more direction
to each of the four principles: independence, neutrality and impartiality, confidentiality, and informality. Table 6.1 lists some examples of this operationalization
of the *Code of Ethics* as represented by the *Standards of Practice*.

The third primary document of the IOA is the *Best Practices* guide, which "is
intended to provide guidance to Organizational Ombudsmen in practicing
according to IOA *Standards of Practice* to the highest level of professionalism
possible." As the *Standards of Practice* are broad explanations of the *Code of Ethics*,
similarly, the *Best Practices* document provides more detail to the *Standards of Practice*, but *only* to the organizational ombudsman.

Recall from Chapter 5 that the classical ombudsman is organized by statute
and operates by the direct language of that statute. The organizational ombudsman's role is probably therefore more loosely structured. One example of best
practice from the *Standards* relates to standard 2.2 (see Table 6.1):

> All members of the specified community served by the Ombudsman may voluntarily seek services from
> the Ombudsman Office and will be treated with respect and dignity. The Ombudsman should assure
> access impartially, including to people with disabilities, people who need language interpreters, or
> people whose work hours require flexibility in scheduling appointment times.

Who is qualified to be an ombudsman? Gadlin (2000) indicates that the first
university ombudsmen were "truly amateurs" (p. 40). However, there is general
consensus that anyone who is serving as an ombudsman should possess "integrity,
ability to be fair and sympathetic, willingness to be critical of the powers that be,
etc., along with knowledge of the rules, procedures, and culture of the institution
within which they were assuming the ombudsman role" (p. 40). These individuals
also need to be skilled at dispute resolution and mediation. One question often
asked is whether an individual serving as an ombudsman should be an attorney.
The usual answer is no, unless there are specific guidelines that require someone

---

[2] In fact, most ombudsmen are simply faculty members who are generally well respected and therefore trusted
to "have the right instincts" and "do the right thing." Few ombudsmen are the kinds of trained experts referenced by Dunn.That is why the word "perhaps" is used in the text.

[3] Our own university Ombudsman sees both students and faculty (and staff), and there have been discussions
in the Faculty Senate that question whether an Ombudsman can fairly represent equally both faculty and student if each has contacted the Ombudsman regarding the same issue. In our case (and in many universities),
the Ombudsman is also a faculty member and there at least seems to be an altered balance of power certainly
from the student perspective. But obviously, many universities have agreed that a different Ombudsman may
better serve the faculty, and for example, at Duke University, the Faculty Ombudsman is a two year appointment and is elected by the faculty (*Duke Today*, 2010).

Table 6.1 Examples of Specific IOM Standards of Practice

IOM'S STANDARDS OF PRACTICE			
Independence	**Neutrality/Impartiality**	**Confidentiality**	**Informality**
The Ombudsman Office and the Ombudsman are independent from other organizational entities.	The Ombudsman is neutral, impartial, and unaligned.	Communications between the Ombudsman and others (made while the Ombudsman is serving in that capacity) are considered privileged. The privilege belongs to the Ombudsman and the Ombudsman Office, rather than to any party to an issue. Others cannot waive this privilege.	The Ombudsman functions on an informal basis by such means as: listening, providing and receiving information, identifying and reframing issues, developing a range of responsible options, and—with permission and at Ombudsman discretion—engaging in informal third-party intervention. When possible, the Ombudsman helps people develop new ways to solve problems themselves.
The Ombudsman holds no other position within the organization which might compromise independence.	The Ombudsman strives for impartiality, fairness and objectivity in the treatment of people and the consideration of issues. The Ombudsman advocates for fair and equitably administered processes and does not advocate on behalf of any individual within the organization.	The Ombudsman does not testify in any formal process inside the organization and resists testifying in any formal process outside of the organization regarding a visitor's contact with the Ombudsman or confidential information communicated to the Ombudsman, even if given permission or requested to do so. The Ombudsman may, however, provide general, nonconfidential information about the Ombudsman Office or the Ombudsman profession.	The Ombudsman as an informal and off-the-record resource pursues resolution of concerns and looks into procedural irregularities and/or broader systemic problems when appropriate.

Adapted from International Ombudsman Association Standards of Practice (2009).

with a law degree, usually a state statute. For example, in Indiana the new Ombudsman for the Department of Child Services requires that the ombudsman have either a law degree or a master's degree in social work (Evans, 2009). This ombudsman position, because it is created by state stature, is therefore an example of a classical ombudsman. Similarly, Fallberg, Mackenney, and Óvretreit (2004) indicate having legal training is very important because it is necessary to arrive at settlements between parties. Nevertheless, understanding the concept of due process and having some alacrity and familiarity with the law are likely very valuable and helpful. Above all else, moreover, an irreproachable reputation and the highest ethical standards are two character traits that are essential in individuals serving in these roles (Harrison, 2004). Table 6.2 lists the typical requirement for a typical organizational ombudsman.

Overall, the university ombudsman is an important position, and faculty may benefit when there is an individual who is specifically employed to address the diversity of faculty concerns. Ohio State University (OSU) provides an example of a traditional faculty ombudsman, who does the following:

- Serves as an adviser to faculty to assist them in determining the viability of their complaints and issues.
- Directs faculty to appropriate offices, committees, and university rules and policies.
- Serves when appropriate as an informal mediator of early-stage complaints, to mediate as an impartial party rather than as an advocate for faculty involved in complaints (OSU, 2010, para. 1).

Using a slightly different model, Texas Tech University employs two ombudsmen, one for staff and a separate one for students, and faculty complaints are heard by the staff ombudsman if the complaint is human resource–oriented or heard by the student ombudsman office if it relates to a student issue (Texas Tech, 2010). Finally, it should be mentioned that the American Association of University Professors (AAUP) was founded in 1915 and remains the leading organization dedicated to the promotion and protection of the academic freedom and rights of university faculty (AAUP, n.d.). Most colleges and universities follow general AAUP guidelines found in the *Redbook—AAUP's Policy Documents and Reports* (2006), especially its procedures for hiring, promotion, and tenure; other institutions use the *Redbook* as a resource even if they do not follow it.

Table 6.2 General Job Description Requirements for Position of Ombudsman

CRITICAL SKILLS AND CHARACTERISTICS
1. Communication and problem-solving skills
2. Decision-making/strategic thinking skills
3. Conflict resolution skills
4. Organizational knowledge and networking skills
5. Sensitivity to diversity issues
6. Composure and presentation skills
7. Integrity

ACCOUNTABILITIES
1. Dispute resolution/consultation and referral
2. Policy analysis and feedback
3. Community outreach and education
4. Establish//maintain office of the ombudsperson

EDUCATION AND WORK EXPERIENCE
1. Varies, usually mostly a bachelor's degree, but an advanced degree is often desired and based on the setting of the ombudsperson
2. A work history that indicates the above characteristics and function of this job have been previously demonstrated

Discussion of Case

The case study, although it is quite complex, in reality is an example of the layers of detail that ordinary academic nursing administrators encounter every day. Indeed, this author was recently queried by a new interim academic department chair who was requesting a very straightforward answer to a question, and the response began with "rarely ever is the decision-making process of a department chair very black and white." In this case study, the levels of complexity are not surprising, especially in a very large nursing organization. The first question asked was, How would you first proceed? Certainly, administrators knew the department chair must adhere to a few key leadership/managerial tenets if she was to be both ethical and responsible in the conduct of her administrative duties: (1) there are always two sides to any story—wait until you hear both before you jump to conclusions; (2) faculty members will disclose what they want you to know, and not disclose what they want to hide or not reveal or keep private (not public); (3) your job is to serve the good of the organization, treat everyone fairly, and ensure they obtain whatever process if "due"; and finally, (4) you are being paid to exercise your best judgment; otherwise there would be someone else in your position, or it would not exist.

Here, all pediatric faculty (both undergraduate and graduate) knew of this resignation, and yet no one formally expressed a personal interest in the position to the department chair or even associate dean. Instead, a senior faculty member went to advocate for another, a process often observed in academia, with faculty members not asking *directly* for what they want and instead expressing their desires or wishes *indirectly* and even through others. In the absence of anyone stepping forward to volunteer for this position (and work involved), the administrators were challenged to fill the position quickly and ensure a smooth transition to a new academic term. Expressing these facts of life to Dr. Solheim demonstrated honesty and a certain transparency, and Dr. Solheim would have been forced to agree with them, if not with the way the emergency was resolved.

The second question was, Have you followed the university policy on hiring or violated a required faculty hiring protocol? What do you think?

In this case the university human resource policy does not direct that senior nursing coordinator positions be posted, as these are not line administrative positions, such as department chair or associate dean. Further, even with a faculty resignation there is no assumption that there is a budget allocation for a new hire. That would need to be determined by the dean. That there was a formal announcement of the resignation (although not required in this case) was at least arguably sufficient notice for any interested candidates to express their interest in the position to the respective academic nursing administrator.

Although Dr. Solheim had the right to file a complaint with the university ombudsman, the question remains whether she was exercising good judgment in doing so. Academia is no different from the corporate world when it comes to give-and-take in the workplace, and there are often consequences of being or not being a team player or in being an agent who helps maintain or improve organizational morale or one who tends to contribute to negative organizational morale. Dr. Solheim is going to need the support of the department chair and the associate dean for promotion, and she is not using good emotional intelligence if she thinks she acts without consequence. This is not to insinuate that she should not report violations of due process[4] if they are indeed founded, but she should evaluate very seriously if the charges have real merit and how the issue is best addressed without damaging her own institutional reputation. More important, there is a strong case that Dr. Solheim was acting very independently and even interfering.

By the same token, there is reason for the faculty to protect its interests in shared governance and its place at the hiring and appointments tables. Going to an ombudsman does not require the process to be nasty or adversarial; it can create a better process for *the next time* an emergency like this occurs. If that had been the way that Dr. Solheim presented the issue, it would have demonstrated maturity and commitment to the organization. If this had been her objective, however, consider whether she should have raised that point with the department chair directly—and only petitioned the ombudsman if the chair declined to consider the issue that way.

WHEN TO CONTACT THE UNIVERSITY COUNSEL

University counsel is available to answer questions about the law, to provide guidance and interpretations about dispute resolution processes, and to help university clients resolve problems. But university counsel is counsel for the university, not for any particular member of the faculty, and not "for" one member "against" another. Typically, requests for legal assistance are best made by a department chair or associate dean, so faculty members should think about going to their supervisors first. If you view your issue as serious and rising above the specific jurisdiction or powers of the ombudsman (remember, this is not a legal course of action), you will need to consider where your complaint is best heard by going through the chain of command or even using an ethics hotline most universities maintain. With most confidential or anonymous ethics hotlines, your claim can be reviewed by someone with independent authority to decide whether it ought to be reviewed by university counsel.

---

[4] As noted in several other chapters, the words "due process" mean different things and can vary greatly in meaning between private and public institutions. The implications are more formal in public institutions because of constitutional prohibitions on "the state" depriving people of "property or liberty" interests "without due process of law. Private institutions can also commit themselves to fair procedures, and those procedures are what is "due," but they are not protected by the constitution.

Findings and Disposition

In this case it was unfortunate that Dr. Solheim did not choose instead to report her complaint to the school's or department's faculty affairs committee—first, because a complaint to the university ombudsman can take the issue away from those who should "own" it, involve an outsider unnecessary to resolution, and complicate the process by injecting different processes and even participants. Perhaps she should have also consulted with some of her other senior colleagues to determine what the proper action should be. Perhaps she could have asked the dean if she felt this was a due process violation or if the appointment followed accepted university procedures for "emergency" hiring. It is unknown whether this was done, but it might have allowed her more time to reflect on a course of action and to more carefully weigh the impact of a variety of strategies to communicate her displeasure.

The third question posed in the case study was, When you either meet with the ombudsman or provide your side of the case in writing, what will you say or write? What do you think you should say about how you handled this complaint?

In this case, there was no formal meeting between the ombudsman and the department chair. Instead he simply called her and she reiterated the human resource policy on faculty hiring and indicated this was not an administrative level appointment that required a formal posting procedure. She also indicated that an e-mail had gone out to all faculty about the individual's resignation but due to the emergent nature of a replacement with just weeks before the beginning of the term, an administrative decision was made by the dean and herself to not convene a formal search committee. However, had anyone expressed formal interest in the position, then that person would have been considered. With that, the ombudsman thanked the department chair and made a note to personally check with Human Resources and the associate dean to verify if there really were specific policies on emergent faculty hiring.

As for the disposition of this case, the DNP graduate was hired and was ultimately very successful in her role, but she was not welcomed warmly. It took her longer than it should have to become integrated, and she experienced ongoing resentment from the other pediatric faculty. Although her competency allowed her some breathing room, residual individual issues remained to some extent with the other pediatric faculty. The ombudsman later asked HR and the associate dean whether there was any internal policy regarding the appointment of senior course coordinators. Upon the associate dean's reply (and HR's confirmation that no procedural hiring policies were violated) that these appointments were always made internally and that formal search committees are rare and not the ordinary process by which these positions are filled, the ombudsman concluded that the appointment had not violated any rule or procedure, and in a meeting with

Dr. Solheim he explained all of this to her. The ombudsman also called the department chair and associate dean, advising them of his determinations and that he was closing his file. He cautioned them that they must guard against taking any action that could be interpreted as retaliation against Dr. Solheim, especially as she would soon be considered for promotion. Last, a senior colleague of Dr. Solheim (after the fact) did mention to her in conversation that she really must be more careful about "stirring up trouble," and although Dr. Solheim was defensive, she realized that perhaps she was the only one damaged in this altercation. She subsequently decided to request a delay in her application for full professorship by a year to help heal her relationships with the administrators who would evaluate her.

The way this case ended serves to remind that people who utilize the ombudsman must be assured that there will not be any adverse consequences (retaliation) toward those who invoke it. The fact that Dr. Solheim was not comfortable with proceeding was her decision; but if she had decided to proceed with her candidacy for promotion, the associate dean and department head would have had to be scrupulously fair. Any "no" vote by them could well have been alleged to be retaliation for having filed the charge.

Relevant Legal Case

DePree v. Saunders 80, No. 08-60978 (5th Cir. 2009)

Dr. DePree, a tenured professor at the University of Southern Mississippi, sued the university's president and various administrators and faculty members after he was removed from teaching duties in August 2007 and evicted from his office in the College of Business. The Interim Dean of the College of Business had written the president and stated Dr. DePree had contributed, according to court records, to "an environment in which faculty members and students do not feel safe to go about their usual business." He was accused of engaging in negative and disruptive behaviors and criticized as the only accounting professor who had failed to "engage in the scholarly or professional activities necessary to be labeled 'academically-qualified' or 'professionally-qualified' by the University's accrediting agency, AACSB [Association to Advance Collegiate Schools of Business]." Eight letters from other faculty in the department confirming these allegations accompanied the interim dean's letter. Upon receipt of the letter, the president notified Dr. DePree that he was relieved of all his teaching duties and service requirements to the university, not permitted to enter the College of Business except to retrieve personal items, and to continue his scholarship with continued access to the university computer system and library. The president then instructed the provost to investigate the charges and requested the university ombudsman investigate the charges and submit a report.

DePree filed a lawsuit with the district court within 3 weeks of the letter and complained these actions were in retaliation for maintaining a Web site critical of the university and some of its administrators and faculty and because he complained to the College of Business' accrediting agency (AACSB) about the school. In his suit, DePree claimed First Amendment retaliation, due process violations, and various state law claims. The ombudsman delivered a report to the president in December 2007 and recommended that DePree have a mental health examination to assess his fitness to teach, that he had to produce sufficient scholarly work to the satisfaction of independent evaluators, and that the restrictions by the president remain in place.

The district course granted summary judgment in favor of the defendants and denied DePree's motion for temporary and permanent injunctive relief. Further, the district court denied a temporary restraining order against the defendants in suit. On appeal to the Fifth Circuit Court the issues of First Amendment retaliation, due process violations, and various state law claims were again evaluated.

On the First Amendment retaliation, the appeals court indeed remanded DePree's injunctive claim based on First Amendment retaliation for further development chiefly because the appeals court could not determine whether the president could impose discipline on the plaintiff if indeed the discipline was retaliatory and the Web site comments and letter to the AACSB were protected speech. Second, the actions by the president preceded the late report by the ombudsman. However, the First Amendment charges against all parties aside from the president were dismissed because recommendations for a course of action against DePree were not described and the president alone enforced the penalties on the plaintiff. In discussion, the court admitted that these issues of protected speech were complex. Is Web site material or a letter to an accrediting body written by a tenured professor "protected speech," and did the university indeed retaliate because of these behaviors? There is no access to the eight written letters, but there is a statement of the court that this issue was difficult to ascertain.

On the due process claim, DePree claimed a violation of the due process clause because the university prohibited him from teaching and denied him further access to the College of Business. As stated in this ruling "The threshold requirement of any due process claim is the government's deprivation of a plaintiff's liberty or property interest" (*DePree v. Saunders* 80, 2009, p. 1). This claim was rejected because the plaintiff's salary and title continued and there was nothing contractual that indicated every professor had to teach as part of his or her professorial role, and therefore the court ruled he had no constitutional property right to teach. Although it is unclear whether the plaintiff had a right to enter the building, the court did affirm the university had a right to reassign or transfer an employee. It is this temporary and permanent restriction to the building that may have been evaluated as potentially retaliatory as part cause for the remand on the First Amendment retaliation claim, but there is no certainty. There is no indication that the plaintiff was provided office space (normally accorded to a tenured professor) somewhere else to conduct the scholarly work he was required to produce.

On the alleged state violations, all were dismissed for various reasons. Because his salary continued he could not claim breach of contract, and because this claim appeared in a later legal response, not the original brief, it was dismissed. Further, state charges of tortuous interference with business relations, intentional infliction of emotional distress, breach of contractual duty of good faith and fair dealing, defamation, and assault were all dismissed against all defendants mostly from lack of genuine material fact to support the allegations. The assault charge was interesting. From the court record, according to the plaintiff, the associate dean "aggressively walk[ed] toward [DePree], yelling at [him], repeatedly referring to [him] as a 'son-of-a-bitch,' and shaking papers in his face creat[ing] an apprehension in [DePree] of an imminent harmful or offensive contact." The court did not find evidence of any imminent or harmful contact, and there was no claim of personal injury. Indeed the court indicated there was evidence these two individuals had squared off like this before, and there was no indication that DePree was harmed merely because someone was cursing at him and waving papers in his face.

Summary

In *DePree v. Saunders 80*, we do not know the ultimate outcome of this case. It appears, however, the plaintiff maintained his salary and title, but there was acknowledgment by the court that at this appeal there was some concern that there *may* have been retaliation against the tenured professor for activities that were protected speech. We are likewise concerned that severe penalties were enacted *before the ombudsman's report*, and barring the faculty from entering the College of Business building permanently without any indication of alternate office space seemed extreme.

Overall, as this chapter is focused on the role of the ombudsman for faculty, we are faced with a few questions. Could the ombudsman have been better utilized? Why did it take 4 months for the ombudsman to conduct an investigation and prepare a final report? Could the president have taken some intermediary disciplinary measures while the investigation was ongoing? Could the plaintiff have gone to the ombudsman himself? How would that have operated? Could the ombudsman have fairly done both tasks (serve the faculty member by hearing his complaint and conduct the investigation as requested by the president)? We do worry about this when we see models in which one ombudsman sees faculty, students, *and* staff. Is it possible there was someone else better prepared to conduct this investigation, perhaps one of the university's staff attorneys? The better strategy might have been to have used the ombudsman to prepare a report *before* the severe penalties were first enacted.

If you are a faculty member or seeking to become a faculty member, it is wise to find out if your respective university or college has an ombudsman and what type—one who serves faculty only or one who serves the full university community. It may also be important to consult your university Web site or faculty handbook and determine the functions of the ombudsman. If you are a faculty member and you have an issue that you believe needs to be resolved, you will need to decide what is the best avenue for your claim—human resources, office of equality, the next person on your administrative chain of command, the university attorney or the ombudsman. Determining who is best to handle your issue is critical. Each has its own timetable, process, and consequences. It is worth taking the time to consider all your options and consult individuals who will give you confidential, wise counsel and consider your best course of action.

CRITICAL ELEMENTS TO CONSIDER

- Do you have a university ombudsman? What kind? Whose claims does he or she hear?
- What is the best office to hear your claim – office of the ombudsman, equality, another person in your administrative chain of command (dean or provost perhaps), or human resources? Or does your issue require hiring your own attorney?

HELPFUL RESOURCES

- International Ombudsman Association
  http://www.ombudsassociation.org/
- Organizational Ombudsman Blog: Independent, Neutral, Impartial, Confidential, & Informal
  http://organizationalombudsman.wordpress.com/

References

Alcover, C-M. (2009). Ombudsing in higher education: A contingent model for mediation in university dispute resolution processes. *Spanish Journal of Psychology, 12*(1), 275–287.

American Association of University Professors. (2006). *AAUP's policy documents and reports* (10th ed.). Washington, DC: AAUP.

American Association of University Professors. (n.d.). History of the AAUP. Retrieved October 25, 2010, from http://www.aaup.org/AAUP/about/history/

Dawson elected faculty ombudsman: Professor to serve two-year term. (2010). *Duke Today*. Retrieved September 20, 2010, from http://www.dukenews.duke.edu/2010/05/ombudsman .html*DePree v. Saunders 80, No. 08-60978 (5th Cir. 2009)*

Dunn, A. (2010). Officials consider creating ombudsman office: Proposed ethical concerns department to take legal requests from faculty. Spectator.com (Seattle University). Retrieved September 20, 2010, from http://www.su-spectator.com/news/officials-consider-creating-ombudsman-office-1.1112224

Evans, T. (2009). DCS ombudsman codified, but that's just the beginning. *Indy.com*. Retrieved September 22, 2010, from http://www.indy.com/posts/dcs-ombudsman-codified-but-that-is-just-the-beginning

Fallberg, L., Mackenney, S., & Øvretreit, J. (2004). *Protecting patients' rights?: A comparative study of the ombudsman in healthcare*. Cambridge, MA: Radcliffe.

Gadlin, H. (2000). The ombudsman: What's in a name? *Negotiation Journal, 16*(1), 37–48.

Harrison, T. (2004). What is success in ombuds processes? Evaluation of a university ombudsman. *Conflict Resolution Quarterly, 21*(3), 331–335.

International Ombudsman Association. (2007). *Code of ethics*. Retrieved September 19, 2010, from http://www.ombudsassociation.org/standards/Code_Ethics_1

International Ombudsman Association. (2009). *Best practices*. Retrieved September 19, 2010, from http://www.ombudsassociation.org/standards/IOA_Best_Practices_Version3_101309.pdf

International Ombudsman Association. (2009). *Standards of practice*. Retrieved September 19, 2010, from http://www.ombudsassociation.org/standards/IOA_Standards_of_Practice_Oct09.pdf

Ohio State University. (2010). Faculty ombudsman. Retrieved October 25, 2010, from http://ombudsman.osu.edu/

Organizational Ombudsman Blog. (2010, September 9). Ombudsman and ADR position. Retrieved October 25, 2010, from http://organizationalombudsman.wordpress.com/

Texas Tech University. (2010). Ombuds office. Retrieved September 19, 2010, from http://www .depts.ttu.edu/ombuds/

CHAPTER 7

Due Process Issues for the Student

CASE STUDY

Due Process for Students

Your role: You are Dr. Jane Mahoney, Course Coordinator for Nursing of Children. You are responsible for the oversight of two theory/didactic sections of 40 students each as well as the oversight of 10 clinical rotations with 8 students in each clinical group.

You receive an e-mail from a BSN-accelerated nursing student, Jeremy Johnson, who is in his third semester of study (out of four semesters), contesting his clinical failure. The clinical faculty member, Doris Russert, told you that Mr. Johnson has anger management issues. Professor Russert reports that Mr. Johnson had an outburst at the nurses' station on a busy pediatric floor and that she has awarded Mr. Johnson a clinical grade of Unsatisfactory for unprofessional behavior. She also states that he had an anger management issue in clinical conference and left the conference abruptly.

When you meet with Mr. Johnson, you note that he is 6 feet 6 inches tall and is built like a professional football player. Mr. Johnson claims that the clinical faculty member changed the time of the clinical day and did not notify him. He states that he expressed frustration at the nurse's station but did not have an outburst. He also tells you that Professor Russert did not observe him and was not on the unit at the time. He begins to cry and tells you that he is being treated like a monster because of his size.

Questions

- What questions do you need to ask Professor Russert?
- What documentation do you need to review?
- What is your best course of action?

Due Process: Legal Principles and Review of the Literature

It is crucial that clinical faculty understand the student's right to due process (Whitney, 2009). *Due process* is one of the most complicated subjects in American law: it fills casebooks and is the subject of semesters of study in law schools. The two simple words *due process* express the notion that whenever a state agency does something that results in harm to an individual, it must first follow a process that is fairly designed to produce a fair result to that person. Exactly what process is due to the individual varies from case to case, and depends on many different factors. But in very general terms, the right of due process equates to fairness (Johnson, 2009).

The Fifth and Fourteenth Amendments of the United States Constitution guarantee citizens "due process of law" and seek to ensure fairness in the application of governmental authority to citizens. *Substantive due process* is fairness on the merits of the subject, and *procedural due process* is fairness in the way that the merits are addressed. The Constitution does not protect every interest that citizens may have. For example, we have no right to a job, nor do we have a right to be protected from people who are mean or who upset us. In fact, just the opposite is true: the right of free speech means that other people have the right to say things that make us unhappy, and most of us (e.g., those without collective bargaining agreements or tenure) can be fired for no reason at all. What the Constitution protects are *property and liberty interests,* and in actual *cases and controversies*—and as you might expect, lawyers have been fighting about the meaning of those words for centuries.

The Constitution has another limitation in that it only protects citizens from government action. This means it applies to public universities, but whether it applies to private universities "depends" (as lawyers say)—for example, on whether the conduct involved government funding or a specific federal right (e.g., the right to be free of racial discrimination). In the private university context, however, there is a complex matrix of state laws—codified in constitutions, statutes, and administrative codes, or expressed in judicial decisions—that in general terms result in the same bottom line. One of the principles judges use to examine corporate behavior is called the Business Judgment Rule. It is a principle of deference. It recognizes that judges do not know as much about a business as the person doing that job, and means that a judge will not substitute her judgment for that of the businessperson as long as the businessperson reached the decision through a reasonable process. In the context of a university, the test is frequently whether the faculty's decisions have been careful and deliberate (Smith, McKoy, and Richardson, 2001).

What a due or "reasonable" process is often depends on the outcome: the greater the impact on a third person, the better the process should be. Grading performance in a single class can be more subjective and involve fewer protections (perhaps no process is due for that) than deciding to expel a student from the program. The process does not have to be perfect and the decisions do not have to be right, but the process must be fair. The two concepts that are fundamental and always looked to are *notice* and *opportunity to be heard*: Did the student know it was happening, and did she get the chance to tell her side of the story to someone who was independent and had no stake in the outcome?

In education, the nursing program or college satisfies these essential requirements by stipulating in writing—in the form of policies and procedures—what performance is expected, what constitutes misconduct, and the process that will be followed in imposing a punishment—a deprivation of liberty or property. Students have these interests. They have paid money and given up their time for an education, and they have the expectation (based on written and oral promises from the university) that they will receive a degree as long as they perform satisfactorily. Applied to students, *due process* means that before their interest in earning a degree is injured, they will know why. In particular, the procedural guidelines should ensure that students are given the opportunity to be heard, the opportunity to review the charges and evidence against them, the opportunity to appear before an impartial decision-maker, and the opportunity to appeal the decision (Lindsay, 2005; Roth, 2007).

Applied to a university's clinical settings, *due process* has been interpreted to mean that a student has ample opportunity of notice of misconduct, is given suggestions for improvement, and is advised of the consequences for failure to improve (Johnson, 2009). It is to be predicted that there will be disagreement about whether this process was followed, and that is why documentation is essential. Lawyers like to say, "If it's not in the record, it didn't happen." They do so because writing something down at the time it happens is considered by everyone to be proof (1) that it was important and (2) that it happened. It is far easier to conclude that a punishment was properly imposed (and due process accorded) when there is ample documentation by the faculty and notice to the student with recommendations for improvement and information regarding the student's right to appeal (Suplee, Lachman, Siebert, et al., 2008). Recording students' activities on each clinical day by keeping meticulous anecdotal notes concerning accomplishments, performance issues, and discipline conferences clearly satisfies the obligation (Smith et al., 2001).

The considerations for *substantive* due process are the same: they specify what is expected and the rules by which performance will be judged. Standards for theory, clinical objectives, and performance must be provided to students at the start of each semester. Students must be informed that their student status is analogous to all nurses in maintaining a professional standard of care as delineated in the American Nurses Association's Code of Ethics (Johnson, 2009). Students' practice expectations should be addressed in the course syllabus to include respectful behavior, communication, and clinical preparation, as well as professional responsibility to faculty, professional nursing staff, ancillary clinical employees, patients, and families (Whitney, 2009). Conduct that is not within acceptable limits should also be addressed in the nursing student handbook, course syllabi, and clinical evaluation tools. Students and faculty reflect the image of the educational institution. A breach of expected conduct, whether covert or overt, reflects poorly on the nursing program and can place the institution in a precarious predicament (Johnson, 2009).

Universities are free to define what constitutes misconduct—that's the so-called business of education in which courts do not want to get involved. Misconduct can range from emotional outbursts, incivility, and lack of integrity to acts of poor judgment. In the clinical setting, students may demonstrate misconduct by being unprepared for clinical assignments, disrespecting staff and patients, and displaying an inability to manage the stressors related to clinical performance (Smith et al., 2001). Misconduct by student nurses may jeopardize the health and welfare of patients. To ensure that the college or university pass students who provide safe nursing care, faculty have a legal responsibility to convey unsatisfactory grades to students who are not capable of meeting standards of nursing practice; in doing so, faculty must also remember to provide due process to students at the same time (Smith et al., 2001).

Students must know the expected behaviors as well as the consequences if they fail to meet them in the very beginning of their clinical rotation (Kolanko, Heinrich, Olive, et al., 2006). Faculty versed in the concept of fairness and just decisions regarding clinical evaluations are responsibly acting for the public they serve (Smith-Glasgow and Dreher, 2006). When misconduct failures or dismissals are enacted, several steps must be taken by the clinical faculty to ensure the student's right to due process is maintained (Johnson, 2009). The steps are as follows:

1. The college or university must have clear policies regarding the student conduct and appeals processes.
2. The student is entitled to written notice of any charges against him or her.
3. The student is provided sufficient opportunity to rebut the charges.
4. The student has a right to select an adviser (if stipulated in the program or college policy).
5. The student has a right to confront his or her accusers.
6. The student has a right to present evidence to an impartial body.
7. The student has a right to have an adequate and accurate record of the proceedings.

This is the full panoply of procedures that *could* apply to a deprivation. Whether all of the procedures *should* apply is a matter of discretion for each university to decide on its own. The key point is that there should be something in writing to describe the fair process that a student can follow when he or she contests the fairness of a decision and that the process is fair given the importance of the decision to that student.

Discussion of Case

In this chapter's case study, the consequences to the student are severe and the process of reviewing the imposition of the penalty needs to be scrupulously fair. This requires a thorough investigation of the facts. In this situation, Dr. Mahoney, the course coordinator, would need to meet with Professor Russert, the clinical faculty member, to get the full story. The key facts are what actually happened at the "anger management incident," what parts of it Professor Russert personally observed, and who were independent witnesses to it. Dr. Mahoney would also need to review the clinical evaluation form and related clinical documentation to see if it was both accurate and adequate. If Professor Russert was present for the incident in question, then Dr. Mahoney would ask her to explain the behaviors that she witnessed in detail and to summarize all of her verbal and written communications with the student since that time. Dr. Mahoney would also note if Mr. Johnson had any other incidents of clinical or academic misconduct. She would carefully review the nursing program student handbook, clinical course failure policy, syllabus, and clinical evaluation form for clarity and the student appeal policy. Dr. Mahoney would also meet with Mr. Johnson again to ask follow-up questions and remind him of his ability to consult the office of equality if he felt that he was the victim of improper discrimination because of his size.

⚖ WHEN TO CONSULT THE UNIVERSITY COUNSEL

Consult the university attorney when you are confronted with a new and difficult situation, or if you want to review high-stakes policies such as clinical misconduct, clinical failure, or clinical dismissal policies.

Findings and Disposition

After conducting an investigation, it was found that Professor Russert was not present when Mr. Johnson had his alleged "anger management incident." She had heard that Mr. Johnson had an outburst from the unlicensed assistive person who was at the nursing station at the time. There was no incident report or anecdotal notes documenting the incident. The faculty member had relied on the verbal account of the unlicensed assistive person only and had no written evidence of the incident from the person who witnessed the event. Professor Russert had documented what was communicated to her on the clinical evaluation form and clinical warning form. Furthermore, Professor Russert had not met with Mr. Johnson to hear his account of the incident. Professor Russert also interviewed the clinical assistant and learned that Mr. Johnson's large stature was a concern to her, and exaggerated her response to his actual conduct. No one else witnessed any improper event, although there were others in the area who presumably would have heard or seen something if it had been inappropriate.

The unlicensed person communicated that Mr. Johnson appeared frustrated when he found that his clinical rotation had been changed to an afternoon rotation. He clenched his fists and stated loudly, "I can't believe this!" He did not direct his anger toward any one individual. There were no anecdotal records delineating any acts of clinical misconduct. Furthermore, Dr. Mahoney reviewed the nursing program student handbook, syllabus, and clinical evaluation tool in reference to the incident.

After considering the facts and consulting with the department chair, Dr. Mahoney overturned Mr. Johnson's clinical failure on the basis that he had not been afforded due process. She determined that Mr. Johnson's behavior did not warrant a clinical warning and failure but rather a counseling session related to professional conduct. Dr. Mahoney met with Professor Russert and explained how her actions had violated the student's due process rights, and she was admonished to consult the course coordinator before issuing a clinical failure to any student on conduct grounds, as well as the need to follow policy related to clinical documentation. Dr. Mahoney confirmed this in writing, which was placed in Professor Russert's file.

PREVENTION TIPS

- Offer faculty development sessions on clinical evaluation and due process.
- Remember the importance of first finding out all the facts.
- Follow written policies and guidelines outlined in the student handbook.
- Have evidence that students have read clinical expectations—such as a signed statement indicating that they have read the handbook.
- When an incident occurs, document deviations from policy and have faculty and students develop a plan with specific follow-up date and consequences of failure to satisfactorily complete the plan.
- Have students read the documentation, have a chance to put their version in writing, and sign the form indicating they are aware of the documentation—they do not have to agree with the documentation; however, there does need to be evidence that they have read it.

Relevant Legal Cases

Board of Curators of the University of Missouri v. Horowitz, 435 U.S. 78 (1978)

Regents of the University of Michigan v. Ewing, 474 U.S. 214 (1985)

Landmark cases have set precedents for misconduct dismissals and adherence to due process. In 1978, the U.S. Supreme Court found for the University of Missouri, sustaining dismissal of a medical student for clinical deficiencies (*Board of Curators of the University of Missouri v. Horowitz,* 1978). In this particular precedent case, a medical student was dismissed for deficiencies in clinical performance. The Court determined that clinical evaluation of inadequacies was sound because the university adhered to standards of due process. The Court applied the principle of judicial deference in this case, respecting the authority of the university's decision regarding the deficiency misconduct. This landmark case situated universities in authoritative posture, imposing that no court should intrude into academic decisions regarding student performance (Parrot, 1993). The Court did not overturn the clinical evaluation, given that the university granted the student cumulative information of academic deficiencies and consequences of same (*Missouri v. Horowitz,* 1978).

Substantive due process was supported in Ewing's case, when the evaluation process of the student to meet clinical performance was upheld and deferred to the faculty member's judgment (*Michigan v. Ewing,* 1985). In this case, the student filed suit to stay a dismissal on the grounds that the university did not grant him due process privileges. The Court found that the university did not depart from accepted academic norms (Smith et al., 2001). The above two cases were decisive contributors to the *Morin v. Cleveland Metro General Hospital* (1986). Morin's case challenged dismissal of the nursing student for misconduct and unsafe clinical practices. The student's case was filed complaining the dismissal was arbitrary and capricious; however, the court of appeals upheld the student's dismissal, citing precedence of case law set by *Missouri v. Horowitz, 1978* and *Michigan v. Ewing,* 1985.

Summary

When a student receives feedback and evaluation of clinical misconduct, clinical faculty members will be held to a standard of fairness when investigations are made concerning whether a fair process was followed. In this chapter's case study, the clinical faculty member was not reasonable and rushed to quick and unfair judgment of clinical misconduct that should have been avoided, and would have been had the faculty member actually provided the student with an opportunity to be heard. In the appeals process, the course coordinator followed a thoughtful process that resulted in evidence that supported the student's appeal. The complete absence of any notes in the student's record made it impossible to impose any remedial action fairly, and confirmed that there had been no evidence that formative evaluations had taken place. As a result, the record demonstrated that due process had not been provided to the student. Dr. Mahoney did decide to require the student to undergo additional training in appropriate behavior. You may have noticed that the record did not include any other mention of "improper outbursts," and this one was only arguably that. But Dr. Mahoney's decision was reasonable, and the harm inflicted on the student was slight. For that reason, it is extremely unlikely that any judge or jury would interfere—rather, the law would support the business judgment that Dr. Mahoney had made, because she followed a process that was due.

Imagine what would have happened in this case if Dr. Mahoney had not overturned the clinical failure. The student would have been dismissed from the program and filed a lawsuit. A judge or jury would have seen just how carelessly Professor Russert had acted, how arbitrarily the university had allowed this to happen, and how summarily the student had his career in nursing ended with such a devastating comment about his character. It is not difficult to predict the outrage that the court would have expressed—and that means the verdict and award of money damages against Professor Russert and the university, compensating the student for the university's defective and unfair conduct, could well have been very high.

Due process, in short, protects not just the student. It protects the faculty member and the university as well.

CRITICAL ELEMENTS TO CONSIDER

- As a faculty member, you must provide the student with an opportunity to be heard before rushing to summary judgment.
- Consult academic policies related to clinical failure prior to informing the student verbally or in writing.
- If you are a novice faculty member, consult an experienced faculty member to review your documentation.
- If you are an experienced faculty member or academic administrator, educate new faculty about students' due process rights.
- Provide the student advanced notice of a clinical failure.
- Maintain daily evidence-based anecdotal documentation.
- Document student behavior in an objective manner including, date, time, location, witnesses, and action taken.
- Remember: Most cases related to clinical misconduct or performance issues have been upheld by the courts as long as due process has been afforded to the student and the nursing program followed its own policies.

HELPFUL RESOURCES

The American Nurses Association's Code of Ethics can be found at http://www.nursingworld.org. Click on the **Nursing Ethics** header, and then **Code of Ethics for Nurses.**

References

Board of Curators of the University of Missouri v. Horowitz, 435 U. S. 78 (1978).

Johnson, E. G. (2009). The academic performance of students: Legal and ethical issues. In D. M. Billings & J. A. Halstead (Eds.), *Teaching in nursing. A guide for faculty* (pp. 33–52). St. Louis, MO: Saunders.

Kolanko, K., Clark, C., Heinrich, K., et al. (2006). Academic dishonesty, bullying, incivility, and violence: Difficult challenges facing nurse educators. *Nursing Education Perspectives, 27*(1), 34–43.

Lindsay, C. L., III. (2005). *The college student's guide to the law.* Dallas, TX: Taylor Trade Publishing.

Parrott, T. E. (1993). Dismissal for clinical deficiencies. *Nurse Educator, 26*(1), 33–38.

Regents of the University of Michigan v. Ewing, 474 U. S. 214 (1985).

Roth, J. (Ed.). (2007). *Higher education law in America* (8th ed.). Malvern, PA: Center for Education and Employment Law.

Smith-Glasgow, M. E., & Dreher, H. M. (2007). Legal issues in student supervision. *ADVANCE for Nursing, 9*(18), 37–41.

Smith, M. H., McKoy, E., & Richardson, J. (2001). Legal issues related to dismissing students for clinical deficiencies. *Nurse Educator, 26*(1), 33–38.

Suplee, P., Lachman, V., Seibert, B., et al. (2008). Managing nursing incivility in the classroom, clinical setting, and on-line. *Journal of Nursing Law, 12*(2), 68–77.

Whitney, K. M., (2009). Managing the learning environment: Proactively responding to student misconduct. In D. M. Billings & J. A. Halstead (Eds.), *Teaching in nursing. A guide for faculty* (pp. 227–237). St. Louis, MO: Saunders.

CHAPTER 8

Due Process Issues for the Faculty

CASE STUDY

Due Process for Faculty

Your role: You are Ellen Shapiro, the Director of the Undergraduate Nursing Program. Professor Alice Fink, the Adjunct Faculty Coordinator, reports to you.

Professor Jean Kelly is an adjunct assistant professor at your university. She had been a full-time assistant professor for approximately 25 years there, teaching primarily women's health nursing until she retired in 2005. Professor Kelly has been teaching OB clinical at Holy Spirit Hospital for the last two quarters.

The director of the OB unit at Holy Spirit Hospital, Roz Hartman, contacts your adjunct faculty coordinator, Professor Alice Fink, and tells her that she does not want Professor Kelly to return to Holy Spirit Hospital. She tells Alice that it is "all about Jean" and that Jean's skills are rusty. She does not provide any details. As requested, Professor Fink removes Professor Kelly from the clinical site and in the next term, she does not assign her to teach OB clinical at Holy Spirit Hospital or any other clinical site.

You receive a call from Professor Kelly. She is outraged by having been "fired" and advises you that she will take legal action against you and the university for lack of due process and against Roz Hartman for defamation. She states that she and her students have not made any errors and that she has been diligent with care and documentation. She tells you that she believes that Roz Hartman does not like her because she has been an advocate for her students, and this is just retaliation against her. She also tells you that the decisions have made it impossible for her to earn additional income.

Questions

- How would you proceed?
- Did Professor Alice Fink react appropriately to Roz Hartman's news about Professor Kelly?
- Is Professor Kelly correct? Does she have a legitimate grievance?
- Has Roz Hartman defamed Professor Kelly?

Due Process for Faculty: Legal Principles and Review of the Literature

In this country, no one is guaranteed a job. Under the common law, employees hold their jobs "at will," meaning that employers can fire their employees whenever they decide, for whatever reasons they decide. Over time, exceptions have been made to this principle, both by judges and by legislatures, and voluntarily by employers and employees, who can change it for themselves through contracts, either on a personal level or for a group (e.g., union contracts). In academia, a university's relationship with a member of the faculty will typically be governed by the terms of the person's appointment (a contract) and of the rules and procedures applicable to faculty (e.g., policies and faculty handbooks).

The first legal principle applicable to faculty personnel actions is that both private and public colleges and universities must abide by terms of employment contracts with faculty (Poskanzer, 2002). The second is that faculty are typically protected by considerations of due process, which is one of most difficult concepts in the law, as explained in Chapter Six (which should be reviewed in this context). In academia, a college or university typically stipulates in writing the procedures by which personnel decisions affecting faculty are made, and these become part of the faculty's rights and protections. In cases of adverse action by a college against a member of the faculty, such procedural guidelines should ensure that faculty are given the opportunity to be heard, are provided in writing both the charges and the evidence of the charges against them, and are given the opportunities to appear before an impartial decision-maker and to appeal the decision (Lindsay, 2005; Roth, 2007).

It is important that administrators understand faculty members' *property rights* in their employment (and expectation of continued employment) and their *procedural rights* to the manner by which those property rights can be modified or taken away. Due process is the notice and procedural right that a person has when a vested interest in the person's property may be taken away. This right may be provided by the federal or state constitution, by federal or state law, by university policy or procedure, or by contract. Failure to follow procedures outlined in the faculty handbook or appointment letter does not necessarily constitute property interests; rather, failure to do so constitutes a breach of contract. The violation of the procedure may constitute a denial of due process, or it can simply be an error that is without material consequence.

As noted above, the phrase *due process* means that administrative decisions affecting significant personal rights must be carefully and deliberately made. In many universities, grievance policies and procedures exist to afford faculty their due process rights. The only legal consequence of having a property or liberty interest implicated is that the faculty member must receive due process before a deprivation of such interests (Poskanzer, 2002). A property or liberty interest, and a right to due process, does not ensure that administrators will make the best decision or the right decision; the denial of an interest or right does not automatically mean that there will be liability or a remedy.

The American Association of University of Professors (AAUP) also works to protect the due process rights of all members of the profession: full- and part-time teachers; tenured and contingent faculty; graduate students; librarians; and academic professionals. Furthermore, the AAUP establishes and maintains standards for academic due process and for faculty participation in academic decision-making, and it participates in precedent-setting court cases involving academic freedom and tenure issues. *Guidelines for Good Practices: The Excellence of Instruction in Institutions that Employ Part-time and Adjunct Faculty* (1997) has been developed by AAUP and includes some guidance related to adjunct and clinical faculty. For example, the *Guidelines* states that the university will provide the following:

- Long-term planning, whenever possible, to provide for extended terms of appointment consistent with institutional needs, thereby also providing sufficient job security to encourage and support continuing involvement with students and colleagues
- A provision with each appointment of a clear contractual statement of expectations and assignments including in-class teaching and other responsibilities such as course preparation, student advisement, and service
- Sufficient notice of appointment or reappointment to enable adequate course preparation
- A provision of orientation, mentoring, and professional support and development opportunities
- Regular evaluation based on established criteria consistent with responsibilities
- An opportunity for appeal or grievance in the event of allegedly substantial violations of procedure, discrimination, or denial of academic freedom
- Access to all regular departmental communication (AAUP, 1997)

These are, by their terms, only "guidelines" and not requirements. Moreover, few universities and colleges have adopted the AAUP *Guidelines* as their own. As a result, these are provided by way of example, and not as authoritative.

Discussion of Case

In this chapter's Case Study, Professor Kelly complained that she was denied an appointment for two reasons: first, on the merits, the reports of inadequate performance were inaccurate (and perhaps intentionally false); second, the university itself harmed her by not conducting the full and fair investigation that it owed her as a matter of due process. She was alleging that Professor Fink was not reasonable and rushed to judgment, harming her, before investigating the facts or giving her a chance to present the truth, thereby violating her due process rights. Professor Fink listened to Roz Hartman's opinions and acted on them without any supporting evidence or documentation related to Professor Kelly's job performance, despite Professor Kelly's decades of good service. By terminating Professor Kelly's teaching contract (or, more precisely, by failing to renew it for another term), Professor Fink deprived Professor Kelly of her property interest as a clinical faculty member (expected employment) without notice or opportunity to be heard.

Because Roz Hartman serves as director of the OB unit at Holy Spirit Hospital, she has the right and authority to comment on Professor Kelly's job performance in her capacity as the unit's administrator. Therefore, offering her professional opinion regarding Professor Kelly to the university's adjunct faculty coordinator would be considered appropriate and is entitled to conditional protection as long as the statements are made in good faith. Otherwise, they could constitute defamation.

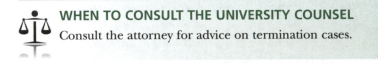

WHEN TO CONSULT THE UNIVERSITY COUNSEL
Consult the attorney for advice on termination cases.

Findings and Disposition

The director of undergraduate nursing programs asked to meet with Professor Fink and asked why she had decided not to reappoint Professor Kelly. She asked to see Professor Kelly's personnel and academic files, and noted that there were no deficiencies appearing in that record. She also did not find any indication that Professor Kelly had performed poorly as a teacher in the most recent terms, nor that her students were performing their duties poorly. She did not find evidence of any other deficiencies. Reviewing this with Professor Fink, she also pointed to Professor Kelly's long, productive career and many prior favorable teaching evaluations at the university.

Professor Fink was new in her role and unaware of Professor Kelly's previous full-time status at the university. Professor Fink admitted that her decision to terminate Professor Kelly's contract was based solely on the criticisms made by Roz Hartman. Although Roz Hartman and the Holy Spirit Hospital had the right not to allow Professor Kelly to work in (or teach at) their facility, they did not have the right to discriminate against her on the basis of her age; however, not enough was known about the reasons. In any event, that was between Professor Kelly and the hospital. After a discussion, it was agreed upon that Professor Kelly would be offered a clinical rotation at another hospital and that she would have an opportunity to respond to the concerns raised by Roz Hartman. Professor Fink was required to apologize to Professor Kelly for not allowing her an opportunity to address Roz Hartman's concerns; and both her error and the apology were noted in Professor Fink's file. Professor Kelly is serving as a clinical faculty member at another hospital and is receiving favorable reviews from the clinical agency personnel.

PREVENTION TIPS

Educate faculty and staff with administrative/supervisory appointments about faculty due process rights and university policies and procedures related to termination practices.

Relevant Legal Case

Gunasekera v. Irwin, No. 07-4303 (6th Cir. 2009).

In 2004, Dr. Jay Gunasekera was the Moss Professor of Mechanical Engineering at the Russ College of Engineering and Technology of Ohio University (OU) and Chair of the Department of Mechanical Engineering, which he had been for 15 of his 20 years at OU. He had graduate faculty status at Russ College, which enabled him to supervise graduate students' thesis work. That year, a student alleged widespread plagiarism in mechanical engineering graduate student theses. Two internal investigations revealed that plagiarism was present in collateral areas of the theses rather than in the analysis or conclusions. Following these probes, Dr. Kathy Krendl, the provost of OU, instructed Dr. Dennis Irwin, the dean of Russ College, to take further action "as appropriate." In response, Dean Irwin asked an administrator and a retired faculty member to investigate the alleged plagiarism. These men prepared a report and submitted it to Dean Irwin and Provost Krendl on May 30, 2006. The next day, Provost Krendl held a press conference to announce the conclusion of the investigations and publicize the findings. As the district court explained, the report found "rampant and flagrant plagiarism in theses" and "singled out three faculty members, including Dr. Gunasekera, for ignoring their ethical responsibilities and contributing to an atmosphere of negligence toward issues of academic misconduct." In response to this report, the university suspended Dr. Gunasekera's graduate faculty status for three years and prohibited him from advising graduate students.

Dr. Gunasekera sued the dean and provost in federal district court, alleging that they and OU had violated his due process rights by (1) depriving him of his property interest in his graduate faculty status without "notice and a meaningful opportunity to be heard" and (2) depriving him of his liberty by "publicizing accusations about his role in plagiarism by his graduate student advisees" without giving him a "meaningful opportunity to clear his name." The district court found against him on a variety of grounds, and Dr. Gunaskera again appealed. This time, the federal court of appeals found in his favor. It observed that Dr. Gunasekera alleged that his loss of graduate faculty status had resulted in a loss of pay (a summer salary research stipend) and benefits (such as a reduced teaching load), which added to the presumption that he had suffered a deprivation of property. Because OU's lawyer admitted that Dr. Gunasekera had not been given either a pre- or postdeprivation hearing, the court of appeals reversed the district court's dismissal of his property interest claim. Notably, the appeals court also held that the dean and provost were personally liable for failing to give Dr. Gunasekera a pre- or postdeprivation hearing for his graduate faculty status because they should have been aware of the hearing requirement.

This decision provides several warnings for administrators. First, it shows that one cannot be safe by delegating an investigation to someone else (as trusted as that person may be), having him or her interview the people involved, and then relying on his or her report. As a compilation of evidence, that report could provide the facts underlying and justifying decisions, but it is not a substitute for the fair process that must be followed to give a member of the faculty his due. Second, it holds individuals personally reliable for deficiencies in the process, because (in effect) they should have known better. This means that administrators must be aware of due process requirements. And third, it shows that seemingly minor things such rank and reputation can and do give rise to "major" rights that the Constitution will protect.

Summary

In the context of state schools, the rights and privileges given to faculty members are property and liberty interests protected by the constitutional requirement of due process; in private universities, they are protected by the university's contractual obligation to follow specified, fair procedures before they are qualified, suspended, or removed. In cases in which faculty are accused of misconduct or inadequate performance, administrators should take care to ensure that the faculty member's due process rights are not violated. Educating faculty and staff who hold administrative appointments about due process policies and procedures is critical. The only legal consequence of having a property or liberty interest implicated is that the faculty member must receive due process before a deprivation of such interests (Poskanzer, 2002).

CRITICAL ELEMENTS TO CONSIDER

- Faculty should have access to all faculty policies
- Review faculty grievance and related policies
- Communicate reasons for termination in writing; evidence allegedly supporting the charge should be contained in this document (Poskanzer, 2002).
- Allow the faculty member (grievant) an opportunity to challenge the grounds for termination.
- A final written dismissal letter should be given to the grievant that states the reason for the dismissal (Poskanzer, 2002).
- Follow your own policies and calendar related to termination and nonrenewal of contracts.
- Faculty should receive adequate notice according to the faculty handbook.
- Educate faculty and staff with administrative appointments about facultys' due process rights.
- Have a consistent, written evaluation process for all full-time faculty and clinical faculty.

HELPFUL RESOURCES

Consult the American Association of University of Professors' Web site (http://www.aaup.org) for their "Statement on Procedural Standards in the Renewal or Nonrenewal of Faculty Appointments."

References

American Association of University of Professors. (1997). Statement from the Conference on the Growing Use of Part-Time and Adjunct Faculty. Retrieved July 10, 2010, from http://www.aaup.org/AAUP/issues/contingent/conferencestatement.htm

Gunasekera v. Irwin, No. 07-4303 (6th Cir. 2009).

Johnson, E. G. (2009). The academic performance of students: Legal and ethical issues. In D. M. Billings & J. A. Halstead (eds.), *Teaching in nursing. A guide for faculty* (pp. 33–52). St. Louis, MO: Saunders.

Lindsay, C. L., III. (2005). *The college student's guide to the law.* Dallas, TX: Taylor Trade Publishing.

Poskanzer, S. G. (2002). *Higher education law: The faculty.* Baltimore and London: Johns Hopkins University Press.

Roth, J. (Ed.). (2007). *Higher education law in America* (8th ed.). Malvern, PA: Center for Education and Employment Law.

CHAPTER 9

Academic Freedom Issues for the Student

CASE STUDY

A Student Claims the Academic Freedom to Deny Her Professor Coauthorship on Class Paper Submitted for Publication

Your role: You are Dr. Fontana, the faculty member who is teaching this RN/BSN course.

Dr. Fontana has been teaching full-time in the undergraduate nursing program for 8 years. She has mentored several undergraduate and graduate nursing students who have published their classroom papers in peer-reviewed nursing journals, the student as the first author and—on most occasions—Dr. Fontana as the second author. Dr. Fontana discloses her authorship policy to every class at the beginning of the year: if a student receives critiques, comments, and feedback on one or two drafts of any paper, and if the paper is then ready for publication, that student is free to seek publication as the sole author. However, if a student writes a paper that still needs work after two drafts, and if the student is willing to work with Dr. Fontana on the paper after the course is formally over, then Dr. Fontana requests second authorship.

At the beginning of the new semester, Dr. Fontana was assigned to an RN/BSN course and she disclosed verbally her authorship policy. One of the students decided to write a paper on female circumcision, a subject that Dr. Fontana had studied years ago. Enthusiastically, Dr. Fontana encouraged the student to seek publication of the work and by the end of the term, Dr. Fontana had provided two substantive reviews of the paper and a third review that was more modest, but that did provide additional feedback. As the semester drew to a close, Dr. Fontana was discussing the most appropriate journal to which the article might be submitted when the student announced to her that she had reconsidered and thought she should be the sole author. Dr. Fontana, startled, did reiterate her standing policy, but the student countered that she thought the feedback was minor and did not warrant second authorship. Dr. Fontana disagreed with her assessment and told the student so; the semester came to a close with no resolution of the issue.

Questions

- How would you first proceed?
- Are there any university or departmental guidelines on student/faculty collaboration and copublication?
- Did the student have the academic freedom to seek sole authorship and publication of the article?
- Is there any possible recourse for the faculty member should the student indeed seek publication of the article as sole author?

University Students and Their Academic Freedom: Legal Principles and Review of the Literature

As Kaplan and Lee write in *The Law of Higher Education* (perhaps the leading text on the law in higher education):

> "Academic freedom traditionally has been considered to be an essential aspect of American higher education. It has been a major determinant of the missions of higher educational institutions, both public and private, and a major factor in shaping the roles of faculty members as well as students" (2007, pp. 247–248).

However, they also further elaborate: "Yet the concept of academic freedom eludes precise definition. . . . It draws meaning from both the world of education and the world of law" (p. 248). Questions of academic freedom, often interpreted as issues of free speech, are therefore common in academia. Typically, the most public issues surround an individual faculty member's right to free speech,[1] but there are still occasions when student free speech or academic freedom is debated. For example, whom does the First Amendment (free speech amendment) protect? Does it protect those in both public and private institutions? And does it protect verbal, written, and symbolic communication? Recall what the First Amendment says:

> Congress shall make no law respecting an establishment of religion, or prohibiting the free exercise thereof; or abridging the freedom of speech, or of the press; or the right of the people to peaceably assemble, and to petition the Government for a redress of grievances.

Regarding whom the First Amendment protects, it is important to note that the legal system treats high school students under age 18 and college students age 18 and over very differently, with high school students having greater authority to regulate speech than universities.

As early as 1965, Schodde wrote advocating for a free student press, freedom of speech, the rights of students to hear controversial speakers on campuses

---

[1] In a technical sense, universities have a right to determine who may teach, what may be taught, and who may be admitted to study, and so it is the university that has academic freedom more than an individual professor, and this was affirmed in 2008 in *Stronach v. Virginia State University* (Roth, McEllistrem, D'Ogostino, & Brown, 2009).

from any sides of a respective issue, the right of due process *for students* when accusations of university policies' violations are alleged, and even a rebellion to the principles of in loco parentis[2]—in which the college student's right to privacy (and academic freedom) and the rights of the parents intertwine, especially when parents are providing financial support in whole or in part. To Schodde, actions supporting in loco parentis were improper for college age adults. To this day there are still ongoing residual issues despite the erosion of in loco parentis, as the social pendulum swings toward individual college student rights and away from parental rights and parental notification.

Another critical issue when determining whether a college student's First Amendment freedom of speech is breached is to return to a founding principle that exists within the amendment itself: "The rules in the U.S. Constitution only apply to *government actors*. Private entities, and therefore private colleges, don't have to live by them" (Lindsay III, 2005, p. 121). In other words, the constitutional protections on freedom of speech for a private college are not codified as they would be at a state-supported college (thus a government entity). Nevertheless, any university, private or not, is usually reticent to abridge constitutional rights that might lead to very negative publicity. Further, as most private colleges and universities usually are recipients of some types of federal monies or aid, they can voluntarily become subject to government regulation.

What sorts of communication does the First Amendment protect in academia? One of the most highly visible high school student free speech cases was *Tinker v. Des Moines Independent Community School District*, 393 U.S. 503 (1969), in which students were found to have the right to wear black armbands to a public school as an expression of opposition to the Vietnam War. The Supreme Court concluded this was a form of "symbolic speech" and "closely akin to pure speech" and that this form of speech in high school students was protected unless school administrators could show that it would cause a substantial disruption of the school's educational mission. The court ruled that high school students do not "shed their constitutional rights when they enter the schoolhouse door." But the Court did note that school administrators have far greater ability to restrict free speech than governments do.

Another widely publicized case involving freedom of verbal speech of college students occurred in 1993 and received national attention. In this case, Eden Jacobowitz, a freshman at the University of Pennsylvania, was trying to write an English paper in his dorm room, but he was disturbed by noise from below his window coming from a group of female African-American students celebrating

---

[2] The doctrine of in loco parentis is a time-honored legal opinion borrowed from English common law, which "by placing the educational institution in the parents' shoes, the doctrine permitted the institution to exert almost untrammeled authority over students' lives" (Kaplan & Lee, 2007, p. 16).

their sorority's Founders Day. His first response was to yell out "Please keep quiet!" (shadowu@world.std.com, 1998, p. 1). As the noise continued, 20 minutes later he yelled out, "Shut up, you water buffalo. If you want a party, there's a zoo a mile from here" (p. 1). Within weeks the university administrative judicial inquiry officer filed charges of racial harassment against Jacobowitz. He was given an option of a settlement or an academic plea bargain or of facing a judicial hearing and possible penalties up to and including expulsion. After very contentious public charges and countercharges, Penn officials later offered to dismiss the charge of racial harassment if Jacobowitz would apologize, attend a racial sensitivity seminar, agree to dormitory probation as long as he lived on campus, and accept a temporary mark on his record (until his junior year if he had no further infractions) that would brand him as guilty. Jacobowitz claimed his use of the phrase *water buffalo* was not used as a racial epithet, and for that reason he declined the settlement, and Penn went forward with the formal charges that he had violated its code of conduct.

What Penn did not expect was the intense national spotlight that would shine on the university, putting its speech code (and the conduct of all the Penn administrators) under severe scrutiny. The American Civil Liberties Union (ACLU) became involved, and a federal lawsuit was filed by Jacobowitz against certain Penn officials, including the school's president. With a highly publicized, now international case causing harm to the reputation of this Ivy League school, an offer was made to Jacobowitz that he simply apologize for the remarks. In turn, the women would drop the case. The case thus came to a close, and Penn conducted an investigation concerning why this episode escalated so. The code of conduct regulating freedom of speech was subsequently dropped and later reissued in a revised form. Penn established a Committee on Open Expression with very specific guidelines, and the current *PennBook* states that individuals or groups violate the Guidelines on Open Expression if:

a. *They interfere unreasonably with the activities of other persons. The time of day, size, noise level, and general tenor of a meeting, event or demonstration are factors that may be considered in determining whether conduct is reasonable;*

b. *They cause injury to persons or property or threaten to cause such injury;*

c. *They hold meetings, events or demonstrations under circumstances where health or safety is endangered; or*

d. *They knowingly interfere with unimpeded movement in a University location.*

Finally, people are constantly reminded not to take academic freedom and First Amendment protections to *write freely* for granted or to minimize their importance. Remember the case of the Jordanian university student who was jailed for writing a poem (which he denied doing) that was critical of Jordan's king (Joyce & Kevlin, 2010). In the United States, the right to criticize leaders dates to before the Constitution and the case of John Peter Zenger, the printer, who criticized the King of England. But it is routinely tested, on a variety of grounds, and always, always for "good reasons."

As evidenced by the issue of the black arm band, the shouts from a college dorm window, and an undergraduate student's writing, these are all forms of expression that warrant a discussion of whether they are protected by the First Amendment and the principles of academic freedom or not. Whether the undergraduate student in this chapter's case study was exercising her constitutional right to publish her paper without her professor is actually another example of both the complexity of this First Amendment case that is addressed in *DePree v. Saunders,* No. 08-60978, (2009) and Kaplan and Lee's admonition that the principles of academic freedom both traverse the social system of higher education and jurisprudence (2007).

Discussion of Case

In this chapter's case study, Dr. Fontana learned that her student intended to publish her class paper independently. At first, Dr. Fontana was quite distressed by the student's decision, as she had given the student substantive feedback on two drafts and subsequently the student had asked for a third round of assistance, which triggered the policy and her right to be identified as a coauthor. In Dr. Fontana's view, she had provided feedback on three drafts, was very pleased with the quality of work, and was looking forward to the student publishing the work with her coauthorship. This had never happened before, and so Dr. Fontana was concerned whether she had done anything to make the student react, in her view, so unprofessionally. She asked herself whether her standing policy could in any way be perceived as improper. Dr. Fontana decided to search the Internet to see if she could find any publishing guidelines that could instruct her. She did realize, however, that communicating her policy orally to students might not have been "strong enough," especially as it was announced so early in the year, before the paper-writing process started.

The second case study question is, Are there any university or departmental guidelines on student/faculty collaboration and copublication? In this case, Dr. Fontana's college did not, and this episode later compelled her to spearhead the development of such a guideline. A quick literature review search on the Internet found very little direction for nursing faculty facing copublishing issues, but an article by two biology professors, "To Co-Author or Not to Co-Author: How to Write, Publish, and Negotiate Issues of Authorship With Undergraduate Research Students" (Burks & Chumchal, 2009), did confirm that there are real negotiating strategies to take with undergraduate students and also risks to faculty who undertake this kind of scholarship. There certainly were no signs during the semester that there were any relationship issues between the student and Dr. Fontana and so, with the semester at an end and the manuscript graded and returned, Dr. Fontana contemplated what the best course of action would be.

WHEN TO CONTACT THE UNIVERSITY COUNSEL

It would be unlikely that a student who claims his or her academic freedom has been violated by a professor would contact the university attorney, but there is absolutely nothing that would prevent the student from asking. University counsel is likely to get involved if the question is related to an article that is being readied for publication (when intervention and advice can solve a situation before it becomes a problem) and also when an alleged violation *has already occurred* (e.g., the student and faculty are fighting over a journal submission); even here, university counsel will perceive the adverse effects of claims and litigation and will be inclined to intervene to protect the university's interests.

In this chapter's case study, it is recommended to negotiate with the individual professor if there are coauthorship disputes. If that does not resolve the issue, the student has the option of going through regular administrative channels (e.g., department chair, associate dean, or dean) or going directly to the ombudsman. Filing a lawsuit directly against the faculty is an option, but that should be a last resort, for which university counsel will provide advice.

If the case of alleged academic freedom violation has already taken place, the decision tree is more complex. If it involves ideas or a product that has led to patents or inventions (less common in nursing), then the stakes (and future possible income) are higher. If the student claims plagiarism of something in print, first contact the alleged offending faculty member, and ask him or her to contact the journal editor in question, and either retract the paper or acknowledge the authorship omission and request adding the student as coauthor (even as first author). It is unlikely that the student will only request an addition of an acknowledgement. If the faculty member refuses, the student can contact the journal or file a complaint. Most universities have a committee on scientific misconduct, and the student can file a claim with that committee. The functions of the Committee on Scientific Conduct for the University of Maine, for example, can be found at http://www.umaine.edu/research/vice-president-for-research/committee-on-scientific-misconduct/. A simple Internet search will provide the procedures of similar committees at various universities. If the alleged action has already taken place (an article is under review, but it has not been published) and the student has subsequently graduated, it is unlikely that departmental channels can effectively resolve the issue or whether the ombudsman office can technically still be used (i.e., the student is now a graduate), but those avenues could be considered. In case of loss of royalties and revenues from patents, individual legal recourse is likely an option.

Findings and Disposition

If Dr. Fontana had not thought much about her efforts on this manuscript or had not believed in its potential for publication, she might have just let the issue go. However, Dr. Fontana genuinely felt her effort and direction were substantive and in the end decided it would actually be unethical for the student to submit the work to the journal, falsely representing the work as solely her own. Dr. Fontana, therefore, e-mailed the student to inquire whether she was still committed to publishing the article and whether she had given her argument that indeed she (as the teaching faculty) had met her guidelines for coauthorship. After about 2 weeks with no answer from the student, Dr. Fontana e-mailed the student again and finally got a response.

The student informed her that she had considered what Dr. Fontana had said at the beginning of class about coauthorship, but reminded her that her guidelines were not written on the syllabus. She further declared in her e-mail that she had given the situation much thought and determined that the amount of feedback given did not warrant coauthorship, despite Dr. Fontana's feedback on the first two drafts and the "most minor of feedback" on the third draft, as she put it. She said she had already submitted the paper for publication and had listed Dr. Fontana in the acknowledgments and stated she thought that was a better representation of Dr. Fontana's efforts. This leads to the third question: Did the student have the academic freedom to seek sole authorship and publication of the article?

Dr. Fontana was convinced that the student was unethically misrepresenting the work as her own, and she simply could not accept the student's actions. True, her policy was not contained in the syllabus, where, in retrospect, it might better have been, but the student never denied being made fully aware of the policy. After much thought and consultation with a fellow colleague (who did not necessarily agree with Dr. Fontana's proposed course of action), Dr. Fontana decided to mail a certified letter to the student declaring that if the student did not contact the editor herself and request that the article be pulled, she would contact the state board of nursing in which the student was licensed and file an ethics complaint against her. After that, she wrote that she would also contact the editor and declare the submission unethically submitted, an action that would certainly cause the editor to pull it. Shortly thereafter, Dr. Fontana received a curt e-mail from the student simply stating that she had pulled the article. To confirm this, Dr. Fontana contacted the editor and indeed verified that the article had been rescinded by the student. Without disclosing any further information, Dr. Fontana thanked the editor for the information.

The fourth question is, Is there any possible recourse for the faculty member should the student indeed seek publication of the article as sole author? Do you agree with the actions or recourse that Dr. Fontana took? Would you have acted differently?

Dr. Fontana decided that in the future she would always include her copublishing guidelines on her syllabus and thought it might be in the college's best interest to devise a publishing policy that would protect both faculty and student intellectual property interests. Several months later, Dr. Fontana did an Internet search to see if the manuscript had been published elsewhere. It had not.

It is also important to note that the actions taken by Dr. Fontana were not supported by her colleague. It is entirely debatable whether the actions of this RN would constitute an ethical charge against her right to practice according to the respective state nurse practice act. It is entirely possible that the student could also pursue countercharges. Although the strategy taken by Dr. Fontana worked in this case, it seems a high-risk course of action. On the merits, if the paper were publishable, the result of the way this misunderstanding was handled and resolved is that important, new knowledge was not shared.

Relevant Legal Case

Ogindo v. Binghamton, No. 07-CV-1322 (N.D.N.Y. 2007)

In this complicated legal case, the argument that a doctoral student had the academic freedom to publish his work without crediting his dissertation adviser became a point of contention and litigation. In *Ogindo v. Binghamton,* a doctoral student in chemistry sued his professors over intellectual theft. In 2007, Charles Ogindo filed a suit seeking $200 million in compensatory damages and $2 million in punitive damages and attorney fees against Binghamton University; his former dissertation adviser, John J. Eisch; the former and current chemistry department chair; and the director of graduate studies.

After successfully completing his oral examinations and all coursework toward his PhD in chemistry, Ogindo never completed his dissertation as his adviser, Dr. Eisch, had disciplined and ultimately dismissed him from the program for poor performance in the laboratory and unacceptable scholarship. Ogindo filed the lawsuit only when he discovered that two papers on two experiments he was involved with had been published without naming himself as coauthor or acknowledging his contributions (Swartz, 2007). One of the experiments was his dissertation experiment, for which Dr. Eisch had criticized his results, only to reverse himself later and admit the student was right after all.

This story is complex, but charges of academic theft or plagiarism of graduate students by professors, and specifically academic advisers (in this case, the doctoral student's dissertation chair), are not uncommon, according to the prestigious *Chronicle of Higher Education* (Bartlett & Smallwood, 2004). Generally lawsuits or formal complaints stem from the following:

1. Questions over jurisdiction, mainly from state-funded universities
2. Questions over internal processes, especially due process

3. Fear of reprisal and professional fallout, especially when the accused is a well-known professor (Bartlett & Smallwood, 2004)

In this case, there was a very tenuous relationship between the student and his graduate adviser. Around April 2005 the student had completed all requirements for his doctorate except his dissertation, alleged that his adviser would not approve his proposed dissertation experiments and instead wanted him to forge data on another experiment led by Eisch and Dutta (another doctoral student). Ogindo attempted to replicate Dutta's experiment, but was unable to do so. Ogindo alleged he was being asked to forge unreplicable results, and Eisch subsequently attempted to get Ogindo removed from the laboratory. An appeal to the director of graduate studies allowed Ogindo to return under probationary status, and eventually Eisch confirmed Dutta's data indeed could not be replicated, and Ogindo agreed to work with another former student. In January 2006, Ogindo applied for a part-time teaching position at another state university but needed Eisch's permission to take the job because he was in dissertation advisement and was being funded under a Clark Fellowship. Eisch refused to support the job offer, indicating it would interfere with the struggling student's full-time commitment as a doctoral student. In late January, Ogindo requested his probationary status be repealed because his initial claims about the viability of Dutto's data had been confirmed. Eisch denied the appeal but affirmed that Ogindo's work product had improved but that he would have to sustain this progress.

In July 2006, Eisch sought to terminate Ogindo's participation in Eisch's research program. Ogindo again appealed to the director of graduate studies and sought possession of his laboratory notebooks, which was granted. Ogindo proceeded to submit several manuscripts to various journals based on his experiments, but without his adviser's approval. Because it is unusual for graduate student work in chemistry to be authored without the graduate adviser, the editors of these journals contacted Eisch, who confirmed he had not authorized the manuscript submissions. Eisch filed a complaint against the student with the graduate progressions committee (GPC) who ruled that "Mr. Ogindo on three instances submitted work for publication or presentation without Professor Eisch's knowledge or consent. The GPC believes these acts constitute serious professional and ethical transgressions" (Justia US Law.com, 2010, p. 5). The GPC recommended termination from the PhD program, but the chemistry department faculty tabled the recommendations and worked out a compromise whereby an outside reader would independently evaluate the student's dissertation work. If the evaluator affirmed the quality of the work, then the student would be allowed to defend the dissertation. If not, he would be offered to resubmit it as a master's thesis. The student agreed to drop his grievance against his adviser and accept these terms, but retained the right to renew his claim.

In September 2006, Ogindo requested that a new dissertation committee be reconstituted, and in November he submitted another draft of his dissertation. In December the dissertation committee rejected the dissertation and gave the student until February 22, 2007, to revise it. Ogindo submitted a new draft on February 5, 2007, but his new adviser found it unacceptable and wanted a complete rewrite rather than a corrected copy. Subsequently, the Cornell University professor (the selected outside reader) completed his evaluation of Ogindo's work but found "the dissertation in no way constituted a Ph.D. thesis" (Justia US Law.com, 2010, p. 6). On May 25, 2007, Ogindo was informed his work did not constitute a PhD, and he was offered the opportunity to complete a master's thesis. Ogindo refused the offer, and requested his grievance be reinstituted and he be allowed to defend his dissertation. He was informed he could not reinstate the grievance because the terms of the grievance had been completed and his insistence that he be allowed to defend his dissertation was again denied.

In July 2007, Ogindo became aware that his adviser Dr. Eisch had coauthored a paper published in the *European Journal of Inorganic Chemistry* that mirrored his own work. As Ogindo's name was not included as a coauthor or contributor, he filed a lawsuit against the defendants in New York State Supreme Court alleging breach of contract, fraud, and promissory estoppel,[3] but his lawsuit was dismissed on October 24, 2007.

Later that fall, Ogindo requested registration for one credit of independent study to maintain the continuous registration required of doctoral candidates. Because his fellowship funding had been discontinued, the student was obligated to pay the one credit tuition himself, which he ultimately failed to do. In December, Ogindo refiled his lawsuit in the federal court, alleging federal causes of action including substantive due process, copyright infringement, and patent infringement as well as discrimination and retaliation. In March 2008 he was warned by the graduate director that he was in danger of being formally dropped from the university (remember, the offer for the master's thesis was still on the table) if he did not maintain his continuous registration with a full tuition payment. As he could not technically register for spring courses because he had not paid his fall tuition bill, he was dismissed from the university on March 26, 2008, for nonpayment and noncontinuous graduate registration. In June 2008, Ogindo amended his federal court complaint. On October 17, 2008, the court dismissed all claims of substantive due process, copyright infringement, patent infringement, breach

---

[3] The legal term *promissory estoppel* means "legal rule of evidence (and not a cause of action) which (1) prevents a party from making an allegation or denial that contradicts what it had previously stated, or what has been legally established, as the truth, (2) supports a claim for damages of the party that had a good-faith reliance on a misleading representation of another party" (BusinessDictionary.com, 2007, p. 1). In other words if someone makes a promise and an individual acts on the intent of the promise (regardless of whether the promise is valid), then the promise itself cannot be revoked for purposes of the actions of the individual claiming promissory estoppel.

of contract, promissory estoppel, educational malpractice, and fraud claims. The plaintiff's remaining claims alleging (1) discrimination on account of his race and/or national origin; (2) retaliation for plaintiff's assertion of a right protected by 42 U.S.C. § 1983; and (3) a violation of his right to due process of law, were reviewed and also summarily dismissed in January 2010.

Summary

This chapter examines how academic freedom is much more than just a professor's right to express unpopular points of view, in public or in the classroom. The principles of academic freedom extend to students, too, and apply broadly to words, symbols, dress, lifestyle, and actions—to newspapers, the "public square," and to the Internet. But the right to speak is not without bounds.

Frause has written:

> While the First Amendment may allow for the unabashed type of conduct that exists in some Internet circles (e.g., hurtful, anonymous comments), the practice of falsely representing another person's ideas as your own—plagiarism —is still unethical, and in some cases, illegal (2010, p. 1).

Although the court ruled against the graduate student, it remains obvious that these issues are very difficult for students to win (although certainly not impossible) because of the power differential between student and professor or student and university. Complicating all this is the academy's need for alternative revenue sources, and the desire to control what "results from" the exercise of inquiry on campus. In the case of *Ogindo v. Binghamton* the findings of the contested experiments and the revenue from possible patents in the biotech industry might have been significant, meaning that the financial stakes for both student and university could have been high. The student made one major mistake, which turned out to be fatal: initially seeking independent publication of the experiment articles himself and without his adviser. This procedural error caused him to "lose" on the merits. Finally, as mentioned in this chapter's case study, Dr. Fontana did not have a published standard college/department coauthorship policy at the time of this case. Other subsequent and similar cases led to the development of a coauthorship policy, which can be found in the appendix.

 CRITICAL ELEMENTS TO CONSIDER

- College-age students 18 and above have a constitutional right to freedom of expression, but that freedom only limits government actors. Private institutions have greater rights to limit free speech.
- There is no "academic freedom" for students to publish work product independently of their professors who have had substantive input into that intellectual work product. If a student is going to turn a class

Continued

CRITICAL ELEMENTS TO CONSIDER—cont'd

assignment or paper into a publication, she or he should first ask this question: "Is this work completely my own or have I had assistance with it in first draft or revision?"

- The next step is to consider whether there is an official coauthorship policy for student and faculty in your university, college, department, or on the course syllabus. That should be the best guide for how to next proceed.

- Our view is that coauthorship between student and faculty ought to be encouraged and welcomed, not discouraged or resisted by the student. The best science today is team science and not the product of a single individual, viewpoint, or effort.

- Further, editors, especially nursing editors, really do not want to publish student papers unless they reach a very high bar. A journal editor would not publish anything that looks as though it is a class assignment. Journals have very specific guidelines and missions, and all successful submissions ultimately published in respective journals have met the standards set by the editor and the journal's editorial board. Having faculty review and participate helps students exceed this bar. In short, two heads are typically better than one.

- Nursing students (particularly undergraduate students, but also graduate students) are often at an advantage when their submission is coauthored by a faculty member, especially one with a doctorate. It gives the manuscript gravitas that otherwise may be missing, especially when the student is technically not a licensed nurse.

- Students are encouraged to question professors, civilly and constructively, who profess the policy that anything written in their class may warrant the option that the professor be listed as second author. These policies, unless they adhere to acceptable coauthorship standards and policies, may be unethical, and for this reason knowing what coauthorship policies exist is very important. Challenges to policies should be made up the chain of command, and in a respectful way, with the argument that the university's intention should be to encourage and reward (by recognition, when deserved) innovation and creative thinking, not burden it.

- There are also guidelines for coauthorship that are found on journal Web sites, and when a manuscript is submitted, often each author's

CRITICAL ELEMENTS TO CONSIDER—cont'd

exact contribution must be attested to. For example, the *Journal of Clinical Nursing* has very specific guidelines that state the following:

ALL named authors must have made an active contribution to the conception and design and/or analysis and interpretation of the data and/or the drafting of the paper and ALL must have critically reviewed its content and have approved the final version submitted for publication" (2000-2010, p. 1).

- Further, the journal noted above and many others adhere to the definition of authorship designated by the International Committee of Medical Journal Editors (ICMJE). According to the ICMJE criteria, established authorship or coauthorship must be based on substantial contributions to conception and design of, or acquisition of data or analysis and interpretation of data; drafting the article or revising it critically for important intellectual content; and final approval of the version to be published (2009, p. 1).
- Our view is that copublication between students and faculty ought to be a positive experience, but students should not be taken advantage of in the scholarship of publishing enterprise, and adherence to best practices in copublishing will ensure this. Academic freedom of students (not just faculty) must be protected.
- Last, respective faculty guidelines (that do not, of course, violate any institutional policy) should appear on any course syllabus.

HELPFUL RESOURCES

- First Amendment Center: First Amendment Schools
  http://www.firstamendmentschools.org/freedoms/speechfaqs.aspx
- Student Press Law Center: Test Your Knowledge of the First Amendment
  http://www.splc.org/falawtest/
- Exploring Constitutional Conflicts: Free Speech Rights of Students
  http://www.law.umkc.edu/faculty/projects/ftrials/conlaw/studentspeech.htm
- Foundation for Individual Rights in Education (FIRE)
  http://www.thefire.org/
- American Civil Liberties Union (ACLU)
  http://www.aclu.org/

References

Authorship. (2000–2010). *Journal of Clinical Nursing*. Retrieved November 1, 2010, from http://www.wiley.com/bw/submit.asp?ref=0962-1067

Bartlett, T., & Smallwood, S. (2004, December 17). Four academic plagiarists you've never heard of: How many more are out there? Chronicle.com. Retrieved October 31, 2010, from http://chronicle.com/article/Professor-Copycat/18418

Blacker, D. (2007). *Democratic education stretched thin: How complexity challenges a liberal ideal.* Albany: State University of New York Press.

Burks, R. L., & Chumchal, M. M. (2009). To co-author or not to co-author: How to write, publish, and negotiate issues of authorship with undergraduate research students, *Science Signals,* 2(94), 3.

DePree v. Saunders 80, No. 08-60978 (5th Cir. 2009).

Frause, B. (2010). Thwarting the rise of plagiarism. Public Relations Society of America. Retrieved November 1, 2010, from http://prsay.prsa.org/index.php/2010/10/28/halting-rise-of-plagiarism/

International Committee of Medical Journal Editors. (2009). *Uniform requirements for manuscripts submitted to biomedical journals: Ethical considerations in the conduct and reporting of research: Authorship and contributorship.* Retrieved September 1, 2011 from http://www.icmje.org/ethical_1author.html

Joyce, R., & Kevlin, N. (2010). Jordan: Student jailed for writing poem. Universityworldnews.com. Retrieved October 27, 2010, from http://www.universityworldnews.com/article.php?story=20100911064405442

Justia US Law.com. (2010). *Ogindo v. Binghamton University et al*—Document 100. Retrieved September 1, 2011, from http://law.justia.com/cases/federal/district-courts/new-york/nyndce/3:2007cv01322/70116/100

Kaplan, W. A., & Lee, B. A. (2007). *The law of higher education* (4th ed.). San Francisco: John Wiley & Sons.

Koster, K. (2010, August 1). DOL issues wider, more liberal interpretation of "parents" under FMLA. Employeebenefitnew.com. Retrieved October 27, 2010, from http://ebn.benefitnews.com/news/dol-issues-wider-more-liberal-interpretation-of-parents-under-fmla-2683992-1.html

Lindsay, C. L., III. (2005). *The college student's guide to the law.* Lanham, MD: Taylor Trade Publishing.

Ogindo v. Binghamton, No. 07-CV-1322 (N.D.N.Y. 2007). Retrieved October 22, 2010 from http://docs.justia.com/cases/federal/district-courts/new-york/nyndce/ 3:2007cv01322/70116/100/

PennBook. (2009). Guidelines on open expression. Retrieved October 27, 2010, from http://www.upenn.edu/provost/PennBook/guidelines_on_open_expression

Roth, J. A., McEllistrem, S., D'Ogostino, T., et al. (2009). *Higher education law in America* (10th ed.). Malvern, PA: Center for Education & Employment Law.

Schodde, S. (2006). Background: NSA's academic freedom policies. In E. G. Schwartz (Ed.), *American students organize: Founding the National Student Association after WW II* (pp. 396–397). Ann Arbor, MI: American Council on Education.

shadowu@world.std.com. (1998). Chapter 1: The water buffalo affair. Retrieved from http://www.shadowuniv.com/waterbuffalo/wball.html September 1, 2011.

Swartz, D. (2007). Binghamton University doctoral student sues professors over intellectual theft. Africaresource.com. Retrieved October 27, 2010, from http://www.africaresource.com/index.php?option=com_content&view=article&id=448:binghamton-university-doctoral-student-sues-professors-over-intellectual-theft&catid=136:race&Itemid=351

Storch, J. (2009, September 17). In loco parentis: Post – Juicy Campus. InsideHighered.com. Retrieved October 27, 2010 from http://www.insidehighered.com/views/2009/09/17/storch

Stronach v. Virginia State University, No. 3:07CV646-HEH, 2008 WL 161304 (E.D. Va. Jan. 15, 2008).

Tinker v. Des Moines Independent Community School District, 393 U.S. 503 (1969).

University of Pennsylvania. *Policies and Procedures, 1990–1991.*

Academic Freedom Issues for the Faculty

CASE STUDY

An Undergraduate Nursing Faculty Member Claims It Is a Violation of Her Academic Freedom to Be Forced to Use a Certain Textbook for Class

Your role: You are Dr. Drayton and you are the course chair for NURS 101: Professional Issues in Nursing, taught during the sophomore year in a BSN program.

As the fall semester is about to begin, you are informed that that there will be four sections of NURS 101 taught with 25 students in each section. A new faculty member has been hired, Dr. Joy, and so as course chair you send an e-mail in early July informing the four faculty teaching this course (including Dr. Joy) that you have gone ahead and ordered the textbook for the course. You also tell them that in the next few weeks you will be scheduling a course meeting so the group can plan for the logistics of the course in the fall. You subsequently receive an e-mail from Dr. Joy informing you that she has selected an alternative text for her section. You politely e-mail her that the standard policy of the undergraduate nursing program is that all nursing sections have the same textbook. She replies that it is her academic freedom to choose her own text and that as long as she meets the objectives of the course, there really should not be a problem with her using a separate text.

Questions

- How would you first proceed?
- Is Dr. Joy correct that a faculty member's right to an individual course textbook selection falls within the domain of academic freedom?
- What do you think is the rationale is for the policy of using the same text for all sections of one course?
- Can this issue be resolved to avoid discord among team teaching faculty in this course?

University Faculty and Their Academic Freedom: Legal Principles and Review of the Literature

The tenets of academic freedom have been mostly associated with university faculty, but as discussed in Chapter 9, these issues are pertinent for college-age students as well. This chapter will examine, however, the often confusing issues surrounding what actually constitutes "academic freedom" in the classroom.

The American Association of University Professors' (AAUP) classic "1940 Statement of Principles on Academic Freedom and Tenure with 1970 Interpretive Comments" states the following:

1. Teachers are entitled to full freedom in research and in the publication of the results, subject to the adequate performance of their other academic duties; but research for pecuniary[1] return should be based upon an understanding with the authorities of the institution.

2. Teachers are entitled to freedom in the classroom in discussing their subject, but they should be careful not to introduce into their teaching controversial matter which has no relation to their subject. Limitations of academic freedom because of religious or other aims of the institution should be clearly stated in writing at the time of the appointment.

3. College and university teachers are citizens, members of a learned profession, and officers of an educational institution. When they speak or write as citizens, they should be free from institutional censorship or discipline, but their special position in the community imposes special obligations. As scholars and educational officers, they should remember that the public may judge their profession and their institution by their utterances. Hence they should at all times be accurate, should exercise appropriate restraint, should show respect for the opinions of others, and should make every effort to indicate that they are not speaking for the institution (AAUP, 2006, pp. 3–4).

Underlying these three principles is the central thesis that teachers (in this case they are speaking about university or college professors, no matter what their rank) are entitled to freedom in the classroom in discussing their subject. This principle does not indicate that controversial statements cannot be made in the classroom, but that they should have some direct context to the course and the relevant course readings.

As the First Amendment is interpreted, *speech* is not just the spoken word (including the right *not* to speak), but the written word and symbolic acts (Lindsay III,

---

[1] Of or pertaining to money.

2005). What you will need to determine in this chapter's case study is whether freedom of speech can somehow be determined to also extend to an individual faculty member's right to select a respective textbook for his or her course.

As made clear elsewhere in this book, even the First Amendment is not absolute. There are kinds of speech that are not protected, and reasonable regulations can be imposed in certain circumstances. Speech that can be "banned" includes that which is intended to incite lawless actions or panic or threat of public safety (e.g., one cannot stand in an auditorium and jokingly yell Fire! (*Gitlow v. People,* 268 U.S. 652, 1925),[2] obscenity (*Roth v. U.S.,* 376 U.S. 254, 1957);[3] or speech that is judged to be defamatory or libelous (*New York Times v. Sullivan, 376* U.S. 254, 1964).[4] Finally, the term *commercial speech,* which first entered the judicial vernacular in 1971, is different from *public speech* and can be regulated to ensure it is not false (Cásarez, 1998).

One of the more recent cases that received both national and international attention concerned University of Colorado Department Chair and Ethnic Studies Professor Ward Churchill. Mr. Churchill was a tenured professor but without a doctorate—facts that would become important in his later dismissal case. He wrote an essay on September 12, 2001, very critical of the United States in light of the attacks on New York City on September 11, 2001. Although the essay at the time did not draw much attention, his expanded comments were included in his 2003 book, *On the Justice of Roosting Chickens: Reflections on the Consequences of U.S. Imperial Arrogance and Criminality.* In 2004, Churchill was supposed to give a speech at Hamilton College in upstate New York, but after a political science professor saw his name on a roster of future speakers, a maelstrom arose, particularly after the student newspaper reprinted Churchill's 2001 essay (Schreker, 2010). His speech was eventually canceled by university officials, and thereafter the controversy surrounding Churchill's printed comments led to the cancellation of most of his other university speaking tour events, often for expressed reasons of "safety and security of our students, faculty, staff, and the community in which we live" and for "credible threats of violence" (Schreker, p. 3). Lost in the debate was Churchill's overriding thesis that the promise of equality as prescribed in the Declaration of Independence had largely gone unfilled (Briley, 2005).

---

[2] In *Gitlow v. People* (1925) it was determined one could not falsely yell Fire! if there was no fire and if such speech would cause panic and potential injury to others.

[3] In *Roth v. U.S.* (1957), the first real legal standard for judging obscenity, it was determined whether, to the average person, applying contemporary community standards, the dominant theme of the material, taken as a whole, appeals to prurient interest. However, as we have seen in the courts since this ruling, communities are not monolithic and what perhaps is obscene in one community may not be in another.

[4] In *New York Times v. Sullivan* (1964) a constitutional prohibition was announced in which for the first time it was codified that a public official could not recover damages for a defamatory falsehood relating to his official conduct unless the public official could prove that the statement was made with "actual malice"—that is, with knowledge that it was false or with reckless disregard of whether it was false or not. Defamation or libel, although both serious, remain difficult ultimately to prove.

A debate took place in the United States and abroad about whether Churchill had a right to free speech (academic freedom). Ultimately, the University of Colorado (a state-funded institution) came under enormous pressure from politicians and constituents in that state, and a committee was empaneled to investigate the quality of his scholarship and research, arguably in response to the allegations of a few about plagiarism and research misconduct. In May 2007, the president of his university set in motion the procedures to dismiss or fire Churchill on the grounds of plagiarism and research misconduct, but Churchill claimed that was subterfuge for the attack on his right to free speech and institutional guarantee of academic freedom (Jaschik, 2007). After reviews by two separate committees—a Committee on Scientific Misconduct and a second committee required to address his tenure—the university's board of trustees voted 8–1 to terminate his employment. Churchill immediately filed suit in state court, and after an almost 2 years, a jury rendered a verdict in his favor of a dollar on April 2009 for violation of his First Amendment right to free speech. This verdict was set aside a year later by the court of appeals (Schreker, 2010) on the grounds of immunity, but it remains pending as the courts consider other issues.[5]

What is often lost in the discussion surrounding academic freedom is that the courts almost always rule that "the right to academic freedom belongs to universities and not to individual professors" (Roth, 2009, p. 150). It is this principle that is most likely to affect the discussion between Dr. Drayton and Dr. Joy. A few recent cases illustrate the point.

In *Stronach v. Virginia State University,* Dist. Court, (E.D. Virginia, 2008), mentioned briefly in Chapter 9, a physics professor's grade of D assigned to a student was overturned by the department chair when the chair sided with the student, who claimed the professor had in error given him higher grades on two quizzes (the student sent in faxed copies of his quizzes). The professor claimed the student had doctored the grades on the quizzes. He sued in federal district court, claiming violation of his academic freedom because administrators had retaliated against him for testifying for another professor who had sued the university. VSU officials asserted that they had a right to change the grade without the professor's input or consent and the court agreed, dismissing this claim. It did so saying, "Significantly, the Court has never recognized that professors possess a First Amendment right of academic freedom to determine for themselves the content of their courses and scholarship, despite opportunities to do so" (2008, p. 6). An *untenured* professor's right to assign grades was rejected in *Lovelace v. Southeastern Massachusetts University,* 793 F. 2d 419 (Court of Appeals, 1st Circuit, 1986) and

---

[5] On November 29, 2010, the Colorado Appeals Court ruled that the University of Colorado Board of Regents was largely immune from being sued by Churchill either for (1) its handling of his case or (2) for any First Amendment violations; and the court specifically stated that it did not see its ruling limiting the rights of other faculty members. It was reported that Churchill plans to again appeal the decision, and thus this case continues (Jaschik, 2010).

similarly the claim of a *public* university professor that the First Amendment right to expression gave him personally the right to assign grades was rejected in *Brown v. Amenti*, 247 F. 3d 69 (Court of Appeals, 3rd Circuit, 2001). Although not precisely on point, the courts' logic in these cases is almost certainly fatal to a professor's claim to have the "First Amendment right" to select the textbooks for his or her class or section thereof.

Discussion of Case

How would you first proceed? Remember, your new faculty member is resisting using the same textbook as the rest of the team. Dr. Drayton was very displeased that this issue had surfaced. Many years ago faculty were individually choosing their own texts, pledging that they would all adhere to covering the same course objectives. However, Dr. Drayton recalled there was dissention among students who on course evaluations panned one text and praised another. She also recalled those course team meetings were always disjointed because different texts presented information in different ways, so that developing a coherent outline of content was always a cumbersome process. Aside from the different textbooks (and complaints about their variable cost), Dr. Drayton also had to deal with complaints about how *Professor X* gave three tests whereas *Professor Z* gave only two.

Despite the practical difficulties, Dr. Drayton and other faculty members had always subscribed to the belief that these faculty choices and decisions about teaching and conducting their respective courses were all sound issues of pedagogy, important for the faculty members individually to decide, and therefore a matter of academic freedom. In short, she was sympathetic with Dr. Joy on a personal level, if not an administrative one.

Is Dr. Joy correct that a faculty member's right to an individual course textbook selection falls within the domain of academic freedom? Arising out of this longstanding discord, a faculty decision had been made years ago that to increase the quality of the nursing program and increase NCLEX scores, the faculty must work more closely together and move toward consensus on the standardization of the curriculum.

Actually, discussions concerning the standardization of nursing curriculum have been ongoing for years. In 1981, Nichols called for more standardization, but it was in the context of requiring a baccalaureate degree for entry level into professional nursing. Koithan (1994) later documented nursing's obsession with standardizing both baccalaureate and associate degree education that resulted in an overemphasis on training rather than educating nurses. More recently, Clavreul (2008) wrote:

> A nationwide, standardized nursing curriculum at both the associate and bachelor levels would allow nursing students to move effortlessly between schools, and in turn, allow nursing schools to fill vacant seats where appropriate. Far too often, a student drops out and that seat remains vacant (para. 12).

Clavreul's concerns are geared toward better upward mobilization of nurses from lower educational ranks to higher ones, particularly when Aiken and colleagues (2009) have documented that only 6% of nurses having an associate degree go on to achieve a master's or doctoral degree, whereas 20% of nurses prepared at the BSN level do. Further, more upward mobility of nurses (which would likely be enhanced by more national standardization of curricula) is necessary to realize the goal for nursing recently announced by the Institute of Medicine in *The Future of Nursing: Leading Change, Advancing Health* (2010). The report calls for an increase in the number of nurses prepared at the baccalaureate level from 50% to 80% by 2020 and for doubling the number of nurses having a doctorate by 2020. Much of the necessary standardization of nursing that will be needed to achieve these goals can be still be done in the context of innovation and by close alliance to the strategies also recently outlined in *Educating Nurses: A Call for Radical Transformation* (2010).

Dr. Drayton was indeed fortunate that, years before Dr. Joy joined the faculty, a policy was developed and approved by full nursing faculty vote. The policy called for individual course chairs to oversee the text selection for each respective required baccalaureate nursing course in consultation with the other faculty team members who were teaching the course. In other words, this policy did not give the course chair unilateral power, but enabled the course chair to lead the textbook review process, moving the group faculty team to consensus, and end by taking a vote on which text or texts to select. It was also determined that for required courses in which there was more than one faculty member teaching the course, each semester one syllabus template would be agreed upon.

The third question in the case study is: What do you think is the rationale for the policy of using the same text for all sections of one course? Subsequent implementation of this policy immediately changed the dynamics of the students in various course sections, and having one group of students prefer one professor's syllabus requirements (or different text) over another ceased almost immediately. A common syllabus and common text also gave faculty more flexibility and allowed for seamless opportunities for faculty to take over a class when one faculty member was traveling to a conference to present a paper or was to be absent for a short period.

Last, although NCLEX scores had traditionally been excellent, the baccalaureate nursing program administrators worried that the faculty would become complacent and "sit on their laurels" and that this might result in a decline in the scores. This policy was therefore created to ensure more standardization and stability in the program, necessary components if there was to be more psychometric microanalyses of individual course outcomes rather than just on exit HESI scores or NCLEX performance.

Findings and Disposition

Dr. Drayton, being an experienced course chair and longtime nursing faculty member, wanted to solve the problem expeditiously while maintaining the cohesiveness of her coursing team. This leads to the fourth question: Can this issue be resolved to avoid creating discord among team teaching faculty in this course? Instead of choosing to e-mail Dr. Joy again and inform her of the standing policy on textbook selection, Dr. Drayton thought a more personal approach would be best. Martin (2007) discusses how even in a climate in which e-mail is predominant, often face-to-face communication is essential and may be more effective. Dr. Drayton therefore called Dr. Joy and left a message on her voicemail that because e-mail can be so impersonal, they should instead meet so Dr. Drayton could go over some of the background of the reason that textbook selection is handled as a group faculty decision and not an individual one. Dr. Joy agreed to a meeting. After an explanation by Dr. Drayton and a review of the policy, Dr. Joy stated that she honestly did not agree with the policy, because in her previous position this was certainly not the practice, but that she would willingly comply. She was also glad to hear that the policy did not apply to elective nursing courses. She did ask whether the policy applied to master's and doctoral courses, and Dr. Drayton informed her that although there was no set policy for graduate courses, most of the faculty did work together to use common texts, especially for core cognate courses and for specialty courses in which one textbook might be used for a series of courses. Dr. Drayton was glad she handled this issue with a personal touch, and she was proud of her own leadership abilities in handling the matter without involving the department chair.

WHEN TO CONTACT THE UNIVERSITY COUNSEL

If you believe your academic freedom has been or is being violated, document thoroughly first, and then go through all the appropriate channels, especially the chain of command. Again, many faculty members are very confused about what academic freedom actually entails. It should be possible to contact the university attorney for a simple query, but even university attorneys are likely going to operate from a context of what is in the best interest of the university, since that is their first client, not the individual member.

Relevant Legal Case

Sheldon v. Dhillon, No. C-08-03438 RMW (N.D. Cal. 2009)

June Sheldon was a master's prepared biology and microbiology instructor at San Jose/Evergreen Community College. Having taught at San Jose/Evergreen Community College since 2004, Sheldon received a student complaint in August 2007

about a class discussion 2 months earlier regarding the mendelian basis of homo-
sexuality. After an internal investigation in December 2007, the vice chancellor
notified Sheldon in December 2007 that her contract for the spring term 2008
was rescinded, she was to be removed from the senior adjunct faculty roster and
her employment terminated and that this was being done with the approval of the
District Board of Trustees.

Sheldon contested much of the findings of the internal investigation committee. According to Sheldon, after taking a quiz, the student questioned the theory
of the heredity of homosexual behavior. Sheldon answered the student, using the
assigned textbook as a guide for her discussion, and indicated there was a stronger
biological basis for homosexual behavior in men than in women. She also indicated in class that there was substantial debate over the question of
nature versus nurture and did not believe she had engaged in any kind of polemic
at all. According to the student, however, she had made "offensive and unscien-
tific" (p. 3) statements including saying that "there aren't any real lesbians" (p. 3)
and that "there are hardly any gay men in the Middle East because the women are
treated very nicely" (p. 3). Having been made aware of the student's complaint in
September 2007, Sheldon agreed to meet with the biology faculty to discuss mainstream scientific thought on the issue and was subsequently offered a spring teaching contract without mention of the incident. With a teaching contract renewed,
Sheldon declined teaching opportunities at other institutions.

On December 6, 2007, Sheldon received a letter from the dean of the math
and science division accusing her of teaching misinformation in science and
stating that the seriousness of the complaint warranted her dismissal. This was
followed by a letter from Human Resources on December 18, 2007. On July 16,
2008, Sheldon filed suit in federal court for retaliation in violation of her First
Amendment rights (stating her answer to a student question was protected), for
violation of her First Amendment rights of her protected content and viewpoint
of her speech, and for Fourteenth Amendment guarantees of equal protection
and due process.

In its ruling the court held that free speech as a private citizen is protected
but not necessarily the speech of public employees in their work capacity, citing
the case of *Ceballos v. Garcett,* 361 F.3d 1168 (Court of Appeals, 9th Circuit, 2004).
"There is some argument that expression related to academic scholarship or
classroom instruction implicates additional constitutional interests that are
not fully accounted for by this Court's customary employee-speech jurisprudence"
(*Id.* at 425). The court allowed the professor to pursue her First Amendment
claims, and in July 2010 the case was settled, with the community college district
agreeing to pay her $100,000 and to remove from her file any reference of her
dismissal (AAUP, 2010).

Summary

This chapter has demonstrated that the domain of faculty academic freedom is not nearly as as expansive as is sometimes presumed. It is actually private citizen speech that is protected by the First Amendment and not necessarily speech conducted by employees, even when the employer is a university or college. Furthermore, it is likely the university, not the faculty member, that is entitled to the freedom from constraints. The courts give great deference to educational institutions to conduct their educational enterprise without great interference from the courts, and that includes deciding what is taught in the classroom.

The AAUP historically has been a great advocate for the rights of academic freedom for faculty, but even that organization did not intervene formally in the Ward Churchill case because in the end he was not dismissed (technically) for his September 11 essay, but instead for faulty scholarship. However, it is not implausible that he was indirectly fired for his speech, and the actions that took place (analogous to a witch hunt, perhaps) occurred in a highly politicized environment. However, several faculty bodies did meet, investigated charges extensively, and all produced lengthy summaries and findings, all of which indicates some degree of due process did take place (Fourteenth Amendment protection).

Finally, in the case of Sheldon, it is perhaps comforting to know that there is some legal precedence by which the content of scholarship of an individual faculty member is protected, particularly if the classroom speech directly pertains to the content of the course directed. Although the court could not determine (indicated this in the ruling) whether the student claim in this case was truthful or the faculty claim was truthful, nonetheless, it seems logical to us that if the community college could have provided confirmation of the professor's classroom speech by other students in the classroom at the time, then the defendant's case would have been much stronger.

If you are taking courses in a history or political science department, it is not uncommon to see political flyers on faculty office doors and bulletin boards. Rarely has an individual faculty member been required to remove the flyers. However, political flyers on nursing faculty offices are likely less common, and there have been directives in which nursing faculty have been particularly discouraged to do this. Is this right or wrong? Do you think a nursing faculty member has a right to put something that is not obscene, defamatory, or libelous, but that is political on an office door? Have more discussions about what faculty academic freedom really means. If your goal is to become a nursing professor, knowledge of its domain of authority will be helpful to you as you acclimate to your academic role.

CRITICAL ELEMENTS TO CONSIDER

- First, remember at its most rudimentary interpretation, the First Amendment right to free speech mostly pertains to the speech of private citizens speaking on public issues, not employees talking about work issues.
- Second, the courts have mostly ruled that freedom of speech rests more in hands of the institution, not of the individual faculty. Your classroom response to questions and classroom commentary is likely protected as long as it is relevant to the course content.
- Departmental policies almost always need to be followed unless there are extenuating circumstances or if you can prove the policy is improper for some reason.
- Collegial faculty relationships are important, and it takes good leadership skills to problem-solve effectively. E-mail has become our default form of efficient communication, but often problem solving will require personal interaction.
- Faculty handbooks can become very important legal contracts. Read yours. Know what is in it. Individual or groups of faculty can request that certain procedures become codified as policy. Informing a new faculty member that some practice is policy rather than a generally accepted practice is more organizationally sound.

HELPFUL RESOURCES

- American Association of University Professors (AAUP)
  http://www.aaup.org/aaup
- American Association of University Women
  http://www.aauw.org/about/
- American Civil Liberties Union (ACLU)
  http://www.aclu.org/
- First Amendment Law Prof Blog
  http://lawprofessors.typepad.com/firstamendment/
- *Journal of Academic Freedom* [online]
  http://www.academicfreedomjournal.org/

References

Aiken, L., Cheung, R. B., & Olds, D. M. (2009). Education policy initiatives to address the nurse shortage in the United States. *Health Affairs, 28*(4), w646–w656.

American Association of University Professors. (2006). 1940 statement of principles on academic freedom and tenure. In *AAUP's policy documents and reports* (10th ed.). Washington, DC.

American Association of University Professors. (2010). Legal cases affecting academic speech: *Sheldon v. Dhillon*. Retrieved November 8, 2010, from http://www.aaup.org/AAUP/protectvoice/Legal/

Author. Retrieved November 6, 2010, from http://www.aaup.org/NR/rdonlyres/EBB1B330-33D3-4A51-B534-CEE0C7A90DAB/0/1940StatementofPrinciplesonAcademicFreedomand Tenure.pdf

Benner, P., Sutphen, M., Leonard, V., & Day, L. (2010). *Educating nurses: A call for radical transformation*. Stanford, CA: Carnegie Foundation for the Advancement of Teaching.

Briley, (2005, February 10). Ward Churchill's comments—and the general's. HHN: History News Network. Retrieved November 6, 2010, from http://hnn.us/articles/10146.html

Brown v. Amenti, 247 F.3d 69 (3d Cir. 2001).

Cásarez, N. B. (1998). Don't tell me what to say: Compelled commercial speech and the First Amendment. *Missouri Law Review, 63,* 929.

Ceballos v. Garcetti, 361 F .3d 1168, 1180 (9th Cir. 2004).

Churchill, W. (2003). *On the justice of roosting chickens: Reflections on the consequences of U.S. imperial arrogance and criminality.*

Clavreul, G. M. (2008). Should nursing school curriculum be standardized? Workingnurse.com. Retrieved November 7, 2010, from http://www.workingnurse.com/articles/Should-Nursing-School-Curriculum-Be-Standardized

Institute of Medicine. (2010). *The future of nursing: Leading change, advancing health.* Committee on the Robert Wood Johnson Initiative on the Future of Nursing, at the Institute of Medicine. Washington, DC: National Academies Press.

Jaschik, S. (2007). Ward Churchill and academic freedom. insidehighered.com. Retrieved November 6, 2010, from http://www.insidehighered.com/news/2007/05/30/Churchill

Jaschik, S. (2010, November 29). A loss for Ward Churchill—and others? insidehighered.com, Retrieved March 15, 2011, from http://www.insidehighered.com/news/2010/11/29/Churchill

Koithan, M. (1994). Incorporating multiple modes of awareness in nursing curriculum. In P. L. Chinn & J. Watson (Eds.), *Art and aesthetics in nursing* (pp. 145–162). New York: National League for Nursing.

Lindsay, C. L., III. (2005). *The college student's guide to the law.* Lanham, MD: Taylor Trade Publishing.

Lovelace v. S.E. Mass. Univ., 793 F.2d 419, 425 (1st Cir. 1986).

Martin, C. (2007). The importance of face-to-face communication at work. cio.com. Retrieved November 8, 2010, from http://www.cio.com/article/29898/The_Importance_of_Face_to_Face_Communication_at_Work

Nichols, B. (1981). Standardized education for nursing. *American Journal of Hospital Pharmacy, 38*(10), 1455–1458.

Roth v. U. S., 354 U.S. 476 (1957).

Schreker, E. (2010). Ward Churchill at the Dalton Trumbo Fountain: Academic freedom in the aftermath of 9/11. *AAUP Journal of Academic Freedom, 1.* Retrieved November 6, 2010, from http://www.academicfreedomjournal.org/VolumeOne/Schrecker.pdf

Sheldon v. Dhillon, No. C-08-03438 RMW (N.D. 2009).

Stronach v. Virginia State University, No. 3:07CV646-HEH, 2008 WL 161304 (E.D. Va. Jan. 15, 2008).

CHAPTER 11

Student Issues and Conflicts Over Intellectual Property

CASE STUDY

A Master's Nursing Student Discovers Her Faculty Mentor Has Presented Their Joint Work at a Conference Without Giving the Student Authorship

Your role: You are Dr. Goings, the assistant dean and supervisor of the accused faculty mentor, Dr. Perpetua.

As Assistant Dean for Graduate Nursing Programs, you get an e-mail one day from Ms. Ray, a student in the MSN in Innovation and Intra/Entrepreneurship in the Advanced Nursing Practice track. According to the student, she was assigned to Dr. Perpetua for her master's innovation practicum. The student had conceived the idea to open up a nonprofit women's advocacy center in economically deprived neighborhoods to inform women of their rights and services, particularly surrounding health care and personal safety. As her faculty mentor, Dr. Perpetua had assisted Ms. Ray with the development of the project and the supporting business proposal. Unknown to the student, Dr. Perpetua had submitted an abstract to a national conference outlining the proposal, but without giving acknowledgment to Ms. Ray as the primary creator of the idea. Ms. Ray would have possibly never known about this had she not heard about the conference and discovered Dr. Perpetua was actually listed as a conference presenter *of her project.* In this e-mail, the student indicates that she is shocked and upset and is afraid to confront Dr. Perpetua, but she is asking you to do something about the situation.

Questions

- How would you first proceed?
- How will you investigate this case?
- Do you believe the student has been the victim of theft of intellectual property?
- If indeed theft of intellectual property has occurred, what should be the action against Dr. Perpetua?

University Student Intellectual Property: Legal Principles and Review of the Literature

Chapter 9 presented the case of a professor who claimed her contributions to a student's work was misrepresented by the undergraduate nursing student as solely her own. In that case, the student claimed it was her academic freedom to determine whether her instructor deserved coauthorship on the student's paper, and clearly she did not think so. Although that case was presented as a case of an individual student's academic freedom, this case is similar but will be approached from the perspective of intellectual property rights. As mentioned previously, cases of faculty accused of misappropriating the intellectual property of their students (especially graduate students) are unfortunately not uncommon.

What exactly is meant by the term *intellectual property*? According to the World Intellectual Property Organization (WIPO), "Intellectual property (IP) refers to creations of the mind: inventions, literary and artistic works, and symbols, names, images, and designs used in commerce" (n.d.a., para. 1). It can be divided into two categories:

> *Industrial property, which includes inventions (patents), trademarks, industrial designs, and geographic indications of source; and Copyright, which includes literary and artistic works such as novels, poems and plays, films, musical works, artistic works such as drawings, paintings, photographs and sculptures, and architectural designs (n.d.a., para. 2).*

In most universities, particularly research universities, issues surrounding intellectual property rights, especially patent rights, are highly regulated activities because new patent inventions by work-for-hire[1] faculty have the possibility to result in enormous royalties for not only the inventor but also for the university itself. The specifics surrounding university faculty intellectual property rights are discussed in more detail in Chapter 12, but the issue here is a student's right to his or her own creative ideas, inventions, and even prose while enrolled at a university. At first glance, it might appear that this is a very simple issue: "If the student invents or authors it, it belongs to the student!" However, what if the invention took place in a laboratory, very likely the laboratory of a faculty mentor or often a dissertation adviser? What if there were collaborators on the creative project, extremely likely especially in a laboratory setting? Science is no longer a solitary enterprise and therefore it is very unlikely that most graduate student work can be labeled as completely independent, thus resulting in the complexities of authorship and invention.

This is what happened to Eugene Aserinsky, who was a graduate student in 1952 at the University of Chicago. Now he is officially recognized as the individual

---

[1] The concept of *work for hire* is an important legal term. It is a concept in intellectual property law in which the work of an employee is considered to be owned by the employer. Operationally, work for hire is an exception to the copyright concept that the creator of a work is its owner.

who discovered rapid eye movement (REM) sleep when he noted and documented the cyclic occurrence of eye movements during sleep every 90 to 100 minutes in adults (Brown, 2003). However, at the time of the discovery it was coattributed to his PhD adviser (and department chair of physiology) Nathaniel Kleitman, and that incorrect attribution remained common understanding until recently. According to the corrected obituary for Dr. Aserinsky that the *Los Angeles Times* published on August 14, 1998, 20 days after it had incorrectly identified him as the codiscoverer of REM sleep:

> *Emaline Rich, Aserinsky's first cousin, said that Aserinsky made the discovery alone when he was a graduate student at the University of Chicago. She said that Kleitman was listed as co-author of the research paper only because Kleitman was the professor supervising Aserinsky's doctoral thesis. (p. A30)*[2]

The fascinating story of Aserinsky and Kleitman is told by Lynne Lamberg in her short article, "The Student, the Professor, and the Birth of Modern Sleep Research" (2004). This story did not include litigation (as many others have), chiefly because the discovery of REM did not result in the invention of a commercial product or a literary work. In this case the discovery resulted in publication in the prestigious peer-reviewed journal *Science* (Aserinsky and Kleitman, 1953), where Kleitman was erroneously given credit for the discovery as second author.

As mentioned above, current intellectual property is divided into industrial property (which includes, but is broader than inventions) and copyrighted artistic expressions. A more recent case of alleged intellectual property theft by a professor of a student's creative capital[3] took place in 2010 when Seung Won Lee, a graduate student at Parsons, the New School for Design in New York City, claimed he spent 3 years working on a social networking gaming application called Jump-Cell for his graduate thesis (Markos, 2010). His professor, Jinsook Erin Cho, had encouraged him to develop a marketing plan for his idea, and he traveled to his home in Korea to do so. Shortly thereafter, he read a newspaper account of a new application very similar to his, called Rat Busters, which had been developed by his thesis adviser, Professor Cho, with an $80,000 institutional grant from Parsons. After reading that the invention was attributed to Professor Cho and one of his friends, Lee returned to the United States and filed his lawsuit in the New York Supreme Court in Manhattan. Subsequently, Professor Cho filed countercharges, admitting that Mr. Lee had come up with the idea, but arguing that he and his patent colleague had indeed done all the development work at great expense to put the invention to market (Markos).

---

[2] Perhaps even worse, the current Wikipedia citation on sleep doesn't even mention Aserinsky in a discussion of the discovery of REM sleep and instead cites Kleitman and William Dement, a second-year medical student who was also working in this laboratory and who later became one of the leading sleep researchers in the world (Wikipedia, November 16, 2010). The first author on this chapter completed a postdoctoral fellowship in sleep and respiratory neurobiology in 2001–2003 at the University of Pennsylvania, and even I first learned *incorrectly* that REM was discovered by Kleitman *and* Dement!

[3] Students can also be accused of stealing each other's creative concepts as the movie *The Social Network* vividly demonstrates.

At the time this book was published, the case of *Lee v. Cho* had not litigated, but the questions for academic faculty are clear: (1) is it legal to appropriate another's idea (even if it is not yet fully developed) and refine it (as Professor Cho has admitted) for a knock-off patent; (2) is it ethical that, although the professor admits he borrowed the idea, there was absolutely no acknowledgment of the student's contribution; (3) did the university have a policy on intellectual property policy that applied to this dispute; and (4) what could university counsel advise regarding the applicability of U.S. patent law to an inventorship dispute such as this? These questions are considered below.

Copyright is a particular form of intellectual property that is a core concept in academia because it applies to writing (scholarship) and other forms of expression (e.g., software, courseware), and it is the most likely source of misappropriation by students, who claim authorship in prior manuscripts (e.g., course papers). According to the Berne Convention for the Protection of Literary and Artistic Works,[4] most of whose signatory countries belong to the World Trade Organization, copyright extends to the following:

- Books, pamphlets and other writings;
- Lectures, addresses, sermons;
- Dramatic or dramatico-musical works;
- Choreographic works and entertainments in dumb show;
- Musical compositions with or without words;
- Cinematographic works to which are assimilated works expressed by a process analogous to cinematography;
- Works of drawing, painting, architecture, sculpture, engraving and lithography;
- Photographic works, to which are assimilated works expressed by a process analogous to photography;
- Works of applied art; illustrations, maps, plans, sketches and three-dimensional works relative to geography, topography, architecture or science;
- "translations, adaptations, arrangements of music and other alterations of a literary or artistic work, which are to be protected as original works without prejudice to the copyright in the original work; and
- Collections of literary or artistic works such as encyclopaedias and anthologies which, by reason of the selection and arrangement of their contents, constitute intellectual creations, are to be protected as such, without prejudice to the copyright in each of the works forming part of such collections. (World Intellectual Property Organization, n.d.a, Article 2)

---

[4] The Berne Convention principles were actually instigated by Victor Hugo, author of *Les Miserables* among other works, who was concerned about the *droit d'auteur* ("right of the author"), which at the time of his writings meant authorship rights, and copyright did not extend beyond an individual country's borders. Signed in 1886, this agreement has been updated over the years and as of 2007 some 163 countries have signed this document, which is essentially an international trade agreement (Bouchoux, 20008).

Although nursing students (undergraduate and graduate) may not often be involved in issues of patent rights from inventions (however, students in Drexel's MSN in Innovation mentioned in the case and Arizona State University's MHI in Healthcare Innovation are degree programs in which graduate nursing students may actually invent and seek patents), issues of copyright from individual manuscripts (typically course papers) are likely much more prevalent. An important point about copyright is that ideas themselves cannot be copyrighted; however, the expression of ideas can be copyrighted, as was first derived in *Story's Executives v. Holcombe* (1847).

In a 2009 copyright case at San Jose State University, an undergraduate student was taking a course titled "Data Structures and Algorithms." Emanating from a class assignment, the student posted his class work product, in this case computer code, on the Internet (Stripling, 2009). His professor claimed that the student had committed copyright infringement by publishing work product (code) that was connected to his class.[5] In this case the professor argued the purpose of the code was for his class, under his instruction, and therefore he had at least partial claim to it (Stripling, 2009). A commentary on this case actually provides a good summary of the impact of copyright laws on university or college students:

> Students own the copyrights in the works they create at our institutions. As the digital age offers new opportunities to disseminate scholarship, including student scholarship, we need to remember that students own their copyrights (just as professors own theirs) and formulate appropriate policy to respect those rights. (Smith, 2009, para. 3).

Whether in fact the student had any claim to ownership, as university counsel would tell you, depends on the facts; for example, whether the invention was made possible by substantial use of the university's resources, what the university's IT policies state, and whether there was a contractual agreement with a funder/sponsor of research.

Discussion of Case

Recall the first question: How would you first proceed? Remember, you are Dr. Goings, and you are confronted by an accusation from a student against Dr. Perpetua. One of the more central tenants of management and leadership, especially when dealing with conflict resolution, is that there are always two sides to a story. It is easy to be seduced by a salacious story or to come to quick judgments about a claim when you are first presented information or evidence, which at first glance appears convincing and true. However, in any given individual case in academia, what first seems obvious is untrue or far different from the actual reality. Therefore, fact finding directed at both sides (or in some cases there may be additional sides) is essential. This leads to the second question, How will you investigate this case?

---

[5] There were other issues as well, including whether the student had breached the honor code by posting answers (code) to an examination that was already due.

The next step Dr. Goings will take is *fact finding*. She will need to investigate this claim thoroughly before she can best establish to her satisfaction the actual details and facts of the case, which would then lead her to a conclusion and a course of action. Although she already has the initial student claim, Dr. Goings asks the student to provide greater detail and any supporting documents or other evidence that relates to her claim. Once she receives this further explanatory documentation from the student, Dr. Goings knows she will have to do the same with Dr. Perpetua, including having a private meeting with Dr. Perpetua to present her with the accusation, hear her side of the story, and obtain her documentation.

In the meantime, Dr. Goings sends a confidential e-mail to her associate dean, outlining the situation. She opts, however, not to copy or blind-copy any e-mail correspondence (an overused practice in academia) between the student or Dr. Perpetua and herself. It is important for Dr. Goings to be confident that she can handle this situation properly. Moreover, this associate dean has confidence in Dr. Goings, and knows that Dr. Goings will seek her counsel at any point that she decides she needs further administrative assistance. But there is a very important legal reason not to send copies and blind copies. Because claims often lead to litigation, and litigation *always* leads to extensive "discovery," meaning that copies of every e-mail ever sent must be retrieved from everyone who ever saw it, this decision was not only administratively prudent but legally and financially smart.

WHEN TO CONTACT THE UNIVERSITY COUNSEL

If a student believes that he has been a victim of intellectual property theft, the best course of action is to follow the chain of command: approach the professor first, make the case, then go to the department chair and dean if there is no resolution. Sometimes, obtaining advice from the ombudsman can be helpful. If there are real disagreements about "rights," then university counsel can be consulted. Note, however, that the university counsel's client is *the university*, and counsel will say so at the start of the meeting, as giving legal advice to both sides of a dispute could result in later disqualification if the case goes to court. In that case, however, the student will need to retain personal counsel, and if the professor claims a personal interest in the proceeds (separate from the institution), the professor might have to do so as well.

Findings and Disposition

After Dr. Goings received the more formal student complaint, she discerned it was a serious charge. Recall the third question, Do you believe the student has been the victim of intellectual theft? Dr. Goings brought Dr. Perpetua in for a meeting, and Dr. Perpetua did confess that she had sent the abstract in without the student's permission and without properly acknowledging her efforts on it. Incredulous, Dr. Goings asked why she had done this. Dr. Perpetua indicated that she exercised poor judgment, but that the student's work was similar to her own and that the student had developed her work in great part from her direction and supervision. Dr. Goings dismissed these rationalizations and handed Dr. Perpetua a copy of the authorship guidelines of the college which Dr. Perpetua's conduct clearly violated.

Recall the fourth question, If intellectual theft has occurred, what should be the action against Dr. Perpetua? With the admission of misconduct, Dr. Goings informed Dr. Perpetua that she would consult with the associate dean and dean to formulate a penalty for this violation. In the meantime, she requested that Dr. Perpetua write the student a letter of apology (with a copy to Dr. Goings) and offer to meet with the student to discuss the issue. After consultation with both the associate dean and dean, it was decided that Dr. Perpetua would receive a written letter of reprimand that would be placed in her permanent file and would be noted on her annual evaluation. She was further warned that any additional violation of this nature could result in further action against her, up to and including termination.

Relevant Legal Case

S. R. Seshadri v. Masoud Kasraian, No. 97-1610 (7th Cir. 1997)

In this case, Mr. Kasraian was a PhD electrical engineering student at the University of Wisconsin. Professor Seshadri was an electrical engineering professor and Kasraian's dissertation supervisor. From court records it is documented that the two individuals had previously published four joint articles, with Kasraian as first author and Seshadri as second author. Subsequently, Seshadri had requested that Kasraian sign up for a course he was teaching, but the student refused. Whether Seshadri considered the course essential to the program of study for Kasraian or whether the course was to be canceled without adequate enrollment (thus causing anger at the student for refusing to take the class) is unknown. However, shortly thereafter, the two individuals submitted a paper to the *Journal of Applied Physics*, with Kasraian again as first author and the professor as second author, and they both signed a copyright form to the journal in the event the article was accepted and published. A dispute ensued, and the professor wrote the journal editor and requested his name be removed from the article and that the article be rescinded. The professor claimed the submission "was based on certain erroneous information given by" Kasraian ("Student Is Joint Author," 1997, para. 1), and the article was returned to the student.

The student proceeded to revise the article and resubmitted it to the journal, with the professor given an acknowledgment but not second authorship, and the article was accepted for publication. The professor filed academic conduct charges against the student, claiming he (the professor) was the sole author of the manuscript, but the charges were dismissed when the student showed evidence that he (the student) was actually the sole author, not just on the manuscript in question but on the four previous articles as well. For his part, the student charged the professor with academic misconduct, and the professor was suspended from the university for a year without pay and not allowed to supervise graduate students for a year.

The professor then filed suit against the student in federal court in Wisconsin, alleging copyright infringement and theft of intellectual capitol.[6] Ruling in favor of the student, the court dismissed the case on summary judgment, holding that there was probably joint authorship, but the professor had declined authorship on the paper in question and thus there was no copyright infringement. Further, there was no finding that there was a basis for the charge that the manuscript contained erroneous information. The plaintiff appealed to the federal appeals court, which affirmed the dismissal despite the professor's argument that his copyright claim was still valid with respect to future publications.

Summary

Disputes over intellectual property between college students and faculty can be anticipated to involve graduate students and their faculty supervisors, often thesis or dissertation chairs. Conflicts can easily arise when university policies are nonexistent or ambiguous, and when clear directions about authorship are not fully addressed (the more proper term is "negotiated") at the beginning of any joint scholarship enterprise. Students are understandably not well versed in the protocols and procedures, common courtesies and laws that govern the generation of knowledge or intellectual property, but faculty members—even research faculty— are often surprisingly uninformed. A more serious problem is presented by faculty, who may take unethical advantage of their position of power and authority over the student.

Clear college or university guidelines are the first line of defense that protects faculty and students as well as the institution. A best practice is to include a link to the institution's policy on intellectual property on a course syllabus, in order to set a standard for academic integrity, and how joint authorship relationships should proceed and under what criteria. It is often the professor who says, "This

---

[6] The professor also sued the university, claiming that his suspension violated Title VII of the Civil Rights Act of 1964, which prohibits employment discrimination based on race, color, religion, sex, or national origin. He claimed the adverse action was taken against him because of his "creed [which] requires scrupulous honesty in the scholarly pursuit of scientific knowledge." The claim was dismissed because this "creed" did not constitute a "religion." This footnote is provided to show that, when litigation occurs, you can expect the claims to be many and varied and that lawyers are willing to make all kinds of arguments.

is good work. I think it could get published. Would you like me to help you?" It is at that point that a whole host of questions arise and should be addressed: (1) Will the professor suggest he or she be second author? (2) Will the professor procure the college's authorship policy and discuss it with the student? (3) Will the professor decline second authorship even if in the end the professor's contribution is significant? Unfortunately, it often happens that faculty members are discouraged into minimizing their own contributions to student work. If an instructor is giving substantive feedback, and if that instructor's guidance on revisions is shaping the structure of the manuscript, and if in the end the instructor's contribution to the work product is significant, then the student should understand that it would be unethical to submit the work as solely her or his own. That is what academic integrity is all about. Of course, some faculty may simply decline authorship because they do not need the publication or have particular reasons for removing themselves from coauthorship. However, a faculty member should not decline coauthorship simply because he or she does not think it is the right thing to do. Good science and well-articulated ideas (and manuscripts) are often best produced by having multiple sources of input. Finally, lacking the gravitas of a faculty member (particularly one with a doctorate) to help them, students will often find editors very uninterested in publishing their work, especially if they sense it is simply a classroom work product. In the end, student scholarship is copyrighted at its creation and inception, but the tangled web of who owns what then evolves as other individuals add their input to the ideas and words written for possible publication.

CRITICAL ELEMENTS TO CONSIDER

- Student work (intellectual property) is copyrighted at its creative inception. Unlike patents, there are no specific forms to complete, unless copyright registration, which is optional and affords certain additional rights to the copyright holder, is desired.
- If a student is seeking publication of his work or joint work, usually copyright is relinquished to the publisher unless negotiated otherwise.
- Students should procure the authorship policy in their college or university if seeking copublishing with a faculty member.
- Remember, copublishing with a faculty member is a good thing, and if the professor/faculty member is particularly reputable or has a national or international reputation, these kinds of joint scholarly ventures can enhance a student's career immensely.

Continued

CRITICAL ELEMENTS TO CONSIDER—cont'd

- If an author's name is to be included on an abstract or manuscript or any document submitted for peer review, it is that person's ethical responsibility to review the materials with all parties (coauthors) before it is submitted for review and to attest that the authorship (and authorship order) attributed to the respective author(s) is valid.
- Publishing is the only way nursing science can be transmitted in a permanent way. It is the most influential form of showcasing one's ideas and possibly making an impact on the discipline. Nursing students (both undergraduate and graduate) are encouraged to seek out publishing opportunities as they arise.

HELPFUL RESOURCES

- American Bar Association Section on Intellectual Property Law—Law Student and Outreach Programs
  http://www.abanet.org/intelprop/law_student.html
- Harrington, T. (2010). *Intellectual property on campus: Students' rights and responsibilities.* Carbondale, IL: Southern Illinois University Press.
- Whittaker, Z. (2010). Students: All your intellectual property belongs to us. ZDNet.com. Retrieved November 19, 2010, from http://www.zdnet.com/blog/igeneration/students-all-your-intellectual-property-belong-to-us/4648
- World Intellectual Property Organization, "Resources for Students"
  http://www.wipo.int/portal/en/resources_students.html

References

Aserinsky, E., & Kleitman, N. (1953). Regular occurring periods of eye motility, and concomitant phenomena, during sleep. *Science, 118,* 273–274.

Bouchoux, D. (2008). *Intellectual property for paralegals: The law of trademarks, copyrights, patents, and trade secrets* (3rd ed.). Florence, KY: Cengage Learning.

Brown, C. (2003, October). The stubborn scientist who unraveled a mystery of the night. Smithsonian.com. Retrieved November 16, 2010, from http://www.smithsonianmag.com/science-nature/stubborn.html

Lamberg, L. (2004, Spring). The student, the professor, and the birth of modern sleep research. *Medicine on the Midway,* 17–25.

Lemley, M. A. (2008). Are universities patent trolls? *Fordham Intellectual Property, Media and Entertainment Law Journal, 18,* 611–631.

Markos, K. (2010, July 28). Fort Lee man says professor, former friends stole his game design. NorthJersey.com. Retrieved November 16, 2010, from http://www.northjersey.com/news/business/tech_news/99443299_Ex-student_sues_over_rights_to_app.html?mobile=1

Seshadri v. Kasraian, No. 97-1610 (7th Cir. 1997).

Smith, K. (2009, June 26). Openness and academic values. *Scholarly Communications@Duke.* Retrieved November 17, 2010, from http://library.duke.edu/blogs/scholcomm/2009/06/26/openness-and-academic-values/

Story's Executives v. Holcombe, 23 F. Cas. 171, 175 (C.C. Ohio 1847).

Stripling, J. (2009, June 16). Code warrior. Insidehighered.com. Retrieved November 17, 2010, from http://www.insidehighered.com/news/2009/06/16/computer

Student is joint author, not liable for infringement in suit by professor. (1997). *Mealey's Litigation Reports: Intellectual Property.* Retrieved November 17, 2010, from http://cyber.law.harvard.edu/metaschool/fisher/joint/links/articles/mealey.html

World Intellectual Property Organization. (n.d.a.). Berne Convention for the Protection of Literary and Artistic Works. Retrieved November 16, 2010, from http://www.wipo.int/treaties/en/ip/berne/trtdocs_wo001.html

World Intellectual Property Organization. (n.d.b.). What is intellectual property? Retrieved November 16, 2010, from http://www.wipo.int/about-ip/en/

CHAPTER 12

Faculty Issues and Conflicts Over Intellectual Property

CASE STUDY

An Undergraduate Faculty Member Discovers a Graduate Faculty Member Has Used Her Intellectual Property Without Her Permission

Your role: You are Professor Anton, an undergraduate faculty member teaching a junior-level medical-surgical nursing course, and you share an office with Professor Wise, a graduate faculty member teaching in the nurse-practitioner program.

As a new faculty member, you are interested in increasing your scholarly productivity. You agree to write a pharmacology chapter for a new medical-surgical text. You have to research all the latest drug therapies; in addition to writing a narrative, you must also compile very intricate tables that list the drug, its indications, special nursing considerations, and prominent side effects. Professor Wise, who shares an office with you, is teaching in the graduate nurse-practitioner program and has an upcoming lecture to give on oncology-focused primary care.

Professor Wise one day notices the impressive, detailed tables on oncology/cancer drugs that you have compiled for your chapter, and she asks you if she may borrow your tables and take a look at them. As it was a simple request and you wanted to be collegial, you agreed to let Professor Wise review your prepublication materials. Two months later, you are in your joint office and need a paper clip. You wander over to Professor Wise's desk to look for one and see something that looks very familiar. You reach down to more carefully examine the item on Professor's Wise's desk, and what you are stunned to discover is a graduate nursing handout on oncology drugs that is almost an exact copy of your own detailed tables. Further, it has Professor Wise's name on it but no attribution that the tables are your original work. Astonished, you are certain that you had not given Professor Wise permission to use the tables in her graduate course (although you almost certainly would have, had Professor Wise asked), and you are also certain that Professor Wise could not make a case that this was "fair use" of your intellectual property by any stretch of the imagination.

Questions

- How would you first proceed?
- Do you believe that you have been the victim of theft of intellectual property, or was it "fair use" by Professor Wise?
- If indeed intellectual theft has occurred, what should be the action against Professor Wise?

University Faculty Intellectual Property: Legal Principles and Review of the Literature

Chapter 11 discusses the issues surrounding intellectual property that affect university students, but the emphasis there is on graduate student grievances. This chapter focuses on three issues: (1) grievances between faculty when accusations of intellectual property theft of original work are made by one faculty against another, (2) work-for-hire issues, in which the university that pays the salary of individual faculty may claim or have ownership of intellectual property that is completed while the faculty is employed by the university, and (3) how fair use legal practices affect faculty in the classroom. Using this chapter's case study as background, this narrative will focus on these three central issues.

Faculty or Colleague Theft of Original Work

Intellectual property disputes in academia often surround legal challenges to copyright, patents, trademarks, and original work that may not yet have reached the copyright, patent, or trademark application stage. In the case of original work, one of the hallmarks of being a faculty-scholar employed by a university is that the faculty member engages in the production of creative, original endeavors—whether the faculty member is a fine arts instructor, a chemist, an English professor, or a nursing professor. Depending on the 2006 Carnegie university and college classifications, which consider the respective mission of the university and rank them as (1) a university with very high research activity, (2) a university with high research activity, or (3) a doctoral/research university (Jaschik, 2009), the amount of aggregate scholarship expected of the individual faculty member varies.[1] At research universities, the number of publications is associated with an increased likelihood of securing federal research grants, and therefore the institutional pressure on faculty to produce creative endeavors (publications, books, grants, other sources of funding, etc.) is substantial (Ali, Bhattacharyya, and Olejniczak,

---

[1] The criteria and formula used to categorize a university in one of three categories includes the following: research and development spending (in science, engineering, and other areas); the number of postdoctoral and nonfaculty research staff members with doctorates, doctoral degrees conferred, number of disciplines in which the doctorate is conferred; and a per capita calculation to judge the relative importance of research within institutions.

2010). It is this kind of institutional pressure on the production of scholarship that can lead to aggressive, unethical, and even nefarious conduct and intellectual dishonesty up to and including theft.

One of the most public cases of charges of intellectual theft occurred in 1996 in the Department of African American Studies (the first PhD program in the then-new discipline founded in 1988) at Temple University. In that case, the founding department chair, Dr. Molefi Kete Asante, who first articulated the concept of Afrocentric Theory, was accused of misappropriating the intellectual work product of Assistant Professor Ella Forbes, a junior untenured faculty member in his department. According to Boynton (2002), "During his 12 years as chairman, Dr. Asante built the department into a nationally recognized center that promoted his popular ideology, and he enjoyed unchallenged autonomy" (p. 1). Boynton further writes, "He stepped down in 1996 amid charges that he misappropriated a professor's work for a textbook and then denied her tenure when she complained. The conflict was deemed a book contract dispute, not misconduct, but the junior professor was granted a new tenure review, minus Dr. Asante" (p. 1).

The case received international attention because Dr. Asante was regarded as a prodigious scholar and chief architect of this new discipline. The notoriety of the case was inflamed by Dr. Asante, who was reported in the press as having given a speech at a meeting of the United Africa Movement in which he characterized the controversy as a "racist plot" by "white people" and "their agents within our department" for an authorship dispute that was threatening his scholarly reputation (Goodman, 1996).

Although it was not disputed that Asante first recruited Forbes to help him cowrite a high school textbook, Asante and his publisher claimed Forbes had agreed her name would not appear as a coauthor of the textbook unless more than 30% of text was her own work product and that this benchmark was not met (Goodman). For its part, Temple University concluded that this was a contractual dispute and not a claim of intellectual property theft (although it did grant Forbes a second full-tenure review).

Work for Hire

More typically, intellectual disputes by faculty are with their respective employer— the university. In this case, the concept of *work for hire* is usually central to the dispute. As defined in the 1976 Copyright Act (U.S. Copyright Office, 1976) as amended,[2] "work-for-hire" is:

> *(1) a work prepared by an employee within the scope of his or her employment; or (2) a work specially ordered or commissioned for use as a contribution to a collective work:*
>
> - as a part of a motion picture
> - as a part of other audiovisual work,

---

[2] All the amendments to the Copyright Act of 1976 made since 1976 through June 30, 2009, can be found at http://www.copyright.gov/title17/92preface.pdf

- as a translation,
- as a supplementary work,
- as a compilation,
- as an instructional text,
- as a test,
- as answer material for a test, or
- as an atlas (Title 17, Section 101 of the United States Code)

The most important point is to determine whether some type of work product fits with this definition, and a key factor in making that determination is the relationship between the parties. However, the statutory definition is complex, and circumstances under which the principle can be applied vary, which is where university counsel can be very helpful. For instance, what if a professor claims his work on a patent took place in his off-hours and not while he was at work (Jassin, 2010)? The current definition of *work for hire* was established the United States Supreme Court in *Community for Creative Non-Violence v. Reid,* 490 U.S. 730 (1989). In this landmark case, the Court held that to determine whether a work is made for hire, one must first ascertain whether the work was prepared by (1) an employee or by (2) an independent contractor.

As it would be unusual for a full-time faculty member to be employed as an independent contractor (there are cases in which adjunct faculty may be technically hired as independent contractors), overwhelmingly the work product of a faculty member derived as part of his or her employment or role likely falls into this category (Borstoff and Newton, 2006). To resolve some of the complexity surrounding work-for-hire principles for employees (in this case, faculty), particularly for a group of individuals who are encouraged to create, design, invent, and publish all types of works that would fall under copyright, patent, or trademark law, royalty policies are usually established under which the individual faculty directly benefits from the creative work product. In the case of larger revenue-producing inventions or products, the university may also benefit. At Drexel University, the following formula currently applies[3] to most revenue-generating intellectual property that falls within certain work-for-hire boundaries:

1. For the first $10,000 of net income: 100% to the inventor
2. For the next $500,000 in cumulative net income: 50% to the inventors, 25% to the Office of the Vice Provost for Research and Dean of Graduate Policy, 25% to the inventor's Institutional Unit(s)
3. For the next $1,000,000 in cumulative net income: 40% to the inventors, 35% to the Office of Vice Provost for Research and Dean of Graduate Policy, 25% to the inventor's Institutional Unit(s)

---

[3] As the law evolves and as new fact patterns and discoveries arise, so university policies have to change. IT policies are likely to become the subject of significant interest (and perhaps contest) on campuses as universities look to increase "alternative revenue sources" (nontuition revenues), including commercialization of IT.

4. For cumulative net income in excess of $1,510,000: 25% to the inventors, 50% to the Office of Vice Provost for Research and Dean of Graduate Policy, 25% to the inventor's Institutional Unit(s) (Drexel University, 2005)

It is best to be proactive when there are potential revenue sources for an individual faculty member's intellectual property. Faculty members are encouraged to be very familiar with their university's policies on intellectual property. In particular, research universities are certain to have one (and, for example, a technology transfer office or division of technology licensing), as university faculty–generated ideas and inventions can become enormous lifelong revenue sources for colleges and universities (Johnson, 2010). If there is ambiguity and/or reason to create a relationship more appropriate to a particular project, we encourage faculty to reach (negotiate) an understanding with the university as early in the process as possible.

Copyright and "Fair-Use" Guidelines for Faculty

University and college faculty are often faced with confusion over what is proper "fair" and free use of copyrighted works. For instance, if an individual faculty member wants to assign a chapter in a book for students to read but does not want students to have to buy the book for a single chapter, can the professor simply make copies of the chapter and distribute them in class? Educators and others can make "fair use" of copyrighted materials under certain guidelines established in Title 17 of the United States Code.

In *Stewart v. Abend* (1990), the Supreme Court ruled that the principle of fair use relies on the potential for that use to negatively affect the work's potential market or value. In this case, a story, written in 1948, became a famed Alfred Hitchcock movie, *Rear Window* (1954). The author of the original story, Cornell Woolrich, had first sold the short story rights and then the movie rights to that short story. He died in 1968 before the copyright renewal of the book reverted back to the original author, which, according to the first copyright law of 1909 (Sixtieth Congress, 2d Session, 1909) would have done so after a period of 28 years. When the movie was subsequently shown on television, the new copyright holder of the movie rights (which had passed on and were sold after Woolrich's death) sued the production company of *Rear Window*. Mr. Abend, the new owner of the movie rights, sued because the movie was a derivative work of Woolrich. In other words, although the first production of *Rear Window* in 1954 was legal, the subsequent television broadcast in 1971 was not deemed "fair use" of the derivative work even though the author had died and there was a new owner of the original literary rights. In principle, what this 1990 Supreme Court ruling established was that the control of an original piece of work reverts back to the author—or the author's designee or successors[4]—when renewal comes up. This, therefore, protects the author (and the heirs) from being deprived of any future value of the work.

As for faculty, fair use can be evaluated, or tested, based on the following four factors:

1. *The purpose and character of the use, including whether such use is of a commercial nature or is for nonprofit educational purposes* (Roth, 2009, p. 350). In this example, the proposed use is for a nonprofit, educational purpose, which weighs in favor of this being a fair use.

2. *The nature of the copyrighted work* (Roth, p. 350). Works that are primarily collections of facts are typically afforded greater fair use protection than creative works. The type of book that the faculty member proposes copying would need to be looked at in more detail from this perspective to determine if the use weighs in favor of, or against, a fair use determination.

3. *The amount and substantiality of the portion used in relation to the copyrighted work as a whole* (Roth, p. 350). This directive is somewhat vague. Can one-third of the book be copied legally and distributed to the class? Possibly. Can over one-half of the book be copied—likely not. But a case can also perhaps be made that several chapters would be considered "substantial" and thus be disallowed. It may also depend on how many total chapters there are in the book and whether the faculty member copies the same chapters of the book year after year for each section of the class, likely arguing against fair use. Reasonable and prudent judgment must be exercised.

4. *The effect of the use upon the potential market for or value of the copyrighted work* (Roth, p. 350). Is the photocopying by the faculty member depriving the copyright owner of income? This is often an issue that will prompt a lawsuit from a publisher and should be considered very carefully.

These four factors must be considered as a whole in determining whether a particular use is fair use. Applying rules based purely on the percentage of a work being copied, for instance, without due consideration of all four factors is a dangerous proposition. Overall, faculty members are encouraged to be very cognizant of fair use legal principles and to be wary of violating them, as such conduct can be reported by anyone, including a student. The very public prosecution of students who illegally downloaded music from the Internet is clear proof that the force of law in the area of copyright infringement can be perilous (Morley and Parker, 2009).

Discussion of Case

Consider the first question in this chapter's case study, How would you first proceed? Recall that you are Professor Anton and you have just discovered your original work was reproduced under the name of your office colleague, Professor

---

[4] That is, if the original author has died and willed all intellectual property rights to his or her heirs.

Wise. Anton was shocked by the disregard for her hard work that was apparently being passed off as the work of Wise, and Anton immediately thought she had been the victim of intellectual theft again so early in her academic career. Having moved to Buffalo from Alabama only months earlier, a colleague at Anton's previous employer (a large community college nursing program) had notified her that a poster of a human caring program that she had conceived and developed had just been presented by the current community college nursing dean as the dean's own work product. When she heard this, she was shocked and could not understand how anyone could simply take the work product of another and pass it off as her or his own, without any attribution at all. This practice is not so uncommon, and a quick visit to the "Harvard Plagiarism Archive," which has tracked allegations of Harvard faculty accused of plagiarism since 2002, highlights this pervasive issue, even at a leading university such as Harvard *(Harvard Plagiarism Archive,* 2010).

Nonetheless, it seemed only months earlier Anton had sworn to herself that she would never again be the victim of intellectual theft, but here she was confronting almost the very same situation. However, Anton was also very confused about what her best course of action should be. Consider the second question, Do you believe Dr. Anton has been the victim of intellectual theft? Or do you think that this was instead a case of unethical misrepresentation (but not illegal taking) of another author's work because the work was unpublished?

WHEN TO CONTACT THE UNIVERSITY COUNSEL

When it comes to faculty disputes between or among faculty about authorship or percentage of effort on grants or other similar types of concerns, it is best to try to resolve the issue with the individual in question. If one-on-one discussion cannot resolve the issue, then we suggest using the university ombudsman. It is unlikely that the university attorney would be an agent who would be consulted for interfaculty disputes. If using the ombudsman is not is not an appropriate or effective strategy, then going through normal university departmental strategies is suggested. If that fails, try securing your own personal attorney for legal advice. Some inventions or patents (and sometimes creative authorship) can generate huge revenues; therefore, making sure one's own intellectual property interests are protected is essential.

Findings and Disposition

This chapter's case study, like most accusations of intellectual property theft that go unreported, was not resolved in a public way (Siegel, 2008). Professor Anton, as a newly hired untenured assistant professor without a doctorate, was very afraid of what might be the result of such a public accusation of intellectual theft and was not at all certain that she would receive the dean's support. After all, her previous dean had just committed intellectual theft as soon as she left the community college, and she wondered if perhaps the stakes were higher for her now in this new position. She further suspected there was some favoritism by the current dean toward Professor Wise, and Anton was further cautious about taking a very public course of action. Still, she also wondered if she should confront Wise about the work product and see what she had to say. As Anton was still new to academia, she chose perhaps a more painful path, to keep the incident to herself, but she did acknowledge personally that she would never again trust Professor Wise. However, by sharing an office with Wise, it was quite challenging for Anton to keep her feelings hidden, but she did.

Years later, circumstances took a circuitous turn, and despite both professors leaving the small college where the intellectual theft had occurred, Anton and Wise (now both holding doctorates) wound up being employed in the same college in New York City. Dr. Anton had never forgotten what had happened to her years earlier, and she thought her best course of action was simply to maintain some professional distance from her previous colleague, who she still thought had engaged in intellectual dishonesty. As you read the ending to this case, do you think Dr. Anton (then Professor Anton) could have handled her situation differently?

Relevant Legal Case

Board of Trustees of the Leland Stanford Junior University v. Roche Molecular Systems, Inc., Nos. 2008-1509, 2008-1510 (Fed. Cir. Sept. 30, 2009)

In this case, Stanford University undertook a large lawsuit against the pharmaceutical giant Roche, claiming that a laboratory method to detect HIV antibodies was discovered by one of its faculty members on their campus and was owned by Stanford. However, Roche claimed that researcher Mark Holodniy signed a contract with Roche giving the firm the rights to the intellectual property. Again, this is another complicated legal case, and what is important here is who owns the rights to the patent. Is it the inventor in this case, Mark Holodniy? Is it his employer, Stanford University (under original work-for-hire principles and intellectual property policy principles as the primary employer), where he was employed as a research fellow? Or was it Centus (later bought out by Roche), the company with which Mr. Holodniy signed certain contracts that may relate to the work? As an indication of the importance and complexities associated with *Stanford v. Roche* and related cases, the matter has now made its way to the U.S. Supreme Court and awaits final disposition there.

Summary

Intellectual property theft is not necessarily common nor uncommon. It does happen (as evidenced by the Harvard Plagiarism Archive), and most of the cases never reach the level of publicity, much less a lawsuit, but are settled out quietly. Any accusation of intellectual theft, be it a copyright, trademark, or patent dispute, is inherently damaging not just to the individual involved but also to the reputation of the institution. Any faculty member who engages in any creative endeavor that might generate revenue *(any revenue)* is encouraged to read, understand, and be very clear about the institution's intellectual property policy. Further, collaborations with other faculty on projects (written or otherwise) need to be clearly negotiated, written, and signed. If significant revenues are possible, consider having a witness and the signatures notarized.

It is easy to be sympathetic with Anton's actions in this chapter's case study, but it was perhaps the path of least resistance, and therefore the real ethical issues surrounding the actions of Wise went unchallenged. Who gains here? Does society gain when ethical lapses, even potential ethical lapses, are overlooked and individual rights are blurred? Was Anton at fault for not trying, even politely, to address the issue with her officemate? If, upon confrontation, Wise had become defensive and denied using the tables without proper authorization, should Anton have pursued relief within her department or college? What if Wise had profusely apologized and their relationship possibly healed, leading Anton never to have to distance herself and act as though nothing had happened between them? Would either of these actions have been preferable to what Anton ultimately decided to do? Or did she have too much to risk by employing one of these alternative actions? Drexel University has always been particularly vigorous about sensitizing nursing students and faculty to ethical issues and encouraging that they be addressed as early as possible. The question has always been, Will a cheating or dishonest student (or faculty member, in this case) always act ethically (and differently) with his or her patients?" It is actually a very disturbing question to pose, as it is thought that all nurses (including nursing faculty) should act with the highest ethical standards, and faculty are bound to model this behavior if they are going to be authentic in their own professional and academic roles.

CRITICAL ELEMENTS TO CONSIDER

- Before entering into a joint authorship or creative project, negotiate the percentage of effort by all parties and determine what authorship order is agreed on.
- Review any college or university intellectual property policy and determine whether you are in agreement with the said stipulations.

Continued

CRITICAL ELEMENTS TO CONSIDER—cont'd

- Determine whether all classroom materials are being used according to proper fair use policies.
- Our recommendation is that if you have ever had an unsatisfactory collaboration with another colleague (a dispute over authorship order or perhaps a colleague not participating equally in a collaborative effort), you should resolve never to collaborate with them again.
- Before working with a colleague on a large project, first strategize to work together on a smaller project to see if the work chemistry is satisfactory and if the colleague's work ethic is agreeable to you.

HELPFUL RESOURCES

- Copyright Act of 1976
- http://www.copyright.gov/title17/
- "Harvard Plagiarism Archive"
- http://authorskeptics.blogspot.com/
- Fisher, W. (n.d.). Theories of intellectual property, Cambridge, MA: Harvard Law School.
- http://www.law.harvard.edu/faculty/tfisher/iptheory.html
- Washington University Law School Faculty Plagiarism Guidelines
- http://law.wustl.edu/students/pages.aspx?id=1000

References

Ali, M. M., Bhattacharyya, P., & Olejniczak, A. J. (2010). The effects of scholarly productivity and institutional characteristics on the distribution of federal research grants. *Journal of Higher Education, 81*(2), 164–178.

Board of Trustees of the Leland Stanford Junior University v. Roche Molecular Systems, Inc., Nos. 2008-1509, 2008-1510 (Fed. Cir. Sept. 30, 2009).

Borstorff, P., & Newton, S. (2006, April). Independent contractor classification: The challenge of doing it right. *Entrepreneurial Executive.* Retrieved December 9, 2010, from http://goliath.ecnext.com/coms2/gi_0198-415954/Independent-contractor-classification-the- challenge.html

Boynton, R. (2002, April 14). Black studies today. *The New York Times, Education Life.* Retrieved December 8, 2010, from http://www.robertboynton.com/articleDisplay.php?article_id=76

Community for Creative Non-Violence v. Reid, 490 U.S. 730 (1989).

Copyright Act of 1909, Pub. L. 60-349, 35 Stat. 1075, H.R. 28192 (1909). Retrieved December 11, 2010, from http://www.copyright.gov/history/1909act.pdf

Copyright Act of 1976, Pub. L. No. 94-553, 90 Stat. 2541 (1976). Retrieved December 9, 2010, from http://www.copyright.gov/title17/92appa.pdf

Drexel University. (2005). Patent policy (re: Intellectual Property). Retrieved December 11, 2010, from http://www.drexel.edu/provost/policies/patent_policy.asp

Goodman, H. (1996, July 21). Professor depicts dispute as a racist plot. *The Philadelphia Inquirer,* p. B1.

Harvard Plagiarism Archive. (2010). *Authorskeptics* (blog). Retrieved December 11, 2010, from http://authorskeptics.blogspot.com/

Jaschik, S. (2006). The new Carnegie classifications. Insidehighered.com. Retrieved December 6, 2010.

Jassin, L. J. (2010). Working with freelancers: What every publisher should know about the "work for hire" doctrine. Copylaw.com. Retrieved December 8, 2010, from http://www.copylaw.com/new_articles/wfh.html

Johnson, J. (2010, November 1). Stanford patent suit heads to U.S. Supreme Court. *Newsfix: KQED's Bay Area News Blog.* Retrieved December 10, 2010, from http://blogs.kqed.org/newsfix/2010/11/01/stanford-patent-lawsuit-heads-to-u-s-supreme- court/

Morley, D., & Parker, C. S. (2009). *Understanding computers: Today and tomorrow* (12th ed.). Boston: Course Technology.

Roth, J. (2009). *Higher education in America* (10th ed.). Malvern, PA: Center for Education and Employment Law.

Siegel, L. J. (2008). *Criminology* (10th ed.). Belmont, CA: Thomson Higher Education.

CHAPTER 13

Dealing With Student–Student Harassment

CASE STUDY

Student-Student Harassment

Your role: You are the clinical instructor.

Liz Rodriguez, a sophomore nursing major in your clinical group, approaches you. She is very upset. She states that she began dating the former boyfriend of Lindsey Jackson, another nursing student. She states that Lindsey has posted several offensive messages about her on her Facebook page and that each one is getting lots of comments, most of which are nasty, about her. Liz also says that Lindsey had posted several mean comments on Liz's own Facebook page, before she removed her as a friend. Even though she is no longer friends with Lindsey on Facebook and therefore doesn't see her status updates, her friends keep sending her all the nasty comments Lindsey is writing on her own wall. All of this is made worse by the fact that Lindsey's cruel status updates about Liz are so frequent that they are regularly appearing on the top of her friends' news feeds. Liz shows you a copy of one of the wall posts that Lindsey posted before she unfriended her and that Liz had saved on her computer. The message reads, *"I hate Lindsey Jackson, that whore. I am not going to let this slide. I will go crazy and really hurt that b—!"* Liz tells you that the postings are so embarrassing that she just cannot function as a student in the same class with her anymore, and begins to cry.

Questions

- How would you proceed?
- Does the school have any jurisdiction over the Facebook page?
- Does Lindsey Jackson's threatening electronic message fall under the school's published Student Code of Conduct?

Student-Student Harassment: Legal Principles and Review of the Literature

Social media have become the way that students communicate. Some seem to live on their Facebook pages. What they do there is not what they do in the classroom or on campus. Universities should stay away from monitoring student speech, not just because of constitutional protections (free speech), but also because universities do not want to put themselves into the role of Internet police, searching for and responding to instances of improper conduct. That is a role universities could never perform without risk or error; and if such a role is taken on, even for Good Samaritan purposes, there can be liability imposed for failing to perform it with due care.

Broadly speaking, *harassment* occurs whenever offensive or unwelcome conduct affects the performance of a person or persons (Boston College, 2009). If it is expressed against a person in a protected class, harassment can also constitute discrimination that violates local, state, and/or federal laws. The prohibitions are meant to combat decision-making based on stereotypes, and typically include race, sex, age, national origin, religious belief, and sexual orientation. The harasser can be in the same protected class as the victim and can be the victim's supervisor, coworker, or even a nonemployee (e.g., a student or a student's parent). Federal law is often very specific in prohibiting discrimination, as with this statement from the U.S. Department of Education Office for Civil Rights (OCR), which is charged with enforcing Title IX:

> No person in the United States shall, on the basis of sex, be excluded from participation in, be denied the benefits of, or be subjected to discrimination under any education program or activity receiving Federal financial assistance.

The OCR (1997) recognizes two types of harassment in academic institutions: quid pro quo harassment and hostile environment harassment.

> Under the law, there are two kinds of discriminatory harassment—quid pro quo harassment of a sexual nature where someone is threatened with a negative consequence unless certain favors are granted or where someone is seduced by the promise of a positive consequence. The second kind of discriminatory harassment is called hostile environment. Hostile environment harassment may occur whenever someone's offensive conduct has the effect of interfering with another's performance. For example, words or behaviors that put down an individual by insulting an aspect of the person's identity (race, sexual orientation, gender, national origin, etc.) can create a hostile work or study environment for that individual. It is easy to recognize quid pro quo harassment, but hostile environment harassment frequently goes unrecognized or is not acknowledged either by the victim or by the one who is causing the problem. (Boston College, 2009)

Words or behaviors that are considered severe enough to create a hostile environment may be determined by such factors as the nature of the conduct (physical or verbal); the frequency of the conduct; and the degree of offensiveness (Boston College, 2009). Given the fact that so many students at a university, in a college, or participating in the same class can "friend" each other and communicate easily to the whole group at once, social media does have the possibility of adversely affecting the quality of the educational experience.

There is an important question about whether or how harassment might be a precursor to more violent forms of aggression. In spring 2004, two University of North Carolina–Wilmington (UNCW) students were murdered by fellow students whom they knew. In the immediate aftermath, UNCW decided to establish a high-profile, Web-based resource for students who were affected by violence or had concerns about safety. Called *Safe-Relate: Help With Violent or Abusive Relationships,* the Web site linked to the main campus Web site and collected resources on a variety of topics, including sexual assault, stalking, harassment, and resources for key constituencies. UNCW publicized *Safe-Relate* and its associated campus resources to students through a comprehensive safety program for students in new student orientation, as well as in major student publications (Higher Education Center for Alcohol and Other Drug Abuse and Violence Prevention, 2009).

To hold a university liable for monetary damages for harassment, the student would have to demonstrate that university officials had actual knowledge of the student harassment and were deliberately indifferent to the reports (U.S. Department of Education, Office for Civil Rights, 1997). College-wide prevention programs, and procedures by which there can be prompt and direct intervention, are critical in addressing and minimizing student-student harassment. Harassment policies need to be widely publicized, as do the universities' methods for reporting and responding to incidents of harassment.

Discussion of Case

In this chapter's case study, the clinical instructor notified the department chair after speaking with the student, Liz Rodriguez. The department chair consulted with the dean about what action to take in this particular case. The dean of nursing notified the dean of students and the office of public safety after reviewing Ms. Jackson's Facebook page. Given the nature of the Web posting, the public safety officer interviewed Ms. Jackson. It is important to note that the clinical instructor acted as a student advocate and made the appropriate referral; however, the faculty member did not assume the role of counselor. If the student required counseling related to this incident, a referral should be made to the counseling center (refer to Chapter 23, Dealing With Mental Health Issues Among Students).

WHEN TO CONSULT THE UNIVERSITY COUNSEL

Consult the university counsel with complaints of student-student harassment including social media harassment and cyberbullying.

Findings and Disposition

The public safety officer concluded that Ms. Jackson's behavior was inappropriate and offensive; however, Ms. Jackson was not thought to be a physical threat to Ms. Rodriquez. The dean and clinical instructor sought legal advice from university counsel, who advised that the university could not instruct Ms. Jackson to edit her Web site; however, it did appear that the conduct violated not only the students' code of conduct but also the nursing conduct code. Accordingly, the dean of students filed a complaint with the student conduct board, and the clinical instructor did likewise with the Nursing Student Conduct Committee. Ms. Jackson, a 19-year-old sophomore, was determined to be in violation of the Nursing Student Code of Conduct. She was imposed a sanction that entailed writing a 10-page paper on the professional conduct required of a student nurse. Finally, the dean and the clinical instructor met together with the class and discussed the importance of professional conduct on Facebook.

Relevant Legal Case

Summa v. Hofstra University, 2011 WL 1343058 (E.D.N.Y. Apr. 7, 2011)

Kelly v. Yale University, 2003 WL 1563424, 2003 U.S. Dist. LEXUS 4543 (D. Conn. 2003)

In 2006, Laura Summa was hired as a student manager of the Hofstra University football team for a 1-year period that would include the primary fall season and the secondary spring season. Accompanying the team to away games, she was subjected to "relentless sexual harassment" by players on every bus trip. Players teased her for having a relationship with another player, and they created a Web page on Facebook that Ms. Summa described as "intentionally demeaning and sexist, implying that [she] was beastly, overweight, hypersexual, and overbearing." They suggested that she and her boyfriend had sex on the bus and made other offensive comments.

Ms. Summa reported the Facebook incident and other incidents to Coach Cohen. Ms. Summa claims that Coach Cohen tried to talk her out of reporting the incident to Campus Safety, arguing that it would bring negative attention to the football team. Ms. Summa reported the incident, and was ultimately put in contact with the university's Equal Employment officer, Maureen Murphy. Ms. Murphy said that she would arrange sensitivity training for the football team, but this did not occur. One football player, who was dismissed from the team, continued to harass Ms. Summa.

At the beginning of the spring season, Ms. Summa reported to work, to find that Coach Cohen had hired a replacement for her. He told her that he presumed she was not interested in continuing with the position. Ms. Summa alleges that this action was retaliation for her complaining about harassment. Ms. Summa's employment offer to work for the University Relations Office was also rescinded.

Ms. Summa filed suit in federal district court, alleging that the harassment and subsequent retaliation she experienced for reporting the harassment violates Title VII, Title IX, and New York's Human Rights Law. She seeks damages and an injunction against Hofstra's similar conduct in the future.

"Peer harassment may sometimes result in legal liabilities: the harasser may become liable to the victim of the harassment or the institution may become liable to the victim" (Kaplin and Lee, 2007, p. 313). In *Kelly v. Yale University*, Kathryn Kelly had been sexually assaulted by another student, Robert Nolan. Both were divinity students at the time. Throughout the grievance process, Kelly claimed that she made repeated requests for academic accommodations. Kelly asked several professors and administrators for a compromise solution that would allow her to continue her studies. Kelly also requested that Yale University provide some academic planning assistance to her. According to Kelly, Yale never responded to her repeated requests for assistance. Kelly also claims that she repeatedly requested alternative housing during the pendency of the grievance procedures. At the time of the assault, Kelly and Nolan lived in the same dormitory. Because she no longer felt safe living there, Kelly requested that the university provide her with alternative housing. Several weeks after Kelly filed her complaint, Yale provided Kelly with a room in the guest quarters at the Divinity School. However, Kelly alleged that she obtained this alternative housing only after a professor, Margaret Farley, intervened on her behalf. With the exception of one phone call, Kelly never had any contact with Nolan following the sexual assault incident, nor did she claim she was harassed by him after that date. Kelly eventually withdrew from all of the classes during the fall semester. As a result, she completed her course work at the Divinity School one semester later than expected. The court ruled that Kelly had a cause of action against Yale University when she remained vulnerable to possible future harassment due to the university's unwillingness to provide academic and residential housing accommodations pending Mr. Nolan's disciplinary hearing. After Yale received notice of the harassing conduct, it had a duty under Title IX to take some action to prevent the further harassment of Kelly.

Social Networking Sites

Snyder v. Millersville University, No. 07-1660 (E.D. Pa. 2007)

In a tangential case pertaining to social networking sites, Stacy Snyder, a 25-year-old graduate student at Millersville University, posted a photo on her MySpace page that showed her at a party wearing a pirate hat and drinking from a plastic cup, with the caption "Drunken Pirate." Her supervisor at Conestoga Valley High

School (where she was student teaching) discovered the page and told Ms. Snyder that the photo was "unprofessional." The dean of Millersville University School of Education concurred, and said Ms. Snyder was promoting drinking in "virtual view of her under-age students." As a result, Millersville University denied Ms. Snyder a teaching degree. Ms. Snyder sued, arguing that the university had violated her First Amendment rights by penalizing her for her after-work behavior. A federal district judge rejected the claim, saying that her "Drunken Pirate" post was not protected speech.

Summary

It should be the intent of all colleges and universities to offer a place where students and faculty can pursue knowledge independent of threats or assaults; at the same time, free speech and the ability to criticize, even unfairly, is core to the mission. Universities are not responsible for what students do off campus, but social media knows no geographic boundary. When what is being done online is adversely affecting the academic mission, a court may hold a university responsible for getting involved. What those duties and liabilities are has not yet been determined. However, it is likely that a university will not be found liable if it acts reasonably under the circumstances to address the situation as it affects the university community according to standards that are appropriate for its mission (e.g., codes of conduct that require civility among classmates). The university must fairly and impartially review all harassment charges and deal with such matters in a confidential and professional manner. The college/university should also prohibit any behavior that is in retaliation to an individual who files a harassment complaint. University administration is responsible for publicizing and implementing a stringent sexual and racial harassment policy in addition to educating all constituencies in promoting a zero tolerance for student harassment. Finally, students need to be educated about the dangers of social networking sites and the Web site content's longevity (Rosen, 2010).

CRITICAL ELEMENTS TO CONSIDER

- Consult the appropriate university official (dean of students, office of equality officer, office of public safety, or legal counsel) based on your university policy.
- Develop a nurse code of conduct.
- Educate students about the dangers of social networking sites and the requisite professional behavior that is required on such sites.
- Offer a Web-based method for submitting complaints (American Association of University Women, 2005).

CRITICAL ELEMENTS TO CONSIDER—cont'd

- Have a designated person or student affairs office to contact if someone is a victim (American Association of University Women, 2005).
- Provide information about the college's student/sexual harassment policy on the college's Web site (American Association of University Women, 2005).
- Review the American Nurses Association's *Code of Ethics for Nurses.*
- Provide educational materials on the college's Web site related to harassment, addressing, for example, actions that an individual can take to stop harassment (Boston College, 2009).
- Implement an on-campus sexual assault advocate program to provide victims with accessible resources in the event of an attack.
- Design a college Web site that is specifically dedicated to sexual assault and harassment and that provides educational materials related to methods to prevent such attacks.
- Discuss student-student harassment and other forms of harassment at the university's orientation with students and parents.
- Discuss student-student harassment and other forms of harassment in a freshman or university-wide seminar.
- Integrate content on student harassment in the college core curriculum.
- Reinforce educational content and policies on harassment to all student organizations.
- Educate faculty and university officials concerning sexual and other forms of harassment.
- The following is a list of national resources dedicated to the prevention of harassment and sexual violence:
  - The Higher Education Center for Alcohol and other Drug Abuse and Violence Prevention
    http://www.higheredcenter.org/
  - American Association of University Women
    http://www.aauw.org
  - National Center on Domestic and Sexual Violence
    http://www.ncdsv.org
  - Security on Campus Inc.
    http://www.securityoncampus.org
  - Sexual Harassment Support Forum
    http://www.sexualharassmentsupport.org
  - Men Can Stop Rape
    http://www.mencanstoprape.org

Continued

CRITICAL ELEMENTS TO CONSIDER—cont'd

- Feminist Majority Foundation
  http://www.feminist.org/911/harass.html
- National Gay and Lesbian Task Force
  http://www.thetaskforce.org
- Rape, Abuse & Incest National Network
  http://www.rainn.org
- U.S. Department of Education Office for Civil Rights
  http://www.ed.gov/about/offices/list/ocr
- National Women's Law Center
  http://www.nwlc.org
- U.S. Department of Justice Civil Rights Division
  http://www.usdoj.gov/crt
- U.S. Department of Justice, Office on Violence Against Women
  http://www.usdoj.gov/ovw

References

American Association of University Women. (2005). *Drawing the line: sexual harassment on campus.* Retrieved on July 25, 2010, from http://www.aauw.org/learn/research/upload/ DTLFinal.pdf

American Nurses Association. (2001). *Code of ethics for nurses.* Silver Springs, MD: American Nurses Publishing.

Boston College. (2009). *Discriminatory harassment.* Retrieved on July 25, 2010, from http://www.bc.edu/offices/diversity/compliance/harassment.html

Equal Employment Opportunity Commission. (2010). *Harassment.* Retrieved July 10, 2010, from http://www.eeoc.gov/laws/practices/harassment.cfm

Kaplin, W. A., & Lee, B. A. (2007). *The law of higher education* (4th ed.). San Francisco: Jossey-Bass.

Kelly v. Yale University, 2003 WL 1563424, 2003 U.S. Dist. LEXUS 4543 (D. Conn. 2003).

Snyder v. Millersville University, No. 07-1660 (E.D. Pa. 2007).

Rosen, L. D. (2010). *Rewired: Understanding the iGeneration and the way they learn.* New York: Palgrave-Macmillan.

Summa v. Hofstra University, 2011 WL 1343058 (E.D.N.Y. Apr. 7, 2011).

U.S. Department of Education. Office for Civil Rights. (1997). *Sexual harassment guidance: Harassment of students by school employees, other students, or third parties.* Washington, DC: Author. Retrieved July 25, 2010, from www.ed.gov/about/offices/list/ocr/docs/sexhar00.html

Dealing With Faculty-Faculty and Faculty-Administrator Harassment

CASE STUDY

Faculty-Faculty and Faculty-Administrator Harassment

Your role: You are the department chair for the Graduate Nursing Department.

Kim Johnson is a clinical associate professor (nontenured) and the director of Graduate Clinical Education. She previously worked in the Clinical Learning Lab and taught the course Fundamentals of Nursing. Professor Johnson stated that she needed a position with more autonomy and more responsibility. Her former supervisor gives Professor Johnson a favorable reference.

Professor Johnson is not doing a good job assisting students in obtaining clinical preceptors as her job description requires, and she is evasive and passive aggressive when you question her about the status of the online clinical evaluation project that you told her was a priority. You hear from two faculty members that Professor Johnson is speaking badly about you and, further, is making racial and sexual remarks about you and another faculty member, Professor Smith, who is also a person of color. You speak to Professor Johnson and clarify her role and your expectations for professional behavior, but her performance does not improve. Her teaching evaluations are abysmal—predominantly 2s and 3s on a 5-point scale. You also learn that her former supervisor was not forthcoming about Professor Johnson's performance; in fact, she had experienced the same type of behavior.

After several more unsuccessful verbal counseling sessions and written notifications about her unsatisfactory performance, you decide to terminate Professor Johnson as the Director of Graduate Education and give her a written warning that she must improve the quality of her teaching, or face termination of her appointment to the faculty at the end of the academic year. You also find 30 files in Professor Johnson's vacated office that belong to the director of the Clinical Learning

Lab. Professor Johnson had no reason to have these files. The day following delivery of this decision to Professor Johnson, you receive a very aggressive, hostile letter from her via e-mail, containing personal insults. It also attacks and insults Professor Smith and warns that Professor Smith "better be careful," but does not make any direct threats against him or you. You believe the letter demonstrates real racial animus, and it expresses such anger, in such an unrestrained way, that you seriously question her mental condition, and have concerns for your physical safety.

Questions

- How would you proceed? Who should be notified about the letter from Professor Johnson?
- What are the implications when a faculty member (employee) is terminated from an administrative position but remains a member of the faculty?
- What actions should you take in your role as a faculty member?

Dealing With Faculty–Faculty and Faculty–Administrator Harassment: Legal Principles and Review of the Literature

Administrators are responsible for maintaining the quality of the workplace environment, as well as the performance quality of employees. Those who are responsible for the educational mission must also protect and enhance the quality of the academic and research missions, for both students and faculty. But administrators may also be members of the faculty themselves, and entitled to enjoy the benefits and protections that are awarded to faculty. When one member of the faculty attacks others (including an administrator), the situation can become very complex.

Federal and state laws exist to make sure that employees do not have to endure prejudice at the workplace that is based on age, sex, race, pregnancy, sexual preference, and disability. These laws include Title VII of the Civil Rights Act of 1964, the Age Discrimination in Employment Act of 1967 (ADEA), and the American Disabilities Act of 1990 (ADA) (Equal Employment Opportunity Commission, 2010) among others. The law protects everyone, regardless of whether the prejudice arises from the administration, from superiors, from colleagues, or from third parties. Employers have the obligation to protect their employees from such discrimination, and from any form of illegal harassment.

There is liability when the conduct is severe or pervasive enough to create a work environment that a reasonable person would consider intimidating, hostile, or abusive. Such conduct may include slurs, physical assault or threats, intimidation, insults, or interference with work performance. Isolated examples of improper comments, especially made by those who are in no position to affect someone's compensation or conditions or work, typically do not rise to the level of illegality. They can become so when the comments become frequent, managers are aware of them, and management fails to respond and stop them. At that point, the management can be deemed to have "accepted" them and allowed them to "be" the workplace environment.

The American Association of University Women (AAUW) (2005) published a report on sexual harassment at colleges and universities, which defined sexual harassment as "unwanted and unwelcome sexual behavior, which interfered with your life" (p. 8). The study showed that nearly two-thirds of college students experience some type of sexual harassment. "A majority of students experience non-contact forms of harassment—from sexual remarks to electronic messages—and nearly one-third experience some form of physical harassment, such as being touched, grabbed, or forced to do something sexual" (p. 8). Sexual harassment may occur throughout the campus, including in student housing and classrooms. Student-to-student harassment is the most common form of sexual harassment on campus. Eighty percent of the students who experienced sexual harassment on college campuses were harassed by a student or a former student.

Because employers bear the burden related to harassment in the workplace, it is in the employer's best interest to educate employees concerning workplace harassment. There should be unambiguous communication regarding both the types of behaviors that constitute harassment and the specific behaviors that will not be tolerated in the work environment. In the event that workplace harassment is suspected, harassment-reporting mechanisms and harassment policies and procedures need to be clearly identified, including associated reporting documentation required by the university. The university should also conduct faculty education that teaches faculty how to identify behaviors that are consistent with harassment, and it should also emphasize its zero tolerance for workplace harassment (Equal Opportunity Commission, 2010).

PREVENTION TIPS

Prevention is the best action to obviate workplace harassment. Preventive measures are usually in the form of workplace violence prevention programs and human resources policies that prohibit workplace harassment (Kelleher, 1996). To help prevent harassment at your university or college, it is important to establish a code of conduct for faculty and students so that everyone is clear as to what does and does not constitute harassment. Publish the code of conduct both in print and on the Web so that student and faculty can easily access the information. Hold seminars in which the harassment policy is reviewed, and provide antiharassment training to all administrators and faculty.

Failure to address worrisome behaviors could give the harasser the impression that the harassing behavior is tolerated. It is suggested that the faculty member speak to the harasser directly regarding the unwanted behavior and ask for the conduct to cease immediately (Kolanko et al., 2006). Faculty should also be encouraged to report the hostile work environment to a supervisor so that an investigation can take place and prevent the situation from further escalation.

The entire academic community should be educated concerning the triggers that may prompt a hostile work environment. These triggers may include feeling uncomfortable or threatened when a colleague makes a personal, racial, or ethnic slur. The development and implementation of a code of conduct for faculty and students will assist in alerting the academic community what behaviors constitute harassment and of the associated consequences for such behaviors; the code of conduct will also emphasize that the university has zero tolerance for harassment by any member of its community (Kolanko et al., 2006). The code of conduct should clearly communicate to the academic community that unwelcome harassing conduct is not tolerated. Universities can achieve this objective by establishing an effective complaint or grievance process, providing antiharassment training to all faculty and administrators, and taking immediate and appropriate action when an employee or student complains. Universities should strive to create an environment in which students, faculty, and staff feel free to raise concerns and are confident that those concerns will be addressed (Equal Employment Opportunity Commission, 2010).

It is important that all employees, especially those who are faculty and administrators, recognize their obligations to report improper conduct and to do whatever is appropriate to stop the harassment. Failure to act in accordance with these obligations should also be noted in evaluating their job performance.

Discussion of Case

As department chair, you send a copy of the letter to the office of public safety, legal counsel, human resources, and the dean of the school of nursing, alerting all of them to the problem and asking them to review the situation and respond as appropriate. You decide not to share the letter with Professor Smith, seeing no reason to trouble him with it unless there is some other indication of threat. You do call him to see if he is aware of any unusual or objectionable conduct by Professor Johnson. He has heard that Professor Johnson has said inappropriate things but never to him directly or within his hearing.

As a member of the faculty, you file a formal grievance against Professor Johnson so that there is a record on file of your dissatisfaction with her behavior. The office of legal counsel does send Professor Johnson an e-mail to desist all communications with the department chair and Professor Smith. A copy of the letter is sent to the security office.

⚖️ **WHEN TO CONSULT THE UNIVERSITY COUNSEL**
Consult the university counsel with potential or real claims of harassment or discrimination.

Findings and Disposition

After terminating Professor Johnson as the director of graduate education and providing her with a written warning that she must improve the quality of her teaching or face termination of her appointment to the faculty at the end of the academic year, the department chair and dean meet with Professor Johnson to discuss her teaching load and expectations. The dean attends the meeting because the department chair recently filed a grievance against Professor Johnson. During the meeting, Professor Johnson is provided with a faculty mentor to assist her in improving her teaching, which is customary in the college. Professor Johnson is also provided with the college faculty benchmark data on teaching evaluations and is instructed that her teaching evaluations are to be in the range of 3.5 to 5 on a 5-point scale. The university's equality and nondiscrimination policy is outlined to Professor Johnson.

During a 6-month period, there is no significant improvement in Professor Johnson's teaching evaluations. Her faculty mentor, Professor McCormick, states that Professor Johnson is not receptive to constructive feedback. The department chair and dean terminate Professor Johnson and do not renew her faculty contract based on her poor teaching evaluations.

Relevant Legal Case

Gupta v. Florida Board of Regents, 212 F.3d 571 (11th Cir. 2000), cert. denied, 121 S.Ct. 772 (2001)

Dr. Srabana Gupta joined Florida Atlantic University's faculty as an assistant professor of economics in August 1994 on the university's Davie campus. Her position was within the social sciences division of the College of Liberal Arts. During the 1994–1995 academic year, Dr. Rupert Rhodd was the coordinator of the social sciences division for the Davie campus, and Dr. Gupta reported to him.

In *Gupta v. Florida Board of Regents,* Dr. Gupta alleged that Dr. Rhodd sexually harassed her during a 7-month period of time following her arrival at the campus. The supervisor's behavior included twice touching the professor's leg and dress (making comments to her, such as "women are like meat" and "men need a variety of women"; and calling her at home two to three times a week). One morning after a bad thunderstorm the night before, Dr. Rhodd called Dr. Gupta and asked if she needed a ride to a university seminar. During that conversation, he said,

"Oh, you were all by yourself on a dark and stormy night? Why didn't you call me? I would have come and spent the night with you." Dr. Gupta understood Dr. Rhodd's suggestion to mean "that he wanted to [have a] sexual relationship with me." She told him, "Don't talk to me that way. You are talking nonsense." Dr. Gupta complained to several people about his inappropriate conduct, and instituted an informal dispute resolution process in January 1995 through one of the university's sexual harassment counselors; however, that process was discontinued in September 1995 as a result of Dr. Gupta's failure to participate.

Dr. Gupta filed suit in the spring of 1996 against Dr. Rhodd for sexual harassment, and against the board of regents for allowing the harassment and permitting a hostile work environment. She later amended the complaint to allege that the university had retaliated against her (made her working conditions more difficult) after she had complained to the university about Dr. Rhodd's conduct. The jury found that Dr. Rhodd had not harassed her, but found the board liable both for having permitted a hostile environment and for retaliation.

The board appealed the decision. The appellate court began by noting there are two types of sexual harassment claims: (1) quid pro quo, which are "based on threats which are carried out" or fulfilled, and (2) hostile environment, which are based on "bothersome attentions or sexual remarks that are sufficiently severe or pervasive to create a hostile work environment" (Kaplin and Lee, 2007). The court of appeals found no evidence at all in the record to support a claim of quid pro quo sexual harassment. It found that Dr. Rhodd had engaged in conduct that was "bothersome and uncomfortable" for Dr. Gupta, but it was not "physically threatening or intimidating," nor of the type that would "unreasonably interfere with the plaintiff's job performance"; rather, the court termed his conduct "the ordinary tribulations of the workplace." Most of the conduct that was offensive to her was not explicitly sexual in nature, though she interpreted it as such; they also found that it was not "so frequent, severe, or pervasive" that a reasonable person would have found it to constitute sexual harassment or to have felt it created a "hostile environment."

With respect to the retaliation claim, "Dr. Gupta presented testimony that she was subject to the following actions, which she contends are adverse employment actions: (1) she was not given a pay raise despite an above satisfactory evaluation by her supervisor; (2) she was denied an extension on her tenure clock; (3) she was placed on the search committee for a position at the university's Boca Raton campus, which prevented her from applying for that position; (4) she was assigned to teach more credit hours than other professors and to teach classes on three different campuses in the fall 1997 session; (5) she was not assigned to teach a desired class in the summer 1995 second session; (6) Dean White's office intentionally delayed her visa application to the Immigration and Naturalization Service; and (7) the informal resolution process involving her sexual harassment claim was terminated without notice after she missed one deadline."

The court held that charges (3) through (7) did not constitute "adverse employment actions." None of those actions were "objectively serious and tangible enough" to alter Gupta's "compensation, terms, conditions, or privileges of employment, deprive . . . her of employment opportunities or adversely affect . . . her status as an employee." In particular, the court held that a university has the right to assign its professors to teach the classes it needs them to teach and that an action cannot be termed *adverse* if it is corrected as soon as the proper official is made aware of it and before it goes into effect. The court did hold that the first two charges would, if supported, constitute "adverse employment actions" but also found that the university had demonstrated the decisions were made on the merits.

Requiring the plaintiff to prove that the harassment is severe or pervasive ensures that Title VII does not become a mere general civility code. The court had no doubt that Dr. Gupta subjectively perceived the alleged harassment to be unwelcome, inappropriate, and threatening. However, a court will consider four factors in determining whether statements and conduct are sufficiently severe and pervasive from an objective standpoint to alter an employee's terms or conditions of employment: "(1) the frequency of the conduct; (2) the severity of the conduct; (3) whether the conduct is physically threatening or humiliating, or a mere offensive utterance; and (4) whether the conduct unreasonably interferes with the employee's job performance."

The case of *Gupta v. Florida Board of Regents* illustrates that uncomfortable or bothersome remarks are not considered liable. The conduct complained of must be "sufficiently severe or pervasive to alter the conditions of employment and create an abusive work environment." It is this element that tests the spirit of most sexual harassment claims.

Summary

People can say bad things—even things that are racist—without it creating a legal liability for the university or its administrators. For a liability to occur, either the actor must be in a position to influence or affect the individual's quality of employment directly (through punishing behavior such as adverse work assignments or deprivation of benefits) or the conduct must be of such significance and persistence that it adversely affects the workplace to the point at which a supervisor should have done something to stop it. In the absence of one or the other of these situations, the conduct is objectionable and it might violate a code of conduct, but is not illegal.

Universities should note the value that the court's decisions have placed on the existence of "user-friendly" harassment policies and complaint procedures. To minimize liability for harassment, colleges and universities should make their anti-harassment policies and procedures clear, publish and disseminate them as widely as possible, and provide training to potential complaint handlers and faculty, staff, and students (Alger, 1998). Complainants should be treated with respect and compassion, and be given anonymity when possible and protection from retaliation. Respondents should receive due process during the investigation.

CRITICAL ELEMENTS TO CONSIDER

- Consult human resources.
- Establish an effective complaint or grievance process.
- Respond immediately when faculty or staff (employees) or student makes a harassment claim.

HELPFUL RESOURCES

Consult the Equal Employment Opportunity Commission Web site (http://www.eeoc.gov) for information regarding harassment and employer liability.

References

Alger, J. R. (1998, September–October). Love, lust and the law: Sexual harassment in the academy. *Academe: Bulletin of the American Association of University Professors, 34.* Retrieved July 10, 2010, from http://findarticles.com/p/articles/mi_qa3860/is_199809/ai_n8814787/?tag=content;col1

Equal Employment Opportunity Commission. (2010). *Harassment.* Retrieved July 10, 2010, from http://www.eeoc.gov/laws/practices/harassment.cfm

Gupta v. Florida Board of Regents, 212 F.3d 571 (11th Cir. 2000), cert. denied, 121 S.Ct. 772 (2001).

Kaplin, W. A., & Lee, B.A. (2007). *The law of higher education* (4th ed.). San Francisco: Jossey-Bass.

Kelleher, M. (1996). *New arenas for violence: Homicide in the American workplace.* Westport, CT: Praeger.

Kolanko, K. M., Clark, C., Heinrich, K. T., et al. (2006). Academic dishonesty, bullying, incivility, and violence: Difficult challenges facing nurse educators. *Nursing Education Perspectives, 27*(1), 34–43.

CHAPTER 15

Managing Issues of Student Complaints of Discrimination

An Undergraduate Faculty Adjunct Uses a Racial Slur in a Clinical Agency

Your role: You are Dr. Roam, the department chair for the undergraduate nursing program, and Professor Wiley is an undergraduate faculty adjunct teaching her third clinical community health clinical course. Although you have ultimate responsibility for the department, the adjunct faculty (because so many of them are hired each semester) are largely managed by the undergraduate clinical coordinator, Professor Vision.

Professor Wiley is a relatively new adjunct faculty member, and she is to teach a community health clinical course to senior undergraduate nursing students. Professor Wiley has taught for two semesters and her evaluations have been satisfactory, but not necessarily above average. The adjunct faculty are largely managed by the undergraduate clinical coordinator, Professor Vision, and it is her job each semester to assess the adjunct clinical needs for all the undergraduate clinical sections, hire or rehire the proper number of adjuncts from the available adjunct pool, and monitor their performance in the clinical agencies in which they supervise students (including doing their annual evaluation and making decisions to rehire or simply not offer a subsequent semester contract based on poor performance). Professor Vision does not necessarily make site visits to assess them, but she is always available to handle any issues that arise, particularly when course coordinators (full-time nursing faculty who have the ultimate responsibility for each clinical course and who directly oversee clinical faculty on a day-to-day basis during the semester) e-mail her or call her about a problem with a particular adjunct faculty member.

On this day, you have just received a text message from Professor Vision, indicating that she urgently needs to speak to you about an incident in the community health clinical course. She says there are no safety issues involved, but as the issue is confidential in nature, she did not want to discuss it via e-mail. The next day you meet with Professor Vision, and she informs you that one of the students e-mailed her with a complaint against Professor Wiley. The student claims Professor Wiley used the term *wetbacks* in reference to Hispanics in a conversation with another staff member at the community health agency. The student further claimed that two other Hispanic students in the group feared that by reporting this incident they might face harassment (or even clinical failure) from the clinical instructor.

Questions

- How would you first proceed?
- Do you believe Professor Wiley should be punished for this incident if indeed it is found to be true?
- Do you think this incident is essentially rare, or do you believe the adjunct faculty (or even the faculty at large) ought to undergo workplace sensitivity training?
- How will you bring this incident to a close and circumvent any rumor-mongering that might take place?

Complaints of University Student Discrimination: Legal Principles and Review of the Literature

Any discussion of harassment is likely to include discrimination, and vice versa. According to most statutes, discriminatory motives or harassing behaviors due to race, national origin, religion, age, gender, and disability (some locales include sexual orientation) are illegal. This chapter addresses both harassment and discrimination complaints by students in the university setting.

Harassment

Harassment on university campuses has been reportedly mostly based on sex or race; the recent case of an assistant attorney general in Michigan who very publically cyber-harassed and bullied the University of Michigan student body president student because he was openly gay is an example that stretches the contemporary definition and scope of sexual harassment (Jones, 2010). By current definitions, the legal term *harassment* can be defined as physical or verbal hostility toward someone with legally protected status. *Nolo's Plain-English Law Dictionary* defines protected status or class as "a group of people protected by law from discrimination or harassment based on their membership in the group. For example, under federal law, race, national origin, sex, and age are examples of protected classes" (2010, p. 1). There are also state and local laws as well as university policies that prohibit discrimination on the basis of sexual orientation (Lassek, 2010).

One of the most comprehensive operationalized definitions of harassment for the university or college setting appears in the *Foothill-De Anza* (Los Altom

Hills, CA) *Community College District Board of Trustees Policy Manual.*[1] The college indicates unlawful harassment comes in many forms but it has delineated the following:

Verbal: Inappropriate or offensive remarks, slurs, jokes or innuendoes based on a person's race, gender, sexual orientation, or other legally protected status. This may include, but is not limited to, inappropriate comments regarding an individual's body, physical appearance, attire, sexual prowess, marital status, or sexual orientation; unwelcome flirting, whistling, or propositions; demands for sexual favors; verbal abuse, threats or intimidation.

Physical: Inappropriate or offensive touching, assault, or physical interference with free movement. This may include, but is not limited to, kissing, patting, lingering or intimate touches, grabbing, pinching, unnecessarily brushing against or blocking another person, or sexual gestures. It also includes any physical assault or intimidation directed at an individual due to that person's race, gender, sexual orientation, or other legally protected status. It may also include leering and staring.

Visual or Written: The display or circulation of visual or written material that degrades an individual or groups based on race, gender, or sexual orientation, or other legally protected status. This may include, but is not limited to, posters, cartoons, drawing, graffiti, reading materials, computer graphics, or electronic media transmissions.

Environmental: A hostile work environment exists where it is permeated by innuendo or insults or abusive comments directed at an individual or group based on race, gender, sexual orientation, or other legally protected status. An environment may in some circumstances also be hostile toward anyone who merely witnesses unlawful harassment in his or her immediate surroundings, although the conduct is directed at others (Foothill-De Anza Community College District Board of Trustees Board Policy Manual, 2005, p. 1–2).

Sexual harassment is defined by the U.S. Department of Education as "unwelcome [verbal, nonverbal, or physical] conduct of a sexual nature" (U.S. Department of Education, 2001) Sexual harassment is prohibited by Title VII of the Civil Rights Act of 1964 and by Title IX of the Education Amendments of 1972. Sexual harassment is generally broken into two types: quid pro quo harassment and hostile environment harassment (Lindsay III, 2005). Using the revised Department of Education Guidelines, the two categories are defined as follows:

Quid pro quo harassment occurs if a teacher or other employee conditions an educational decision or benefit on the student's submission to unwelcome sexual conduct, [regardless of whether] the student resists and suffers the threatened harm or submits and avoids the threatened harm....

By contrast, [hostile environment] harassment . . . does not explicitly or implicitly condition a decision or benefit on submission to sexual conduct [but does nevertheless] limit a student's ability to participate or benefit from the school's program based on sex (U.S. Department of Education, 2001).

Because students do not ordinarily have control over other students, only faculty and other university employees are charged with quid pro quo harassment, and fellow students are more frequently charged with hostile environment harassment. According the American Association of University Women (AAUW), sexual harassment is still pervasive on college campuses today. From the AAUW's 2006 report, *Drawing the Line: Sexual Harassment on Campus*, statistics indicate 62% of female college students and 61% of male college students report having been sexually harassed at their university, and more than 35% do not tell anyone or

---

[1] Used with permission by the Foothill-De Anza Community College District Board of Trustees.

report these incidents. These statistics are alarming, and indicate that despite the enactment of numerous laws and university polices prohibiting sexual harassment and an apparent "ethic" of equality among the most educated, it is still a significant problem and more campus-based educational programs to protect students need to be pursued.

Discrimination

Discrimination can take many forms. An individual can be discriminated against based on gender, race, religion, ethnicity, sexual orientation, marital status, and disability, but also on weight, height, smoking status, accent, dress, political beliefs, and an endless number of other factors that are not necessarily prohibited by law. In the university setting, the following are laws that prohibit a variety of forms of discrimination: Title VI of the Civil Rights Act of 1964 (discrimination based on race, color, or national origin); Title IX of the Education Amendments of 1972 (sex discrimination); Section 504 of the Rehabilitation Act of 1973, as amended (disability discrimination); Age Discrimination Act (age discrimination); and Title II of the Americans with Disabilities Act (prohibiting disability discrimination by public entities).

In the university setting, charges of discrimination by students generally fall into the category of an individual student claiming a professor, perhaps a department chair or advisor, has discriminated against him or her. The following is a discussion of various types of student discrimination based on a federal protected class, including examples of sexual orientation discrimination that is law in eight states and the District of Columbia.[2] Disability discrimination is discussed in Chapter 21.

Gender discrimination refers to unequal treatment based on an individual's gender. There are two main types of discrimination: disparate treatment and disparate impact (Lindsay III, 2005). *Disparate treatment* is sometimes called *intentional discrimination,* and it occurs when a teacher treats a student differently because of gender—for example, if a faculty member gave higher grades to females than males in a college course. Recently, Dr. Kelly, a tenured Ohio University professor charged with having inappropriate relationships with staff and students for over a decade, resigned instead of facing dismissal and tenure revocation procedures (Pyle, 2010). The final charges that led to the resignation included complaints by female Indian students (the university had an MBA program in India) that Dr. Kelly was giving higher grades to an Indian student with whom he was involved. The other type of discrimination, *disparate impact,* is more difficult to prove because it involves the exclusion of someone or a member of a protected class from a certain benefit. One very public charge of disparate impact discrimination is

---

[2] The states include California, Connecticut, Massachusetts, Minnesota, New Jersey, New York, Vermont, and Wisconsin.

the longstanding argument that the SAT college entrance examination is biased against minorities, and the lower scores they receive bars them from admission to leading universities or colleges (Freedle, 2003).

Another common form of discrimination complaint in higher education is race-based discrimination. Because Title VII of the Civil Rights Act of 1964 prohibits both gender and racial discrimination, graduate students who are serving in any kind of student-employee classification (e.g., teaching assistant) have additional protections under the Equal Employment Opportunity Commission (EEOC), where complaints can be filed but only within 180 days of the harassment or discrimination charge. Every university or college has an EEOC officer, and at Drexel University those duties are handled within the Office of Equality and Diversity. According to EEOC guidelines there are four steps in a complaint process: informal/counseling, formal complaint, appeal, and the final phase starts the judicial process (U.S. Department of Transportation, n.d.). Sydell and Nelson (2000) have pointed out that racism has been shifting from open violent behavior and aggressive racism to unconscious forms of racism. Soyer (2008) more recently confirms this stating that "explicit racism is not common any more in modern colleges and universities. The cultures in these institutions often have certain values that reduce the ethnic inequalities, and the assimilation pressure on the students of color" (p. 2). However, Soyer also indicates the dominant white culture still retains racial hierarchies, addresses apparently racial matters, but resists addressing genuine diversity. Whether this last assessment is centrally valid or merely the interpretation of the author is probably a good discussion point. Finally, there is also the concept of *reverse discrimination*. It is defined as "policies or habits of social discrimination against members of a historically dominant group with an implication of unfairness" (USLegal.com, p. 1). Often these charges are brought by individuals who believe that affirmative action or quota practices are inherently unfair or illegal. The first and most notable reverse discrimination case ruling by the Supreme Court was *Regents of the University of California v. Bakke* (1978) (No. 7811) 18 Cal.3d 34, 553 P.2d 1152. In this historic case, Allan Bakke (a 35-year-old white male applicant to the University of California–Davis medical school) was denied admission although his benchmark admission score was higher than some applicants admitted through a special program that gave preference to those from economically or educationally disadvantaged backgrounds or who were members of a minority group. Writing for the majority in a 5 to 4 vote, Justice Powell wrote:

1. *Title VI proscribes only those racial classifications that would violate the Equal Protection Clause if employed by a State or its agencies.*

2. *Racial and ethnic classifications of any sort are inherently suspect and call for the most exacting judicial scrutiny. While the goal of achieving a diverse student body is sufficiently compelling to justify consideration of race in admissions decisions under some circumstances, petitioner's*

special admissions program, which forecloses consideration to persons like respondent, is unnecessary to the achievement of this compelling goal, and therefore invalid under the Equal Protection Clause (pp. 287–320).

3. *Since petitioner could not satisfy its burden of proving that respondent would not have been admitted even if there had been no special admissions program, he must be admitted (p. 320).*

The issue was again addressed in 2003 when the degree to which race (as an affirmative action remedy) could be used in the university admissions process was again litigated. In two separate rulings, the Supreme Court ruled that race *could be used* in the admissions process, but that it could not be the overriding factor. By a 6 to 3 (*Gratz v. Bollinger,* 2003) vote, the University of Michigan undergraduate admission program was ruled unconstitutional because it used a point system for race in its admissions process. By a 5 to 4 (*Grutter v. Bollinger,* 2003) vote, the university's law school admissions process was upheld as it used a much narrower race factor in its admissions procedures.

Discussion of Case

Recall from this chapter's case study that you are Dr. Roam and your undergraduate clinical coordinator, Professor Vision, has just informed you that Professor Wiley has made an ethnic slur in conversation. How would you first proceed? The first question to ask is, Does your university have an office of equality and diversity? If so, you and your department should know that *their* first call should be made to that office and not to you. The office should be regarded as the experts and its advice sought from the start, as it is likely the office will know best how to proceed. So you would begin by asking Professor Vision if she had made that call. But assume for the moment that your university does not have that infrastructure in place.

Dr. Roam was very disturbed by the "alleged comment," and although she understood the students' fear of exposure and their being potential targets of harassment, she reminded Professor Vision the incident should be phrased *as alleged* until the facts of the case could be fully investigated. Dr. Roam was very adamant that this be handled in the most professional and confidential manner. As posed in the second case study question, do you believe Professor Wiley should be punished for this incident if indeed it is found to be true?

WHEN TO CONTACT THE UNIVERSITY COUNSEL

It is unlikely that a student would contact university counsel for allegations of harassment or discrimination as the EEOC office is specifically charged to hear such complaints. However, it is common for administrators and/or faculty to consult with university counsel as these types of matters arise. Even after consulting with university counsel for advice, the ultimate business decision remains the responsibility of the administrator/faculty.

Findings and Disposition

Professor Vision could not decide whom she should interview first, and so she recontacted Dr. Roam, who said the faculty member should certainly be contacted first and simply, calmly, and constructively questioned whether she had indeed made the comment or not. Dr. Roam told Professor Vision that word (or any hint) of an investigation being conducted without having first given the accused faculty member a chance to present her side of the case would be very detrimental to faculty due process. Professor Vision subsequently asked Professor Wiley to meet so they could discuss the alleged remark she made. Almost immediately Professor Wiley acknowledged her use of the term "wetbacks" in a casual conversation, and she apologized profusely for this indiscretion. She stated it was not meant to be a public but a private conversation but that she was indeed sorry any student had overheard her and had been offended. She also acknowledged that the term was racially charged and inappropriate for a nursing faculty member to use. She offered to personally apologize to the student. Professor Vision informed Professor Wiley that the students involved are somewhat fearful of being harassed by her for reporting this incident. To this, Professor Wiley strongly stated that she would never do such a thing. Professor Vision concluded the meeting and informed Professor Wiley that she would have to speak to Dr. Roam about how this incident should be handled further and that she would get back to her. She did encourage Professor Wiley to write up her side of the story for the record and to include the comments she had just shared with her. What kind of punishment should Dr. Roam enforce, or is the offer by Professor Wiley to personally apologize to the student(s) sufficient?

Upon hearing the facts of the case, Dr. Roam encouraged Professor Vision to complete her interview with the accusing student and to forward her any new information from the meeting. She would then make a decision. She contacted the university counsel and informed her that if there were no additional, extenuating circumstances presented by the student (it was unlikely based on the trajectory of the story) then she would fire Professor Wiley for her conduct. The university counsel agreed but informed her it was best to first receive the written statement from Professor Wiley admitting to the act. Within two days, Professor Vision forwarded the statement to Dr. Roam (there were no substantive changes from the facts first admitted to by Professor Wiley), and so Dr. Roam called Professor Wiley in and terminated her. Dr. Roam was very professional in her delivery and informed Professor Wiley that she had done the ethical and honest thing by admitting to the incident and, although she appreciated the offer of a public apology, the incident in her view was severe. She believed Professor Wiley's credibility in the clinical agency was now significantly damaged and would interfere with the educational mission of the current student and perhaps others in the future who might hear of the incident. She wished Professor Wiley well and Professor Wiley moved on with her life and career without any further action or appeals.

Recall the third case study question, Do you think this incident is essentially rare, or do you believe the adjunct faculty (or even the faculty at large) ought to undergo Workplace Sensitivity Training? Discuss this in class now.

Recall the fourth case study question, How should Dr. Roam bring this incident to a close and circumvent any rumor-mongering that might take place? Indeed, Dr. Roam was concerned about this, and as the department chair she felt it important for her (not Professor Vision) to bring the incident to a close and try to prevent any further gossip or rumormongering to persist. Professor Vision was able to find a last-minute clinical replacement for Professor Wiley, and then she e-mailed the students in the clinical group and informed them that the department chair, Dr. Roam, wanted to meet with them briefly after their next class (and before the next clinical day). Dr. Roam subsequently met with the eight students (along with Professor Vision), and she informed the students that she would appreciate it if the meeting and discussion were kept confidential. She apologized for Professor Wiley, and although not using the details of the incident in her discussion, she reported Professor Wiley was indeed sorry for any offense she had caused. Dr. Roam said they would have a new clinical faculty the following week and that she appreciated the students coming forward. She further iterated she was always dedicated to safe, ethical, and respectful clinical/work environments, and she hoped they would move forward with their clinical rotation with those values in mind; she also urged the students not to participate in any rumors as she considered that most unprofessional. "The incident has been completely taken care of," she said, and then she asked if there were any questions. As the students had none, the meeting was concluded. On her way out, one student came over and said, simply and quietly, "Thank you." Dr. Roam later thanked Professor Vision for the excellent and professional manner in which she had conducted the case and its resolution.

Relevant Legal Case

Underwood v. LaSalle University, No. 07-1441, 2007 WL 4245737
(E.D. Pa. Dec. 4, 2007)

In this case, Starling Underwood, a former undergraduate nursing student at La Salle University, filed a lawsuit against the university alleging the nursing program had dismissed him based on race, and he claimed violations of the Title VI of the Civil Rights Act of 1964 as well as gender and disability discrimination claims under Title IX of the Civil Rights Act, the Rehabilitation Act, and Title II of the American with Disabilities Act.

Mr. Underwood had initially passed nine nursing courses between 2003 and 2004; however, in the spring semester 2005 he received a grade of D in a pediatrics class and an F in a nursing research course. He had initially asked for permission to withdraw from the nursing research class, but he waited until the last day of class to do so, thereby violating the policy on withdrawals and so his request was denied, resulting in an F for the course. LaSalle had a policy to dismiss a student who received two grades lower than a C in any given semester; therefore, Mr. Underwood was dismissed. The university initially moved to pretrial summary judgment, and it was only at this time that Mr. Underwood added claims of gender and disability discrimination based on his claim of poor vision that was not severe enough to qualify him for an accommodation (nor was his disability claim of discrimination from using Ebonics seen as valid).

The court ultimately granted LaSalle University summary judgment as Mr. Underwood had already denied racial discrimination at a previous deposition. His claim to gender discrimination had a 2-year statute of limitations in Pennsylvania, despite being added at the twelfth hour as a frivolous claim, according to the court, and the disability claims were likewise dismissed.

Summary

Harassment and discrimination persist in society—and as is clear from the press accounts of attacks on Muslims following terrorist attacks, not far beneath the surface. Because universities and colleges are microcosms of society at large, it is not surprising that these issues continue to arise in higher educational settings. Just recently it was reported that sexual assault was up 64% in 2009–2010 from the previous year and that 90% of cases go unreported (Department of Defense, 2010). Furthermore, 80% of cases of sexual harassment by both men and women go unreported because cadets (in one of major service academies, the U.S. Air Force Academy) fear reprisals for the disclosure (Department of Defense). These are alarming numbers, and as the military (perhaps like most work environments) is a "top-down" organization, it is obvious that cadets are taking their cues from what is apparently being tolerated in the environment. These statistics make one wonder: What are the statistics *outside the military academies,* and is it possible they are similar or perhaps even higher?

We have administratively dealt with numerous allegations of harassment and discrimination in our tenure as nursing academic administrators. Although this chapter's Case Study did not advance to actual charges of harassment, the students felt vulnerable as a racial minority and their fears of discrimination (or harassment) were well founded. It is prudent not to rush to judgment in any case, and make sure all sides are heard. Students who have very strong feelings that they have been harassed or discriminated against should go to the office of equality and diversity. This does not mean there should be an investigation of very obvious frivolous charges, however. But even here, who should best ascertain that a student's charges are frivolous or groundless? Administrators in respective offices of equality and diversity should be more familiar with the federal due process rights that students from a protected class have when claiming any form of discrimination or harassment. Often it is more efficient for these offices to handle these situations, and they should be skilled at detecting the merits of a complaint. It is also important to note that some complaints are made informally and only made formal when a student seeks to fully document an incident and follow through with all the normal investigative procedures. In the LaSalle University case, it became very obvious to the court that the plaintiff only added gender and disability claims in his lawsuit at the twelfth hour as an addendum to his original claim of racial discrimination.

 CRITICAL ELEMENTS TO CONSIDER

- Students do not have to be subject to harassment or discrimination. There are laws at the federal, state, and local levels and university/college policies that are designed to protect students and effectively deal with illegal conduct.
- Any faculty member should be familiar with the on-campus office that handles EEOC complaints and be ready (even as an adviser) to steer students to that office when appropriate.
- Because charges of discrimination are so antithetical to the academy, so deeply personal, and so easy to make, it is unfortunately the case that faculty members need to be prepared for having such charges made against them unfairly. It is difficult to prepare against them (and not worth the energy or effort) except by acting with respect to all at all times. However, in the event that you sense a particular "agenda" being advanced by a student, sharing your concern with your supervisor and preserving that communication in an e-mail can later document what was really going on.
- If there is discrimination based on sexual orientation, it is important to understand that there are some state and local laws and university policies that prohibit this.
- If a student does not feel safe going through normal academic channels for whatever reason (e.g., sexual harassment), he or she can contact the university public safety, university ombudsman, or the university's counseling center.

(HELPFUL RESOURCES

- American Association of University Women
  http://www.aauw.org/
- American Civil Rights Association
  http://www.aclu.org/
- American Disabilities Act
  http://www.ada.gov/pubs/ada.htm
- Equal Employment Opportunity Commission (EEOC)
  http://www.eeoc.gov/
- Human Rights Campaign
  http://www.hrc.org/
- National Association for the Advancement NAACP
  http://www.naacp.org/content/main/

References

American Association of University Women. (n.d.). *Sexual harassment on Campus.* Retrieved December 13, 2010, from http://www.aauw.org/act/laf/library/harassment.cfm

American Association of University Women (2005). *Drawing the line: Sexual harassment on campus.* Retrieved December 13, 2010, from http://www.aauw.org/learn/research/upload/DTLFinal.pdf

Foothill-De Anza Community College District Board of Trustees Board Policy Manual. (2005). Definition of Harassment and Discrimination, 4640, Retrieved September 4, 2011 from http://fhdafiles.fhda.edu/downloads/diversity/HarassmentandDiscriminationP.pdf

Freedle, R. O. (2003). Correcting the SAT's ethnic and social-class bias: A method for reestimating SAT scores. *Harvard Educational Review, 73*(1), 1–43.

Gratz v. Bollinger, 539 U.S. 244 (2003).

Grutter v. Bollinger, 539 U.S. 306 (2003).

Jones, M. T. (2010, November 8). Anti-gay assistant attorney general in Michigan fired for cyber-bullying. change.org. Retrieved December 12, 2010, from http://gayrights.change.org/blog/view/anti-gay_assistant_attorney_general_in_michigan_fired_for_cyber-bullying

Lassek, P. J. (2010). Sexual orientation added to protected-classes list. TulsaWorld.com. Retrieved December 12, 2010, from http://www.tulsaworld.com/news/article.aspx?subjectid=334&articleid=20100618_11_A1_Amjrtf152022

Lindsay, C. L., III. (2005). *The college student's guide to the law.* Lanham, MD: Taylor Trade Publishing.

Nolo's plain-English law dictionary. (2010). Protected class. Nolo.com. Retrieved December 12, 2010 from http://www.nolo.com/dictionary/protected-class-term.html

Pyle, E. (2010, April 17). OU professor retires after ultimatum. *The Columbus Dispatch.*

Regents of the University of California v. Bakke, 438 U.S. 265 (1978).

Soyer, M. (2008, July). *Factors affecting racial discrimination among college students.* Paper presented at the annual meeting of the American Sociological Association, Boston, MA.

Sydell, E. J., & Nelson, E. S. (2000). Modern racism on campus: A survey of attitudes and perceptions. *Social Science Journal, 37,* 627–636.

U.S. Department of Defense. (2010). *Annual Report on sexual harassment and violence at the U.S. military service academies.* Retrieved December 16, 2010, from http://www.sapr.mil/media/pdf/reports/FINAL_APY_09-10_MSA_Report.pdf

U.S. Department of Education. (2001, January). *Revised sexual harassment guidance: Harassment of students by school employees, other students, or third parties, Part II.* Retrieved December 16, 2010, from http:///www.ed.gov/offices/list/ocr/docs/shguide.htmd

U.S. Department of Transportation. (n.d.). EEO complaint process. Retrieved December 13, 2010, from http://www.dotcr.ost.dot.gov/asp/EEODOT.asp

USLegal.com. (2010). *Reverse discrimination law and legal discrimination.* Retrieved December 15, 2010, from http://definitions.uslegal.com/r/reverse-discrimination/

CHAPTER 16

Managing Issues of Faculty Complaints of Discrimination

CASE STUDY

A Graduate Nursing Faculty Is Accused of Age Discrimination

Your role: You are Dr. Slim, and you teach the pathophysiology course to graduate students in one of the several nurse-practitioner tracks your college offers.

One of your students, Ms. Deal, has been struggling in class and is likely to fail. She might be the oldest student in the class, although you do not specifically know her age. Over the course of several weeks, you notice that Ms. Deal asks questions that make you doubt whether she has any recall of her previous anatomy and physiology courses. In one frustrating moment, the student asks another very basic question (and the eyes of her classmates seem to roll in unison), to which you respond with a bit of exasperation, "Wasn't that covered in your physiology class? It wasn't that long ago you took that class. You really ought to remember that information." Refusing to answer the question, you move on. A few days later, you receive an e-mail marked "Confidential" from the Office of Equality and Diversity. It states that a complaint has been filed against you and asks you to contact the director, Dr. Cynthia, as soon as possible. Quite perplexed and also with a great deal of anxiety, you call Dr. Cynthia, and she informs you that a student has filed a complaint against you for age discrimination.

Questions

- How would you first proceed?
- Do you think you said anything in any way that could lead the student to believe you had discriminated against her?
- What do you think about the process and procedures that the Equal Employment Opportunity Commission (EEOC) representative (Dr. Cynthia) followed?
- Do you think you would have benefited from having a faculty ombudsman?

Complaints of Faculty Discrimination: Legal Principles and Review of the Literature

The previous chapter discussed a broad range of the legal literature that prohibits harassment and discrimination. This chapter provides additional information about the key laws that afford protection from harassment and discrimination:

- **Equal Pay Act of 1963** requires that male and female employees be paid the same for jobs requiring equivalent work
- **Title VII of the Civil Rights Act of 1964** prohibits discrimination in hiring, compensation, terms, conditions, status, opportunities, or privileges of employment on the basis of race, color, religion, sex, or national origin
- **Executive Order 11246 (1965)** requires affirmative action in organizations with 50 or more employees and aggregate contracts of $50,000 or more with the federal government
- **Age Discrimination in Employment Act of 1967** prohibits discrimination against applicants and employees 40 years of age and older
- **Title IX of the Education Amendments of 1972** (amending the Higher Education Act of 1965) prohibits discrimination on the basis of sex by any educational program or activity receiving federal financial assistance
- **Pregnancy Discrimination Act of 1978** prohibits discrimination on the basis of pregnancy
- **Americans With Disabilities Act of 1990** prohibits discrimination against and requires reasonable accommodation for individuals with physical or mental impairments
- **Family and Medical Leave Act (FMLA) of 1993** requires provisions up to a total of 12 weeks per year of unpaid protected job leave for employees under specific conditions
- **Lilly Ledbetter Fair Pay Act of 2009** states the 180-day statute of limitations for filing an equal-pay lawsuit regarding pay discrimination; resets with each new discriminatory paycheck

Equal Pay Act of 1963

The Equal Pay Act of 1963 was one of the first federal statutes that was specifically designed to "level the playing field" in the employment arena by prohibiting discrimination on the basis of factors other than merit. It required that male and female employees be paid the same for equal work for jobs that required equal skill, effort, and responsibility and that were performed under similar working conditions. With women entering war industries in large numbers in World War II and thereafter, it was important that wage inequalities be addressed. Even as late as the early 1960s, newspapers published separate want ads for women and men, and companies would often advertize for a position indicating "male wanted" (Brunner, 2007).[1] Concerning the Equal Pay Act of 1963, Brunner writes, "Demonstrable differences in seniority, merit, the quality or quantity of work, or other considerations might merit different pay, but gender could no longer be viewed as a drawback on one's resumé" (2007, p. 1).

Although it seems incredible that until June 11, 1964 (when the bill was enacted), women could be legally discriminated against in employment, the long reach of this statute has been clarified in such decisions as in *Schultz v. Wheaton Glass Co.,* 421 F.2d 259, 3rd Cir. (1970), wherein the U.S. Court of Appeals for the Third Circuit ruled that a job title could not be reclassified so that a woman would be paid less than a man. In *Corning Glass Works v. Brennan,* 417 U.S. 188 (1974), the U.S. Supreme Court ruled that men could not be paid more simply because men would not work for the same low wages in a specific job to which women might agree.

While "equal pay" has become the new standard, it is clear that disparities between the sexes persist. In employment sectors such as academia, the comparability of positions and duties is sometimes difficult to demonstrate (e.g., comparing faculty in a school of business with those in arts and sciences), and data that might demonstrate disparities are difficult (if even possible) to obtain (Dreher and Smith, 2003). A recent report of female partners at elite law firms indicated they made on average $66,000 less than their male counterparts, with this disparity largely attributed to stereotyping, gender bias, and even bullying and intimidation (Williams and Richardson, 2010).

Title VII of the Civil Rights Act of 1964

An important piece of landmark civil rights legislation, Title VII of the Civil Rights Act of 1964 made it an unlawful employment practice for an employer to:

1. Fail or refuse to hire or to discharge any individual, or otherwise to discriminate against any individual with respect to compensation, term, conditions, or privileges of employment, because of such individual's race, color, religion, sex, or national origin; or

2. Limit, segregate, or classify employees or applicants for employment in any way which would deprive any individual of employment opportunities or otherwise adversely affect status as an employee, because of such individual's race, color, religion, sex, or national origin.

Although it is likely that most Americans have come to view the Civil Rights Act of 1964 as settled law, Kentucky Senator Rand Paul (an ophthalmologist)

---

[1] Technically, this indicates sexual bias in hiring not in compensation, but the likely compensation inequities can be easily imagined.

famously questioned whether these laws ought to apply to *private employers* during his 2010 campaign for senate (Smith, 2010). In reality, private businesses can choose to hire whomever they want, but are only prohibited from discrimination in hiring based on definitions of protected class: race, color, sex, or national origin (Haney López, 2006). Since 1990, the Americans with Disabilities Act has added individuals with disability as another protected class in which employment discrimination is prohibited. But will that prevent an employer from not hiring someone because he or she is fat or slovenly or even ugly? It is likely employers do this all the time. Further, prospective employees also are rarely privy to reasons they are not hired, meaning that even protected class discrimination likely occurs but invisibly and without a damaging paper trail. We do note that the Civil Rights Act of 1964 was additionally amended by the Pregnancy Discrimination Act of 1978 (instituting Title VII of the Civil Rights Act of 1964 changes to prohibit sex discrimination on the basis of pregnancy), and amended by Section 703 to include a clear definition of sexual harassment in 1980.

Executive Order 11246 (1965)

President Lyndon Johnson signed Executive Order 11246 on September 24, 1965, requiring that organizations with 50 or more employees and aggregate contracts of $50,000 or more with the federal government implement affirmative action policies to hire (and retain) minorities and females in proportion to the percentage of minorities and females in the geographic area in which the organization is located and from which it draws its employees (Golden, Hinkle, and Crosby, 2001). The law further requires submission of an annual affirmative action plan outlining goals and timetables for achieving proportionate utilization of both minorities and females. This executive order was amended to include reference to individuals with disabilities by the Rehabilitation Act of 1973, to veteran's status by the Vietnam Era Veterans Readjustment Act, and to age by Executive Order 11141.

Age Discrimination in Employment Act of 1967

The Age Discrimination in Employment Act of 1967 prohibits discrimination against applicants and employees 40 years of age and older and prohibits employers from (1) failing or refusing to hire or discharge any individual with respect to compensation, terms, conditions, or privileges of employment because of such individual's age; and/or (2) limiting, segregating, or classifying employees in any way which would deprive or tend to deprive any individual of employment opportunities or otherwise adversely affect status as an employee, because of such individual's age; and/or (3) reducing the compensation of any employee in order to comply with the act. The act was amended in 1976 to protect people from discrimination based on age in programs or activities receiving federal financial assistance, in 1986 to prohibit mandatory retirement at any age except for certain professions under specific conditions, and in 1990 by the Older Workers Benefit Protection Act (Bolick, 1987).

Americans With Disabilities Act of 1990

The Americans With Disabilities Act (ADA) of 1990[2] was landmark legislation that really updated and modernized the current laws that were designed to protect individuals with disabilities. It further codified the prohibition against discrimination and mandated reasonable accommodation of applicants and employees with physical or mental impairments (or a record of perception of such) that substantially limit one or more major life activities[3] and who, with or without reasonable accommodation, can perform the essential functions of the job. This important legislation is discussed in more detail later in this text.

Family and Medical Leave Act (FMLA) of 1993

The Family and Medical Leave Act (FMLA) of 1993 requires covered employers to provide up to a total of 12 weeks per year of job-protected leave *without pay* to eligible employees to care for an employee's child after birth, adoption, or foster care; to care for an employee's spouse, child, or parent with a serious health condition; or for an employee's serious health condition that prevents the employee from performing his or her job. Under most conditions eligibility occurs when the employee has been employed for at least 1 year, has worked 1,250 hours in the previous 12 months, and has provided 30 days' notice under most conditions (as serious health conditions can arise at any time, employees who have not given 30 days' notice may be required to certify their health condition to their employer) (Chapman, 2002).

Although the FMLA has been viewed by many as progressive legislation, it remains a complex law, and some employers struggle to prevent what many now agree are instances of employee abuse of the law (Fischer, 2007; Martucci and Coverdale, 2004).[4]

Lilly Ledbetter Fair Pay Act of 2009

The Lilly Ledbetter Fair Pay Act of 2009 was signed into law by President Barack Obama. Lilly Ledbetter's story deserves retelling here and explains the origins of the law: Via an anonymous written tip, Ledbetter discovered in 1998, almost

---

[2]Title IX of the Education Amendments of 1972 (which amended the Higher Education Act of 1965) is also an important discrimination law that prohibits discrimination on the basis of sex by any educational program or activity receiving federal financial assistance, but is more applicable to students and not faculty or employees.

[3]According to the revisions made in 2008 to the ADA of 1990, major life activities can be defined as (but not limited to) caring for oneself, performing manual tasks, seeing, hearing, eating, sleeping, walking, standing, lifting, bending, speaking, breathing, learning, reading, concentrating, thinking, communicating, and working.

[4]There are substantial instances of employer abuse of FLMA regulations (Stoddard, 2006).

20 years after she was hired as a Goodyear manager, that she was paid between 20 and 40 percent less than her male counterparts with the same titles and duties. By 2007, a decade after filing a federal discrimination complaint, Ledbetter had become a cause célèbre as her case approached the U.S. Supreme Court.

In a controversial 5 to 4 decision, the court said Ledbetter could sue only for discrimination dating back 6 months from her complaint, making it impossible for her to recover years of lost salary and overtime compensation, to say nothing of her retirement and Social Security benefits that will always be figured on her lower wages (Barrow, 2010, p. 1).The Lilly Ledbetter bill therefore amended the Civil Rights Act of 1964, to provide that the 180-day statute of limitations for filing an equal-pay lawsuit regarding pay discrimination resets with each new discriminatory paycheck.

In summary, although each of these laws may not affect every individual, in totality they are designed to enforce equality in hiring and employment through the United States without any discriminatory barriers. Society is not perfect and, as all these laws have been amended since their enactment, changes in the modern world are likely to require a fluid and responsive judicial system.

Discussion of Case

Recall this chapter's case study, in which you were Dr. Slim and you had just been informed a complaint has been filed against you for age discrimination. The case study's first question was: How would you proceed? Dr. Slim was shocked to be accused of age discrimination. He asked Dr. Cynthia what the specific details of the accusation were, but she would not deliver that confidential information on the phone, and so Dr. Slim made an appointment to review the details of the report filed by Ms. Deal. Later, he read that the student claimed he had said in a very demeaning tone, "So exactly when did you take your last A & P class [anatomy and physiology]?" She further claimed his grading was biased against her and that was why she was performing poorly. Dr. Slim informed Dr. Cynthia that he did not recall using an uncivil or mocking tone in communication with her. He stated he was only trying to discern the length of time of her last course because she wasn't recalling very basic material. He further claimed that all of his tests were either multiple choice or short answer and that it was preposterous that his grading was arbitrary. He indicated the student was clearly failing and grasping at straws. Recall the case study's second question, Do you think you said anything in any way that could lead the student to believe you had discriminated against her? Dr. Cynthia asked this question, and Dr. Slim tried to reflect honestly about it. After considering the possibility that his comment was simply a misunderstanding, Dr. Slim rejected the idea that he was somehow at fault, and he was adamant that he was absolutely fair in his grading of all his students.

WHEN TO CONTACT THE UNIVERSITY ATTORNEY

The presupposition is that in order to use university offices and officials, the individual faculty member must already have been hired by the university; therefore, this would not normally be an option for someone who is not yet employed by the university. If you feel you are being discriminated against for some reason, the best recommendation is to use the office of human resources and its policies first. Of course, if ultimately there is a charge of discrimination that would be handled by the campus EEOC office, then that avenue is also a possibility. The office of the ombudsman should always be considered, especially if there is a charge of, for instance, favoritism that fails to be properly handled through normal administrative channels. Sometimes discrimination, or perhaps "an unfair practice," is unintentional. By bringing the details of the alleged favoritism or other similar issue to the attention of an attentive administrator, the issue can often be resolved. If it cannot, then these other avenues are sensible options.

Findings and Disposition

Dr. Cynthia had two versions of the incident, and she needed to make a determination whether a more extensive investigation was warranted. She asked Dr. Slim if any of his other students were failing or doing poorly in the class, and she asked to see the grade distribution for the class as a whole and the files of the students who were doing poorly. Dr. Slim stated there was only one other failing student, and he volunteered that the student was "white and obviously young or college age." Dr. Cynthia responded that she had not asked for that information, but Dr. Slim snapped, "Oh, I knew it was coming. I told you I do not grade arbitrarily, and in my 20 years of teaching no one has ever accused me of being partial." He further stated, "This is a simple accusation, and I feel as though I am being attacked. Why don't you investigate her as you are investigating me?" Dr. Cynthia tried to indicate calmly that she was simply following normal procedures after a complaint is filed and that she was sorry it was causing him anxiety. She tried to reassure Dr. Slim that her role was to determine the validity of a case fairly and that was what she was doing.

Ultimately, Dr. Cynthia found no evidence of arbitrary grading. She decided not to pursue the student's claim of age discrimination for lack of evidence, and she informed both parties of her decision. She did inform the student of the way that the student could continue to press the charge and also shared her professional assessment that student there was no objective evidence for age discrimination. She met with Dr. Slim and, because he said again that he was not at all happy with the process to which he had been subjected, she specifically cautioned him against taking any action that could be viewed as retaliating against the student because doing so would be a violation of both the law and the university's policies. The matter ended there.

This leads to the third and fourth questions: What do you think about the process and procedures that the Equal Employment Opportunity Commission (EEOC) representative (Dr. Cynthia) followed? Do you think you would have benefited from having a faculty ombudsman? Dr. Slim was convinced that the EEOC process was antifaculty. Although the procedures are designed to be fair to all parties, Dr. Slim thought he would have been in a stronger position if there had been a faculty advocate for him. However, his employing university did not have a dedicated faculty ombudsman but rather one who heard cases from faculty, students, and staff. Dr. Slim was more than convinced that his faculty interests were indeed threatened by simple innuendo or indiscriminant charges from students. Despite escaping the incident unscathed, he still felt a sense of vulnerability that he had not experienced before, and he was uneasy about it.

Relevant Legal Case

Anhalt v. Cardinal Stritch University, No. 04-C-1052, 2006 WL 3692631 (E.D. Wis. Dec. 12, 2006)

The plaintiff Dr. Edward Anhalt had been teaching at Cardinal Stritch University in 1985 as an adjunct professor in the night division of the College of Business, a small private college in Wisconsin. His academic credentials included a master's of science degree in education from the University of Wisconsin–Milwaukee, a doctoral degree in education from Rutgers University in 1978, and several postdoctorate courses at Lehigh University in 1978 and 1979.

In the spring of 2002, a new dean was hired to help prepare the College of Business for the reaccreditation of the university. As part of this process, it was important that faculty credentials be reviewed and that a determination be made that all courses were being taught by faculty with the required credentials. The review pointed out that (1) Dr. Anhalt's doctorate was in education and not in business, (2) he was not working specifically in the field he was teaching, and (3) he did not have 18 graduate credits in the field he was teaching. As a result, his contract was not renewed for adjunct teaching in the College of Business. Instead, he was offered the opportunity to teach two marketing courses in the College of Arts and Sciences.

In preparing for this new teaching assignment (and being unfamiliar with this new college's procedures for ordering books), Dr. Anhalt failed to comply with a policy to have students purchase their books from the university bookstore. Instead he chose to use the process of book ordering as a marketing lesson and had the students purchase their required books through him (he wanted them to differentiate between wholesale and retail pricing). Soon students began calling the financial aid office to have checks issued to Dr. Anhalt to pay for their books. Hearing about this, Dr. Anhalt's supervisor (Ms. Karen Walrath) ordered him to cease this procedure. However, he did not discontinue the procedure, and there continued to be more student requests for checks made to the financial aid office. Ms. Walrath subsequently terminated Dr. Anhalt for violation of the book-ordering policy, but he was allowed to finish teaching his two courses. Upon termination, Dr. Anhalt filed suit in federal court alleging that he was 56 years old and had been fired in violation of the Age and Discrimination Employment Act. The court, however, ruled he had not been fired on the basis of age but for failure to follow the university book-ordering policy.

Summary

Although this chapter has discussed faculty members who are charged with discrimination or who claim they have been discriminated against, the important point is that discrimination may take many forms. Discrimination is illegal if the basis is race, color, religion, national origin, sex, age, disability, and, in some jurisdictions, sexual orientation. Although the nursing case involved allegations of age discrimination by a professor toward a student, the case could have easily been a professor who was not hired or perhaps not promoted for factors a professor might have alleged were discriminatory. Discrimination can be intentional or unintentional—the intention of the actor is not important—because in either case it is harmful and may be unlawful (Rooth, 2007).

In the nursing case introducing this chapter, an accused professor felt much maligned by charges of age discrimination. He felt particularly vulnerable being accused of illegal behavior and came away from the experience wishing he had had a faculty advocate protecting his interests and those of the faculty in general. You should consider his reaction to be the common one: no one likes being accused. Discrimination at its worst is antithetical to the respect and focus on merit that are the hallmark of academia. It violates the promise of the Declaration of Independence (1776), which states "that all men are created equal, that they are endowed by their Creator with certain unalienable Rights, that among these are Life, Liberty, and the Pursuit of Happiness...."

CRITICAL ELEMENTS TO CONSIDER

- Detailed and specific documentation of any alleged act of discrimination are needed. Feelings of hurt and offense can be met only by objective data.

Continued

CRITICAL ELEMENTS TO CONSIDER—cont'd

- Confidentiality when dealing with these issues is critical. Keep the grievance from being overly public or gossipy, especially during the resolution process.
- Illegal discrimination can be intentional or unintentional; it is not the actor's motivation but the effect on the victim that is the law's concern.
- You should be very familiar with all policies within the university that deal with discrimination, how it should be reported, and how reports are handled.
- Legal procedures even within the university setting may take time.

(HELPFUL RESOURCES

- American Association of University Women
  http://www.aauw.org/
- American Civil Rights Association
  http://www.aclu.org/
- American Disabilities Act
  http://www.ada.gov/pubs/ada.htm
- Equal Employment Opportunity Commission (EEOC)
  http://www.eeoc.gov/
- Human Rights Campaign
  http://www.hrc.org/
- National Association for the Advancement NAACP
  http://www.naacp.org/content/main/

References

Americans with Disabilities Act of 1990 (ADA), 42 U.S.C. §§ 12101-12213 (2000). Retrieved December 20, 2010, from http://www.ada.gov/pubs/adastatute08mark.htm#12102

Barrow, B. (2010, October 6). Lilly Ledbetter, women's equal pay activist, tells Tulane audiences the fight is worth it. *nola.com.* Retrieved March 24, 2011, from http://www.nola.com/news/index.ssf/2010/10/lilly_ledbetter_womens_equal_p.html

Bolick, C. (1987). The Age Discrimination in Employment Act: Equal opportunity or reverse discrimination? *Cato Institute Cato Policy Analysis, 82.* Retrieved December 20, 2010, from http://www.cato.org/pubs/pas/pa082.html

Brunner, B. (2007). The wage gap: A history of pay inequity and the Equal Pay Act. Infoplease.com. Retrieved December 19, 2010, from http://www.infoplease.com/spot/equalpayact1.html

Chapman, R. D. (2002). Avoiding the "Bermuda Triangle": Navigating the ADA, FMLA and workers' comp void. *Compensation Benefits Review, 34*(3), 58–67.

Corning Glass Works v. Brennan, 417 U.S. 188 (1974).

Fisher, J. (2007). Reconciling the Family Medical Leave Act with overlapping or conflicting state leave laws. *Compensation & Benefits Review, 39*(5), 4–5.

Golden, H., Hinkle, S., & Crosby, F. (2001). Reactions to affirmative action: Substance and semantics. *Journal of Applied Social Psychology, 31*(1), 73–88.

Haney López, I. (2006). *White by law: The legal construction of race* (10th anniversary ed.). New York: New York University Press.

Martucci, W. C., & Coverdale, B. N. (2004). California's new paid family leave law may start a trend. *Employee Relations Today, 30*(4), 79–87.

National Constitution Center. (n.d.). *The Constitution of the United States.* Philadelphia: Author.

Rooth, D. (2007). *Implicit discrimination in hiring: Real world evidence* (IZA Discussion Paper No. 2764). Available at SSRN: http://ssrn.com/abstract=984432

Schultz v. Wheaton Glass Co., 421 F.2d 259 (3rd Cir. 1970).

Smith, M. E., & Dreher, H. M. (2003).Wanted, nursing faculty! If you think the nursing shortage is bad, the nursing faculty shortage is worse. *Advance for Nursing, 5,* 31–32.

Stoddard, M. A. (2006). *An analysis of the United States Supreme Court and the United States Courts of Appeals decisions on the Family and Medical Leave Act of 1993: Their interpretations of the act as a tool for proper implementation of the act by employers.* Unpublished doctoral dissertation, Spalding University. Retrieved March 17, 2011, from http://proquest.umi.com/pqdlink?Ver=1&Exp=03-15-2016&FMT=7&DID=1068278971&RQT=309&attempt=1&cfc=1

Williams, J. C., & Richardson, V. T. (2010). *New millennium, same glass ceiling? The impact on law firm compensation systems on women. A joint report of the Project for Attorney Retention, Minority Corporate Counsel Association.* Retrieved from December 19, 2010, from http://www.pardc.org/Publications/SameGlassCeiling.pdf

CHAPTER 17

Confronting Academic Honesty Among Students

CASE STUDY
Academic Dishonesty

Your role: You are Dr. Lois Morgan, a faculty member for the Community/Public Health Undergraduate Nursing course.

You teach two sections of an undergraduate community/public health nursing course. Maura O'Brien, a student, tells you that four students cheated on the exam. One student took pictures of the exam with her mobile phone and sent the exam questions to her four friends in the afternoon section. Ms. O'Brien, the student who reported the academic dishonesty violation, asks not to be identified because she is afraid of retribution. You check the four students' grades and note that they have achieved a much higher score on this exam than they had on the previous one.

Questions

- How would you proceed?
- Do you have sufficient evidence for an academic dishonesty violation? What other information would you need?
- Do you need the student who reported the academic honesty violation to testify at the student conduct committee hearing?

Academic Dishonesty: Legal Principles and Review of the Literature

"Academic dishonesty" is a relatively simple term that covers a very wide variety of offenses against the spirit and substance of academia. It can include cheating, collusion, fabrication, false information or misrepresentation, falsification, forgery, plagiarism, and any type of fraudulent academic misconduct. It includes intellectual property theft of published or unpublished materials (Lindsay, 2005; McCabe and Trevino, 1993). Technology has provided more efficient, highly sophisticated and complex methods for cheating, thus facilitating academic misconduct

(Kolanko et al., 2006). But "academic dishonesty" is not limited to intentional misconduct: it also includes less serious errors, even "innocent mistakes" such as failing to give someone credit for an idea or for assistance in writing an article; failing to note where an image, a table, or other data came from; or backdating a work that is entirely original. It's not about the actor's state of mind or intentions; it is only about the integrity of the act.

Academic dishonesty challenges faculty and institutions of higher education because it threatens the core value of the academy: the creation of knowledge. Whatever a person says or writes must be that person's own, unless it is building on or using someone else's idea as a springboard, in which case that other person's contribution must be noted. Any form of dishonesty to obtain a degree or certificate, or even to complete a homework assignment, constitutes a breach of the core value and compromises the integrity of the specific institution and the academic community at large. It is both an absolute and a "slippery slope."

There is a very important social purpose at work here. Universities certify personal achievement and ability. The public relies on those certifications. As a result, universities have a responsibility to the public to ensure that individuals who receive educational credentials from their institutions have met the established criteria and standards to deal with the complexities and challenges in the subject area for which they are credentialed. Awarding a degree to someone who has not earned it and does not deserve it will allow that person to misrepresent his or her abilities to an unsuspecting public, in essence allowing fraud to be perpetuated on innocent consumers. That's why the rule is so strict and the student's intention not an issue: the purpose is to protect the public (and the institution). That is all the more important in areas such as health care, where mistakes can cause severe, long-lasting, and often permanent harm to people.

In an effort to eliminate academic dishonesty, institutions of higher education typically have policies that explain the core values of academia, specify the forbidden deviations, and make it easy to punish students who cross the lines. But what happens when individual teachers "take pity" on a transgressing student and do not act in accordance with the university code? Because academia is a community in which all expect to be (and should be) treated the same, the uneven or ineffective execution of honor codes may result in litigation against the university and its faculty when they are applied according to their terms. It is therefore imperative that universities pay attention to laws relevant to academic misconduct codes when designing institutional policies and executing disciplinary actions against students who violate those policies.

Nursing faculty must be diligent in holding nursing students accountable to higher standards of integrity because empiric findings suggest that nursing students who cheat are more likely to fall short in meeting professional standards or, at worst, place the health and safety of their patients at risk (Schmitz and Schaffer,

1995). Bavier (2009) underscored the need for nursing faculty to view academic dishonesty among nursing students as a matter of life and death because cheating on the part of a nurse can result in the demise of human life. The implications of cheating should prompt nursing faculty to accept their legal and ethical responsibilities as the gatekeepers of the profession very seriously. Strategies to curtail cheating include taking proactive steps to prevent academic dishonesty, teaching and applying ethical standards, acting quickly and with serious purpose to address transgressions, and imposing appropriate sanctions to hold students accountable for acts of academic misconduct.

Discussion of Case

In this chapter's case study, the student who reported the act of academic misconduct (Maura O'Brien) was counseled to consider what she would do as a professional nurse if she observed unethical behavior, such as diverting narcotics, wrongly noting a chart, or abusing a patient. Ms. O'Brien was in her fourth year of study in the undergraduate nursing program and recognized the seriousness of the cheating her classmates had done, and so agreed to be a witness in the student conduct and/or judicial board hearing if necessary. Dr. Morgan reviewed the item analysis of the exam and found that the four students O'Brien alleged to have participated in the mobile phone cheating episode had the same wrong answers, and three of the four had performed significantly better on the final exam than they had on the midterm exam. Dr. Morgan then requested an appointment with each individual student, made them aware of the allegations, and gave each student an opportunity to be heard.

If Maura O'Brien had not come forward, the university would not have known of the cheating or been able to investigate it; had O'Brien not been willing to testify in formal proceedings, then Dr. Morgan might not have been able to successfully press charges because she would not have had a witness to what had transpired unless one or more of the cheating students confessed. It is possible that the university could obtain the students' phone records, but this process guarantees delay, costs, and substantial time investments. Dr. Morgan could also formally charge the students, make them attend a disciplinary hearing, confront them with the test results, and make them testify (perhaps lie) in public. How far is the university willing to go?

⚖ WHEN TO CONSULT THE UNIVERSITY COUNSEL

Consult the university counsel in the development and management of academic honesty policies.

Findings and Disposition

One of the students confessed in the meeting and admitted to receiving a picture of the community/public health exam questions via her friend's mobile phone, and the student named the other students involved in the cheating incident. All four students received a grade of zero for the final examination and were required to repeat the class the following year, thus delaying their graduation. The faculty member was counseled for offering the exact examination to two different class sections in the same semester.

 PREVENTION TIPS

To prevent cheating during a test, faculty members can do the following:

- Offer different course examinations to different sections.
- Prohibit cell phones and personal items from the testing area.
- Require academic honesty tutorial early in the student's academic program.
- Require that students sign an academic honesty statement for each examination (Fig. 17.1).
- Assign seats to students during the test.

Intellectual Honesty Certification

All nursing students, both undergraduate and graduate, are now required to attach the following signed statement to every paper they submit in every nursing course they take. Papers that do not have this signed statement attached will not be graded.

I certify that:

- *This paper is entirely my own work, without any words and/or ideas from other sources (print, Web, other media, other individuals, or groups) being properly indicated (words with quotation marks), cited in text, and referenced. I have not submitted this paper to satisfy the requirements of any other course.*

Student's Signature_____

Date_____

Figure 17.1 Sample of an intellectual honesty certification.

Relevant Legal Cases

Matthew Coster v. Cristina Duquette, AC 30601 (Conn. Super. Ct. 2008).

Nancy Jones v. The Board of Governors of the University of North Carolina, 704 F.2d 713 (W.D. N.C. 1983).

Academic honesty and fairness are core values in the university setting. Although public safety is a core public value, courts will not allow university administrators to rush to judgment in punishing students for cheating unless the record proves that there was in fact cheating. Very few cases of academic dishonesty ever get to court, and even fewer get to the point in court at which a judge issues an opinion; however, in those cases, the courts have made it clear that universities must not rush to judgment when they seek to protect the core value of academic integrity. Two reported cases show how the problem can develop.

In the case of *Nancy Jones v. The Board of Governors of the University of North Carolina*, a nursing student was accused of cheating on an exam. The dean was very upset by the charges and pushed hard for punishment. The student judicial court found the student guilty, largely because of the pressure they received from the dean. The student appealed this decision by filing a Section 1983 lawsuit for the violation of her civil rights in U.S. District Court, arguing that the state of North Carolina had deprived her of property without due process of law. The judge found that there had been substantial procedural flaws in how the university had handled the charges, including the facts that the student had not been told the identity of her accusers, or what the evidence against her was, or even the specific charges against her. Holding that the "balance of hardship" favored the student and ordered her immediate reinstatement pending the final resolution of her case, the judge also held that the chancellor denied the student due process of law by unilaterally imposing punishment without complying with any established procedures. The court's decision was affirmed by the U.S. Court of Appeals when the university took the appeal. The student was not only allowed to complete her course, but was vindicated at a fair hearing and was awarded her degree; the university was forced to pay all of the attorneys' fees and costs of the trial, as well as pay damages to the student for having mistreated her.

The case of *Matthew Coster v. Cristina Duquette* highlights the fact that university internal review boards sometimes get it wrong and underlines that fact that universities need to proceed with care, especially when imposing severe sanctions. Mr. Coster and Ms. Duquette were classmates in a course taught by Dr. Moss at Central Connecticut State University. The final exam was a paper about the holocaust, and students were to place their completed papers in Dr. Moss's mailbox. Dr. Moss concluded that approximately 80 percent of the papers submitted by

Mr. Coster and Ms. Duquette were similar. Professor Moss then met with both students about the similarities, and each denied plagiarizing anyone else's work. Believing Ms. Duquette to be the more able student, he then filed a charge of academic misconduct against Mr. Coster. A detailed comparison of the writing style, grammar, and references used in both papers confirmed the professor's charge of plagiarism, and the university accepted the professor's assignment of fault, charging Mr. Coster with stealing Ms. Duquette's paper from Professor Moss's mailbox, copying it, and then lying to Dr. Moss at the meeting.

A student judicial hearing was held before a three-person panel, which found Mr. Coster guilty of academic dishonesty and recommended expulsion from the university. Mr. Coster appealed the panel's decision to the director of student affairs, who denied the appeal.

Mr. Coster did not appeal the university's decision to the courts. Instead, he filed a civil lawsuit against Ms. Duquette, alleging that she in fact had copied his paper. As part of the litigation, experts were hired and used to examine the electronic evidence of when documents were created and worked on; other documents were produced that supported Mr. Coster's claim that he had in fact worked on the paper. Negative inferences were drawn against Ms. Duquette because she was not able to do the same. On the basis of the evidence submitted, the trial court decided that Ms. Duquette, not Mr. Coster, had cheated, held her liable for conversion, and awarded compensatory and punitive damages against her. Ms. Duquette appealed the decision to the court of appeals, which affirmed the trial judge's decision.

Summary

Empiric findings have identified that contextual factors influence the amount of academic dishonesty that occurs in universities (McCabe and Trevino, 1993). For example, students are less likely to violate academic codes in an environment in which the institution creates a climate that is supportive of academic integrity and has requisite codes and polices in place that affirm those principles. In addition, faculty members need to implement and employ such codes and policies and hold students accountable when there is academic dishonesty. It is imperative that faculty prevent academic misconduct/dishonesty in a proactive manner rather than address academic misconduct in a reactive manner—for example, by discussing the importance of doing one's own work, by making students read and sign an integrity code at the beginning of a course, and by requiring students to sign an integrity warranty whenever they submit a paper or take a test. Detailed policies related to proctoring, academic honesty, and the testing environments will assist with the deterrence of academic misconduct, as will publication of what penalties the student will receive whenever an act of academic dishonesty is discovered. In the event of an academic misconduct charge, the faculty needs to follow the institution's policy while being fair to the students involved (Fig. 17.2).

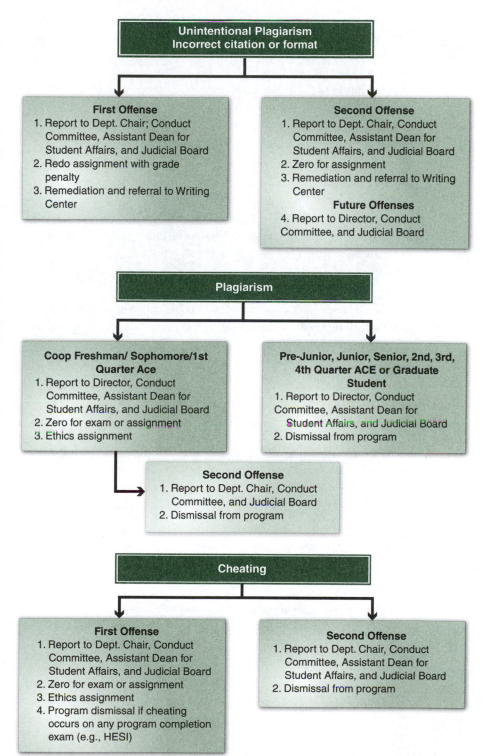

Figure 17.2 Sample academic dishonesty procedure flowchart.
Developed by the Drexel University Nursing Student Conduct Committee, 2008.

CRITICAL ELEMENTS TO CONSIDER

- Develop an academic integrity policy.
- Develop a testing/proctoring policy for faculty.
- Develop a testing policy for students.
- Have students complete an academic honesty online tutorial early in their academic program.
- Consider the use of a software program to detect plagiarism.
- If you are an academic administrator, hold faculty development sessions related to managing and documenting acts of academic dishonesty.
- Provide the student with due process.
- Develop a rubric on how to manage specific academic dishonesty violations so that students are dealt with consistently and fairly in terms of sanctions.
- Establish a student conduct committee to investigate cases of academic dishonesty.
- Develop a test review policy that would include the academic program's position on audiotaping test review, note taking, test question appeal process, and the like.

References

Bavier, A. R. (2009). Holding students accountable when integrity is challenged. *Nursing Education Perspectives, 30*(1), 5–5.

Kolanko, K. M., Clark, C., Heinrich, K. T., et al. (2006). Academic dishonesty, bullying, incivility, and violence: Difficult challenges facing nurse educators. *Nursing Education Perspectives 27*(1), 34–43.

Lindsay, C. L., III. (2005). *The college student's guide to the law.* Dallas, TX: Taylor Trade Publishing.

Matthew Coster v. Cristina Duquette, AC 30601 (Conn. Super. Ct. 2008).

McCabe, D. L., & Trevino, L. K. (1993). Academic dishonesty: Honor codes and other contextual influences. *Journal of Higher Education, 64*(5), 522–538.

Nancy Jones v. The Board of Governors of the University of North Carolina, 704 F.2d 713 (W.D. N.C. 1983).

Schmitz, K., & Schaffer, M. (1995). Ethical problems encountered in the teaching of nursing: Student and faculty perceptions. *Journal of Nursing Education, 34*(1), 42–44.

CHAPTER 18

Confronting Academic Honesty Among Faculty

CASE STUDY

Confronting Academic Dishonesty/Misconduct Among Faculty

Your role: You are the associate dean for research.

Dr. Maura O'Neill, associate dean for academic affairs, appears at your office door and is very upset. Several of the nursing faculty sent her a recent journal article written by Dr. Joan Starski, director of undergraduate nursing programs, regarding the innovative faculty development series at your institution. She claims that Dr. Starski has taken credit for what she in fact had created.

Dr. O'Neill claims that she designed and implemented the faculty development series while she was director of undergraduate nursing programs, and she administered the series for the first five years. Dr. Starski attended some of those sessions. When Dr. O'Neill was promoted to associate dean three years ago, Dr. Starski was promoted to director of undergraduate nursing. She was one of the department's rising stars then and will soon be considered for tenure. Over the past three years, she made some minor changes to the faculty development series, including adding a workshop called "Integrating Scholarship Into Your Professional Life," but Dr. O'Neill continued to have close oversight of the series even when it was under the direct authority of Dr. Starski.

You listen to Dr. O'Neill's concerns and read the journal article. In the article, Dr. Starski takes full credit for the development of the faculty development series and does not mention that the faculty development series is the original work of Dr. O'Neill. Dr. O'Neill does not want to meet with Dr. Starski to address her concerns without another administrator present because Dr. Starski reports to her.

Questions

- As associate dean of research, how would you proceed?
- Whom would you consult for advice?
- Are there university policies related to faculty academic misconduct?
- Does Dr. O'Neill have a legitimate claim against Dr. Starski?

Faculty Academic Misconduct: Legal Principles and Review of the Literature

There are few charges of misconduct that carry with them greater emotion than academic dishonesty, and probably none is more offensive than one brought against a member of the faculty. Cheating by students (covered in Chapter 17) is serious, but they are often new to the academy and always just passing through it; the faculty, by contrast, are its permanent residents. They are not only the guardians of the principle of integrity but have pledged themselves to the community's purpose of exploring new realms and creating new knowledge.

The American Association of University Professors (AAUP) has expressed this "core value" of the academy in its *Statement on Professional Ethics* (2009b). In this passage, it speaks of the "special relationship" that teachers owe to their community:

> *Professors, guided by a deep conviction of the worth and dignity of the advancement of knowledge, recognize the special responsibilities placed upon them. Their primary responsibility to their subject is to seek and to state the truth as they see it. To this end professors devote their energies to developing and improving their scholarly competence. They accept the obligation to exercise critical self-discipline and judgment in using, extending, and transmitting knowledge. They practice intellectual honesty. Although professors may follow subsidiary interests, these interests must never seriously hamper or compromise their freedom of inquiry.*

Regardless of whether a university subscribes to the AAUP, this statement or something like it is important to include in faculty handbooks because it expresses expectations to which faculty should be accountable. There are many ways that faculty can breach these core values. They range from the relatively innocent (e.g., allowing their name to be added to a publication to which they did not contribute), to the negligent (e.g., unintentionally using someone else's work without attribution), to the intentional (e.g., making up data to support a finding, idea, or claim). They are complicated by a variety of factors: the unique environment that makes everyone colleagues, where criticisms of ideas are welcome but not personal attacks; a permanent hierarchy that awards rank and title (and endowed chairs) for achievement, the recognition that comes from receiving substantial research grants and achieving substantial publications; and having centers, doctoral students, or research associates.

In this environment, it is difficult to assert charges, difficult to investigate and review them, and difficult to sanction misconduct when it is found. Sadly, it is probably important these days to have a statement that defines what constitutes academic misconduct and to specify that intention is not relevant to determine whether it has occurred (although it might affect the sanction imposed). This constitutes specific notice of the bad acts and removes the claim of unfairness when a member of the faculty is called to account for misconduct. There is a risk, however: creativity and technology will always produce new ways of pushing the integrity envelope, and absence from a list might be used to prove that it was not intended to be included.

After addressing the types of misconduct for which discipline may be imposed, the university needs to address the process that will be used to determine when a faculty member's conduct meets the definition of misconduct. There must first be an avenue by which someone can report the allegation that guarantees not only safety to the reporter but integrity in the response. The faculty handbooks should therefore specify the person to whom allegations of impropriety should be addressed (e.g., provost, dean, director of research) and how (oral, in writing); guarantee that the identity of the reporter will be kept confidential, and will be protected from retaliation of any kind; and specify the process that will be used to consider the allegation.

Many codes begin with the formal process—the due process that must be followed. But there are several ways that such allegations can be resolved before they become too formal. The first is the investigation that must be made initially to determine if there is reason to invoke the formal process. If the facts are just wrong, then the inquiry can be ended quickly. The facts could also be so clear, and admitted by the transgressor, that an "amicable" resolution (settlement) can be achieved. Mediation is discussed in Chapter 3. The risk here is that the power relationships among the actors (transgressors, reporter, and evaluator) can produce a result that if not regarded as fair or adequate, the integrity of the process can be called into question. Moreover, if the evaluator herself attempts to resolve the complaint and does not succeed, then she must recuse herself from the process thereafter, lest the claim be made that she prejudged the result and corrupted the process.

These are the steps that the university should follow to formally evaluate claims of academic dishonesty by members of the faculty:

1. Notice of the alleged misconduct
2. Opportunity to respond to the charges
3. Review by a faculty body of both the factual allegations and the proposed discipline
4. Progressive discipline, if appropriate to the seriousness of the misconduct
5. Opportunity for higher-level review of the fact-finding and the proposed sanction
6. On unionized campuses, participation by an advocate for the faculty member in hearings or other meetings (Euban and Lee, 2005)

They may, of course, be adjusted to fit the community. These are also just the bare bones of the process: there are very important decisions to be made within each step. For example, does the opportunity to respond include having an attorney participate? Can witnesses be forced to attend? Can the panel impose time limits? Does the hearing have to be set at a time convenient for the respondent? Does it

have to be recorded, or minutes kept at all? Does the panel decide on the punishment, or is it recommended to them by others? If there is a right to appeal, to
whom does it go, and what is the scope of review—plenary (ab initio) or limited
(abuse of discretion)? These are areas in which lawyers and judges will spend
much of their time arguing. If the components of the process itself are delineated
specifically, then the greater the confidence all parties will have when entering
into it, knowing how to conduct themselves—and the greater the deference a
court will give to the result.

WHEN TO CONSULT THE UNIVERSITY COUNSEL

Consult the university counsel when you are creating policies regarding
faculty misconduct. If a faculty member is accused of misconduct, then
consult the university attorney and the office of research for
guidance.

The six steps outlined above are designed to satisfy three essential purposes.
First, they exist to make sure that the university does its best to determine the true
facts of the situation and gives the university its best opportunity to rectify the situation according to its overriding principles. Second, they provide protections to
the individuals who are involved in the process (the complainant and respondent
alike) to reduce the opportunities for arbitrary action and ensure action on the
merits of the case. Third, they permit the community as a whole to determine
what the appropriate sanction is for the bad behavior—a jury of peers, as it were—
allowing the expression of condemnation in the one case to be a reminder to the
community of what is expected. In this way, the process protects the interests of
all of the elements in the academy. This is the fullest sense of what is meant by the
term *due process*. For more on due process with regard to faculty, see Chapter 8.

By its terms, due process responds to the situation, providing the process that
is due in that context. Not all alleged violations will require the same process;
some, in fact, may deserve no process at all (such as a dean's decision not to award
a merit pay increase, to withdraw financial support from a project, or to move a
faculty member to a smaller office); however, deviations from the norm ought to
be understandable and acceptable to the community.

In 1971, a special joint subcommittee of the AAUP considered the question
of sanctions short of dismissal, and enumerated the following lesser sanctions: (1)
oral reprimand, (2) written reprimand, (3) a recorded reprimand, (4) restitution
(e.g., payment for damage due to individuals or to the institution), (5) loss of
prospective benefits for a stated period (e.g., suspension of regular or merit increase in salary or suspension of promotion eligibility), (6) a fine, (7) reduction
in salary for a stated period, and (8) suspension from service for a stated period,

without other prejudice (AAUP, 1970; AAUP, 1971). The AAUP's *Recommended Institutional Regulations on Academic Freedom and Tenure* (RIR) distinguishes between major and minor sanctions, categorizing suspension as major and reprimand as minor.

The AAUP *Recommended Institutional Regulations* provide that major sanctions should not be imposed until after a hearing in which the same procedures apply as in a dismissal case, which include written notice of the charges, a hearing before a faculty committee in which the administration bears the burden of proof, right to counsel, cross-examination of adverse witnesses, a record of the hearing, and a written decision. Regulation 5(c) of the Association's *Recommended Institutional Regulations* states that the administration, before suspending a faculty member, will consult with an appropriate faculty committee concerning the "propriety, the length, and other conditions of the suspension" (AAUP, 2009a). The AAUP further provides that an institution may impose a minor sanction after providing the individual notice and that the individual professor has the right to seek review by a faculty committee if he or she feels that a sanction was unjustly imposed (AAUP, 2009a).

In some instances, progressive discipline is warranted. Universities may consider using discipline short of termination when dealing with a faculty member who has a history of insubordination; inappropriate behavior; or neglect of teaching, research, or service obligations. Using progressive discipline establishes a record of the faculty member's misconduct and the institution's response to the misconduct. In the event that a later decision is made to terminate a tenured faculty member, the university will have a record of progressive discipline—which makes the ultimate sanction look fair to everyone in the community. With that said, universities that have tolerated faculty misconduct for an extended period of time may find it difficult to persuade a court of law that the faculty member's due process rights were protected if misconduct that was tolerated for years suddenly becomes grounds for termination; similarly, it will not look fair if a professor is punished for conduct that had never been punished before and has been exhibited by others in the faculty (even in other colleges, or at other ranks). Prompt, progressive discipline is recommended, as it is also fair to the person involved: it may have the positive outcome of rehabilitating a problematic faculty member, or may lay the groundwork for an eventual termination. In either case, providing intervention before the misconduct escalates into a serious problem for the university is recommended (Euban and Lee, 2005).

There is no requirement that all faculty have the same due process rights. Adjunct or auxiliary faculty are different from tenure-track faculty and are different from tenured faculty. There may be good reasons to distinguish among them in determining the process due. The common right, though, is for the process (and the rights and obligations attendant thereto) to be specified. For example, nontenured or contract faculty are hired only for a distinct period of time and can be given a nonrenewal letter prior to the end of their contract without any process; however, if the review procedures do not differentiate among the types of faculty, the contract faculty could argue that they have the same due process rights. Some contracts require written notice of nonrenewal based on the faculty member's tenure/length of time at the university. Contract faculty ordinarily have a protected property right to continued employment during the life of their contract, and a concurrent right to due process protections if they are subject to dismissal during the period of their employment contract (Euban, 2004).

Discussion of Case

Before referring the faculty academic misconduct case to the university's office of research scientific conduct review committee for review and consideration, you and the dean meet with both faculty members individually. You request that Dr. O'Neill provide copies of the faculty development series that was used during her tenure as director of undergraduate programs when the series was developed. You and the dean compare the faculty development sessions to those mentioned in the article. You also meet with Dr. Starski and ask her to bring copies of the materials that she developed, asking her also to note those areas where she believes she was the originator.

WHEN TO CONSULT THE UNIVERSITY COUNSEL

Consult the university counsel when you are confronted with a new and/or difficult situation related to alleged faculty academic misconduct.

Findings and Disposition

In your meeting with Dr. O'Neill, it is clear that that the journal article authored by Dr. Starski is based on the work of Dr. O'Neill. The description in the journal article is almost identical to the faculty development series developed by Dr. O'Neill. The strong emphasis on mentorship and technology in the article are also the original work of Dr. O'Neill, yet Dr. O'Neill is never mentioned in the article. The article gives the impression that Dr. Starski developed the nursing faculty development series.

When you and the dean meet with Dr. Starski, she is angry and defensive and does not admit to any wrongdoing. She says that she never claimed in the article that she developed the curriculum, but notes that no one (including Dr. O'Neill) had ever written about the program, which she had spent 3 years leading, and no one had ever charted the series the way she did in the article. She speaks to the stress that she is under as a result of being an untenured faculty member who has been directing such an important program for 3 years ("I am the youngest director in this college"), at the very same time that she was being held responsible for generating refereed publications ("What else would you have me write about, if not this important area of faculty development?") and the need to submit her tenure dossier.

You inform Dr. Starski that you have made a complete file of your investigation, including the facts as you found them, and are referring this case to the university's office of research for review and consideration. Two days later, Dr. Starski submits her resignation from the faculty, effective at the end of the academic year. Dr. O'Neill chooses not to pursue an academic misconduct claim with the office of research. She does insist that an erratum be published by the journal citing that the article is based on her original work. Dr. Starski and the journal editor agree to the erratum. You believe that this resolution is fair to the faculty and to the academic community, because the published erratum and the voluntary resignation will send the appropriate message to the community. If Dr. Starski had not resigned, then the scientific conduct committee would have reviewed the case (including the file that you had developed), allowed Dr. Starski to be heard, and considered the imposition of sanctions, as appropriate.

PREVENTION TIPS

Faculty development sessions and faculty policies related to authorship should be available to faculty—addressing that authorship on a publication is usually given to those who are responsible for the intellectual content of a work.

Relevant Legal Case

Newman v. Burgin, 930 F.2d 955 (1st Cir. 1991)

In *Newman v. Burgin* (1991), Professor Anny Newman sought an injunction to preclude Chancellor Burgin and other officials of the University of Massachusetts from imposing sanctions on her for plagiarism. The facts of the case and the way it was handled provide an excellent example of how instances of academic misconduct among the faculty can be addressed.

Professor Newman published a thirteen-page article about a poem ("Suze sina razmetnoga") by a 17th-century Croatian poet, Franjin Gundulic. One of Professor Newman's colleagues in the UMass College of Arts and Sciences, Professor Diana Burgin, thought Newman might have copied parts of it from a 1952 book by Vsevolod Setschkareff. She brought her suspicions to the attention of the Russian department's faculty personnel committee. After translating relevant Setschkareff passages from the German, one of the committee's members (Professor Robert Spaethling) found many similar passages in the book and Professor Newman's article and reported this to the faculty committee. With this finding of good cause to be concerned, the following process occurred:

a. The personnel committee notified the dean of the College of Arts and Sciences about their preliminary finding.

b. The dean called a meeting with Professor Newman, discussed the charge with her, and promised to take no action until he received her written response. She submitted her response to the dean.

c. The dean asked two Slavic-language scholars at other universities to review the article for plagiarism. After doing so, one wrote back that the article contained "exemplary instances of plagiarism." The other said that the work was "indebted to Dr. Setschkareff's major work considerably more than formally acknowledged," but that it would be difficult to show "conscious, deliberate and outright plagiarism," as the author might have suffered simply from "lapses in awareness."

d. The dean asked Professor Newman if she wished to respond. She did not do so.

e. The dean appointed a special committee of senior Arts and Sciences faculty (the "Knight Committee," after its chairman) to investigate the matter formally, making findings and recommend appropriate responses. Professor Newman was permitted to challenge for cause the appointment of any of the committee members. It permitted her to present evidence, to call witnesses, to cross-examine witnesses, and to bring a colleague to help her. Professor Newman submitted letters from six outside scholars of her choice, all of whom concluded that she did not plagiarize.

f. The Knight Committee submitted its report to the dean. It found that Newman had had no "conscious intent to deceive," but that her scholarship had been "negligent" and contained "an objective instance of plagiarism." It recommended "censure" and "no further action."

g. The dean recommended to the university provost that the university "censure" Professor Newman, in essence, by adopting and making public the Knight Committee's findings, and by barring her from participating on certain academic committees (or holding administrative office) for five years. The dean asked Professor Newman to respond.

h. The provost adopted the dean's recommendations and repeated them to the chancellor. Professor Newman repeated her side of the story to the chancellor.

i. The chancellor then adopted, and ordered implemented, the provost's recommendations.

j. Professor Newman filed a lawsuit against the chancellor and the other officials, asking the court among other things to issue an order stopping (enjoining) the implementation of the sanctions.

The basic legal question that the judge had to face is whether the record permits a finding that the university (1) deprived Professor Newman of life, liberty, or property (2) without due process of law. The brief description of that process above shows that, at each stage of the proceedings, the university afforded Professor Newman an opportunity to present her side of the story; it also permitted her to challenge decision-makers for bias, to call witnesses, to see and to criticize the evidence against her, and to see and argue against all tentative recommendations before they became final. In short, the judge concluded that the university had provided Professor Newman with an impressive array of due process safeguards: notice of proposed action, a trial-type hearing in which she was given an opportunity to present proofs and arguments and to challenge the proofs and arguments of others, and a jury of neutral decision-makers who prepared written findings of fact and reasons for their decision. The court granted summary judgment to the university, and the finding was affirmed on appeal. Professor Newman was accordingly sanctioned formally by the university—which had been made far more visible as a result of all the litigation.

Summary

Cases of alleged academic misconduct by faculty must be investigated and resolved because the integrity of the university, its research processes, and ultimately its reputation are in jeopardy if such misconduct (real or perceived) is allowed to exist. "The review of case law, AAUP statements and other policy documents, institutional policies, and the literature on discipline suggests that stating the expected standards of conduct clearly, following the procedures for making decisions concerning faculty misconduct carefully, imposing a degree of discipline that is appropriate to the severity of the misconduct, and giving written justifications for recommendations or decisions made under the faculty handbook or other policies, are critical" (Euban and Lee, 2006, p. 308). Every faculty member is entitled to due process, in which they are given written documentation of their alleged misconduct and evidence supporting the allegation, the chance to refute the allegation, and a trial among neutral-minded peers. This due process also protects all members of the community. A proactive approach to faculty academic misconduct is recommended in the form of explicit policies and faculty development sessions.

CRITICAL ELEMENTS TO CONSIDER

- Universities should develop policies and procedures on scientific misconduct or academic fraud, including a definition of the conduct that must be avoided.

Continued

CRITICAL ELEMENTS TO CONSIDER—cont'd

- Disciplinary sanctions other than dismissal should be identified in the faculty handbook.
- Colleges/departments should review codes of conduct developed by professional associations to determine if they should be included in college/department policies.
- Review policies related to faculty academic misconduct on a consistent basis.
- Have an unbiased, objective committee review and consider the faculty academic misconduct case if consistent with your policy.
- Provide due process to all parties involved.
- Develop department/college authorship guidelines.
- Hold faculty development sessions related to authorship guidelines.

HELPFUL RESOURCES

Visit the American Association of University Professors (AAUP)'s Web site (http://www.aaup.org) for more policies and reports on professional academic conduct for faculty.

References

A v. C. College, 863 F. Supp. 156 (S.D.N.Y. 1994).

American Association of University Professors. (1970). 1940 statement of principles on academic freedom and tenure with 1970 interpretive comments. *Policy Documents and Reports.* Washington, DC: Author. Retrieved July 6, 2010, from http://www.aaup.org/AAUP/pubsres/policydocs/contents/1940statement.htm

American Association of University Professors. (1971). AAUP Joint Commission: Statement on procedural standards in the renewal or nonrenewal of faculty appointments. Retrieved July 6, 2010, from http://www.aaup.org/AAUP/pubsres/policydocs/contents/nonreapp-stmt.htm

American Association of University Professors. (2009a). *Recommended institutional regulations on academic freedom and tenure* (RIR). Retrieved July 6, 2010, from http://www.aaup.org/AAUP/pubsres/policydocs/contents/RIR.htm

American Association of University Professors. (2009b). *Statement on professional ethics.* Retrieved July 6, 2010, from http://www.aaup.org/AAUP/pubsres/policydocs/contents/statementon-professionalethics.htm

Euben, D. R. (2004). *Faculty termination & disciplinary issues.* Paper presented at the 14th annual Legal Issues in Higher Education conference, University of Vermont. Retrieved July 6, 2010, from http://www.aaup.org/AAUP/protect/legal/topics/term-discp.htm

Euban, D. R., & Lee, B. (2005). *Faculty misconduct and discipline.* Paper presented at the National Conference on Law and Higher Education, Stetson University College of Law. Retrieved July 6, 2010, from http://www.aaup.org/AAUP/protect/legal/topics/misconduct-discp.htm

Euban, D. R., & Lee, B. A. (2006). Faculty discipline: Legal & policy issues in dealing with faculty misconduct. *Journal of College & University Law, 32*(2), 241–308.

Newman v. Burgin, 930 F.2d 955 (1st Cir. 1991).

CHAPTER 19

Managing Student Incivility

Disruption in the Classroom

Your role: You are Dr. Advantage, the department chair of the undergraduate nursing program at a research-oriented state university.

One of your new faculty hires, tenure-track assistant professor Dr. Aranthez, is in your office practically in tears. She states that every week in her NURS 300 Pediatric Clinical Nursing course (a course offered in the third quarter of a second-degree BSN program for students who already have an undergraduate degree) Marcia Wolf, a student, persistently tries to find fault with her and does so very publically in front of the large class. Dr. Aranthez states that the student makes very vocal and harsh attempts to correct her if she says anything even slightly contrary to the textbook used in the course. Even when informed that she is putting the content into a contemporary practice context, the student just proclaims loudly that "all of us here want to know who to believe, you or the book, because we only want to get the answer right on NCLEX." Ms. Wolf's comments also appear to embolden the other students. Dr. Aranthez goes on to elaborate that she is trying to be patient with the student and that she is afraid to be too negative in class by correcting her. Further, she states that even if she took the student aside, she is certain the student would badmouth her to the other students and that this would affect her teaching evaluations. Moreover, because she is in a tenure-track position, Dr. Aranthez states that she knows she is under severe pressure to get good teaching evaluations and does not want to do anything that would risk her prospects for a positive tenure review. With three new classes to teach she states she is feeling very anxious about trying to do her best. As the department chair, you know Dr. Aranthez is not only a new PhD, but new to teaching as well and you also know that second-degree nursing students are perhaps the most demanding of all types of nursing students. You are sympathetic and want to help. Finally, Dr. Aranthez concludes her statements to you lamenting, "Maybe I shouldn't have told the class my first day that this was my first lecture as a professor. I was just trying to be honest with them."

Questions

- Is the student being uncivil?
- What further background information should Dr. Advantage seek as it relates to this situation? What do you recommend is the best way for her to regain control of her class and in particular manage the behavior of the uncivil student?
- Do you believe Dr. Aranthez's concerns about the impact of teaching evaluations on her tenure prospects are valid?
- What do you think is a reasonable faculty development program for a new faculty member like Dr. Aranthez?

Managing Student Incivility: Legal Principles and Review of the Literature

Incivility among college students is perhaps just one example of some of the general incivility seen in contemporary society. As Keating wrote in a 2008 article published in the *American Bar Association Journal,* "American society generally has moved away from an ethos in which manners are considered to be important in any endeavor" (p. 1).

Clark and Springer (2007) conducted a study of 36 nursing faculty and 467 associate and baccalaureate nursing students that examined both faculty and student incivility. They reported that in-class student incivility included "disruptions in class,...challenging professors regarding test scores in class, dominating class discussion, carrying on side conversations that disturb other students and sighing to express displeasure with assignments" (p. 25). Out-of-class student incivility included "discrediting faculty, complaining about faculty, and failing to use appropriate communication channels" (Clark and Springer, p. 25). Classroom behavior today is more difficult to manage than ever before. These behaviors, if they occur only rarely, are often fairly harmless and will cause little if any disruption in class or depress the morale of the faculty. But all too often, if these behaviors are not cut off when they first arise, they will spiral out of control if other students adopt or mimic these same behaviors both in and outside the classroom. Faculty members are often advised to ignore the first offense (unless it is blatantly disrespectful and would undermine the authority of the professor), but to intervene firmly and address a second offense privately. The literature has also documented that second-degree or accelerated nursing students have a demonstrable pattern of challenging professors in both the classroom and clinical setting, and this is likely a factor in this chapter's case study, because Dr. Aranthez did not complain of similar behaviors in her other classes (AACN, 2008; Blozen, 2010).

One question often asked is whether this rise in incivility is related to a new generation of students. In other words, is student incivility generational? Suplee et al. (2008) identify that different generational characteristics may contribute to a misunderstanding of expectations between both faculty and students. Johnson and Romanello (2005) have written a very widely quoted article that describes how each generation (see Table 19.1 for a broad list of the contemporary generations) has a distinct set of values, ideas, ethics, beliefs, and learning styles that affect not just students, but instructors as well. It may very well be that having a better perspective on some of the generational characteristics often seen in students (without absolute generalizing) may help faculty members as they teach different generations of students across baccalaureate, master's, and doctoral nursing programs.

Because most college freshmen and sophomores who predominate in 4-year undergraduate nursing programs were born around the early 1990s and are classified as Millennials, it is important to grasp how their development may lead to some of the disruptive or uncivil behaviors seen in the classroom. Frand (2000) first identified the Millennial behavior of "zero tolerance for delays," or what contemporary nursing faculty see as a generation of largely impatient students. This may be significant, particularly for nursing education, if a general tendency to be interpersonally impatient translates to student nurses or (graduates) who are impatient with their patients, particularly those who are chronically ill or older and infirm. This could be very detrimental to the delivery of ethical patient care, a requirement of the 2001 American Nurses Association (ANA) *Code of Ethics for Nurses with Interpretive Statements* (Dahnke, 2009).

Another characteristic highlighted by Delorey (2010) is that Millennials' work and learning styles are more often nonlinear. Growing up in their digitally oriented world, they generally have more respect for the rapid access to information than a deeper reliance on the very validity of the knowledge itself. This phenomenon is perhaps most striking in nursing students' research: they routinely cite Internet sites and Wikipedia entries in scholarly papers without real regard for the validity and accuracy of the information they are citing. This is not to say

Table 19.1 Generational Categories and Characteristics

GENERATION TYPE	YEAR SPAN	GENERAL CHARACTERISTICS
Baby Boomer (or Boomers)	1945–1954	Competitive, committed, independent, loyal
Generation Jones (or Jonesers)	1954–1965	Born with great expectations; disillusioned by coming of age in the 1960s and 1970s—a generational mixture of pragmatists and materialists). President Obama is a Joneser.
Generation X or (GenX-ers)	1965–1980	Self-reliant, resourceful, adaptable, cynical, distrusting of authority, desiring to be defined differently from parents
Generation Y (or Millennials)	1980–2000	Entitled, optimistic, civic minded, team oriented, structured, impatient (zero tolerance for delays), tech savvy, multitaskers

that students are prohibited from using these kinds of citations, as any scholar today has unique and rapid access to all kinds of information on the Web that was previously almost impossible to find. But it is the almost cavalier and lackadaisical use of them that is most problematic.[1] Moreover, we have heard from nursing faculty who have experienced countless numbers of uncivil student complaints about faculty grading that penalizes classroom writing assignments. These assignments sometimes appear to be not much more than Internet regurgitation and "cut and paste", which either borders on or consists of outright plagiarism.

The characteristic feeling of entitlement is perhaps the one characteristic that is the most bothersome and contributes to widespread incivility in the classroom. Alsop (2008) and others have labeled them "trophy kids." Alsop reports that researchers often label them "narcissistic, arrogant, and fickle" (p. vii), but he indicates in reality they have very valuable traits, including the following: (1) often being very socially and environmentally conscious; (2) wanting structure and direction while expecting flexibility in the work environment; and (3) although desiring individual praise and recognition, often being exceptional team players.

With many ADN nursing graduates now immediately returning for their BSN (increasingly without any or limited experience as an RN) to increase their employment prospects (usually because hospitals now commonly hire only BSNs), Millennials now seem to predominate in second-degree programs (American Association of Colleges of Nursing, 2010). Another trend is that brand-new college graduates (also largely Millennials) are immediately returning to college to pursue their second degree in health care—one of the sectors of the economy that has continued to grow during the recent global recession (U.S. Bureau of Labor Statistics, 2009). Nevertheless, many second-degree students (as in this chapter's case study) may be classified as GenX-ers: those born between 1965 and 1980.

According to Sherman (2006), the structure of the American family changed during the formative years of Generation X. This was the first generation in which both parents worked and divorce became more common. They came of age being exposed to massive corporate layoffs (the weak economies of presidents Ford, Carter, and Reagan), and this has led them to value self-reliance and work–life balance. Last, technology underwent major advances during their formative years and became integral to their lives (Sherman).

Swearingen (2004) indicates that because of the societal and economic turmoil in which GenX-ers came of age, they seek autonomy and independence.

---

[1] Although not the focus of this chapter, all students must be given criteria for the evaluation of Web resources for use in their scholarly classroom papers, and Cornell University Library has an excellent link: http://olinuris.library.cornell.edu/ref/research/webeval.html.

However, because their loyalty to an organization may not ensure their long-term employment, as a cohort (a much smaller group than both the Boomers and Millennials) they have become increasingly dissatisfied in the workforce and therefore may change jobs often. Kupperschmidt (1998) defined the following as the most predominant GenX-er characteristics:

- Self-absorbed
- Independent, industrious, and resourceful
- Value fun and balance in life
- Slow to commit long-term to relationships
- Extended adolescence—they remain in parents' homes and resist assuming adult roles
- Boomerang—they leave and return to parents' home for economic reasons
- They marry late to avoid commitment or divorce
- Pluralistic and comfortable with diverse cultures and lifestyles
- Materialistic—practical, seasoned consumers
- Creative, decisive problem solvers
- Flexible, adaptable, and comfortable with change
- Voracious learners
- Innovative risk takers and entrepreneurs
- Value quantity and quality time with significant adults
- Lack basic skills in reading, mathematics, and communication
- Have a cynical, pessimistic, practical, reality-driven worldview
- Have unrealistic expectations for quick solutions to adult problems.

As GenX-ers and Millennials make up the undergraduate population of nursing students (until the next Generation Z), it will be incumbent on nursing faculty to finds ways to educate and socialize them to be professional nursing caregivers who will care expertly for the patients and families who are diverse and who may have complex health needs. The successful nursing professor must make the uncivil classroom civil and also find a way to temper the uncivil student so these interpersonal behaviors observed in the educational setting do not infiltrate their professional careers and negatively affect their delivery of patient care.

Discussion of Case

Recall the first question in this chapter's case study, Is the student being uncivil to Dr. Aranthez? In this case, the student was certainly being uncivil to Dr. Aranthez, and it was because Dr. Aranthez did not immediately correct or counsel the student that she began to lose control of her classroom. What happened instead is that other students began to take their cues from Marcia Wolf and to mimic her behaviors. This "pile-on effect" is likely to occur if disruptive behaviors are not corrected immediately when they arise. Making it worse, Dr. Aranthez waited a long time to seek guidance from her department chair, Dr. Advantage. By this time the damage had been done, and it would be very difficult for Dr. Aranthez (at least in this class) to regain control of her classroom and regain her authority and respect.

Part of the problem is also the fault of the department chair. She knew from experience that second-degree students are perhaps the most difficult of all to teach. Even if she could not assign Dr. Aranthez a different course with another group of students, she should have at least prepared Dr. Aranthez better for this challenging group of students. Youssef and Goodrich (1996) identified that second-degree nursing students have much higher stress levels than do traditional students, and this may contribute to some of the acting-out behaviors so frequently seen in this student population. Further, was a three-course course load in her first quarter of teaching appropriate for a new tenure-track faculty member, especially at a research university where grantsmanship and scholarly expectations are very high? Further, what kind of faculty development did she receive overall to transition her into her new professorial role?

As posed in the second question, What further background information should Dr. Advantage seek as it relates to this situation? Dr. Advantage was not at all surprised that second-degree students were exhibiting these behaviors. She first considered whether a three-course teaching load in her first quarter was really appropriate for a new tenure-track faculty member, especially at a research university where expectations for winning grants and scholarship are very high. She also considered that Dr. Aranthez's faculty mentor was perhaps not the best for this situation. The senior faculty assigned to her was likely a good research mentor, but not at all experienced with undergraduate nursing education, much less mentoring someone to teach second-degree students. Dr. Advantage was also very curious about the quality of Dr. Aranthez's overall faculty development in her transition to her new professorial role and specifically what kind of course orientation she had been provided. Dr. Aranthez said the course coordinator just sent the syllabus around to all the course faculty but that there was no formal meeting of the faculty. She did indicate that the course coordinator had answered all her questions by e-mail, but in retrospect she admitted she was such a novice she did not know the right questions to ask. It was clear that the course coordinator never checked in with her. In short, the situation was very predictable, and the administration had contributed significantly to it.

Dr. Advantage sensed that Dr. Aranthez was very distraught over this ordeal, and she considered what would be the best course of action to recommend to her. She did not want to lose a highly promising faculty member in the first quarter of employment, particularly with the severe nursing faculty shortage in general and shortage of nursing faculty with a doctorate degree in particular (Smith, Glasgow, and Dreher, 2010).

⚖ **WHEN TO CONSULT THE UNIVERSITY ATTORNEY**

Your contact with the university attorney in these cases will generally be through your department chair or associate dean when legal advice is needed for dealing with uncivil students, interpreting a policy, or advising on procedural matters. Faculty safety issues are of paramount importance, and there should be little sympathy for nursing faculty administrators (at every level including dean) who do not take the welfare and safety of their faculty, staff, and students seriously or who dismiss real events as frivolous or believe the faculty to be overreacting. If the issues concern the student's academic freedom in the classroom rather than a violation of the student code of conduct, then getting an advisory opinion from the university attorney is always helpful

Findings and Disposition

The third question posed was, What do you recommend is the best way for Dr. Aranthez to regain control of her class and in particular manage the behavior of the uncivil student? Dr. Advantage thought the best way to address the issue was for Dr. Aranthez to confront the class as a whole because the problem had degenerated from incivility from one student to mimicking behaviors by others. Dr. Advantage instructed Dr. Aranthez to take 5 minutes before the first mid-class break and tell them that she has been bothered by some of the disruptive behaviors (and to list examples without referring to specific students) that she and others have observed in class and that she is no longer going to tolerate them. She should apologize for not addressing this earlier, and tell them that the situation has become so detrimental to the learning environment that she felt the need to establish new classroom etiquette rules,[2] which she is going to enforce. Dr. Advantage then said she should encourage them to make an appointment to see her individually if they had any questions or issues and then move on.

She also told Dr. Aranthez that it helps having this kind of discussion on the first day of any new course. If instances of uncivil conduct arise, she should approach them this way: (1) ignore the first instance of a behavior if it is not entirely uncivil and perhaps give the offending student a stare indicating displeasure

---

[2] In this case, in going forward she would require students to raise their hand and be called on before asking questions, and she would not take more than two questions from any one student during a class period to prevent anyone from dominating the discussion. She mentioned that if students had further questions, they should e-mail her. She also said that she would conduct her class with respect and civility on both sides. Last, if students persisted with loud side conversations, she would ask them to leave the classroom for a second offence during any single class period. If any student questioned her directives, she was to indicate that she had spoken to the department chair, who had fully endorsed these policies.

(nonverbal behavior can be used effectively sometimes, but certainly not always); and (2) take any offending student aside after class and address the issue personally. She further recommended that if the behavior continues, the student should be corrected civilly but sternly in class with comments such as "we need to move on" (for a student dominating the discussion repeatedly), with a reminder of the discussion that she had held with them the first day of class about civility, or "that comment isn't appropriate here in this classroom" (for uncivil comments) or even "I cannot continue class with such loud chatter that is obviously disrupting class for many of you who are here" (for excessive side conversations that do not cease with one verbal warning). Dr. Advantage said she was always willing to come to class and observe quietly to assist Dr. Aranthez with classroom management and ensure the classroom was safe and civil. She encouraged Dr. Advantage to let her know if the suggested strategies did not work, as she would immediately come to class to help her get things back on track.

Finally, the fourth question was, Do you believe Dr. Aranthez's concerns about the impact of teaching evaluations on her tenure prospects are valid? From our experience, these concerns are both real and reasonable, and therefore they are valid. At the same time, though, they are not an excuse not to enforce proper classroom management. If the classroom is disruptive, learning will not take place, and that is the central mission of any university or college. If the professor believes that enforcing proper classroom management policies (that are supported by the chair in this case) may incite some students to write negative comments on course evaluations, then the professor can document or explain any variances on her annual evaluation and include these in a tenure dossier, if necessary. This should not be problematic unless there is a pattern of this happening persistently. The chapter's last case study question was, What do you think is a reasonable faculty development program for a new faculty member like Dr. Aranthez? The senior faculty mentor assigned to Dr. Aranthez might have been excellent for research and scholarship mentoring but very poor for her acclimation to her teaching role, which was predominately with undergraduate students. The recommendation is for department chairs (who usually make these assignments) to be very meticulous about finding the right fit for mentor and mentee, something the literature clearly supports (Waite and Nardi, 2011). There is also nothing wrong with assigning two mentors, one for research development and one more aligned for teaching. A course coordinator must be much more proactive with a new faculty member in a new clinical course. Moreover, not having at least one formal course meeting with all faculty teaching a clinical course before the term begins seems improper, particularly with a new faculty member.

Relevant Legal Case

Jared Loughner and the Tucson shootings (January 2011).

For the legal case relevant to student civility, a recent and highly visible crime is offered. The case is moving through the criminal courts; the defendant is charged with one count of attempted assassination of a member of Congress, Representative Gabrielle Giffords; two counts of killing an employee of the federal government, including the Chief Judge of the U.S. District Court, John Roll; and two counts of attempting to kill a federal employee in a violent act that ended with 6 individuals dead and 14 injured (CBS/AP, 2011).

The story of Jared Loughner and the Tucson shootings began with a series of in-class behaviors at Pima Community College that were so disruptive that Loughner was ultimately dismissed from the school and denied readmission unless he underwent a mental health examination. According to reports, in 2010 the 22-year-old suspected gunman had five run-ins with Pima Community College campus police and was suspended for violating the student code of conduct—ultimately resulting in his dismissal from the college (Donovan, 2011). The five incidents consisted of library and class disruptions, and on September 29, 2010, police discovered one of Loughner's videos posted to the Web site YouTube, in which he claimed the college was illegal according to the U.S. Constitution. On the same day that the video was uploaded to YouTube, reports indicate that:

> ...campus police officers were called to a biology classroom after Loughner began loud outbursts after told by an instructor that Loughner would only receive ½ credit if he turned in an assignment late. His strident comments caused the instructor to call campus police (Santos, 2011, p. 1).

Ben McGahee, a third-year elementary geometry instructor at Pima Community College, complained about Jared Loughner's disruptive outbursts in class, and it took several formal complaints before he was eventually removed from the course (Fahrenholdt, 2011). On the first day of class, the student yelled out a random number in the class and then asked Mr. McGahee "How can you deny math instead of accepting it?" (Fahrenholdt, p. 1) and on another occasion wrote the word "Mayhemfest'" on his math quiz. Pima Community College had a fairly thick file on Jared Loughner, but except for having campus police go to the student's house to inform his father that he had been dismissed from the community college, no formal charges were ever filed against the student and no mental health referrals were ever formally made. One is left to wonder, however, if Loughner's teachers had challenged his behavior when it first occurred and had a system been in place to deal with uncivil behaviors, whether the conduct would have been quickly reported to the appropriate parties for investigation and response.

Summary

We would attest that in the some 20 years each in our academic careers we have seen a rise in incivility in nursing students and nursing faculty alike. However, these patterns of behavior are likely symptomatic of contemporary society that seems less polite and less bound to common courtesy and etiquette than in former times. One may even attribute some of the classroom disruptions (listening to iPods during class, surfing the Web and ignoring the lecturer, or even challenging the professor outright in disrespectful tones) to some of the behaviors exhibited by Millennials. We, however, believe that proper classroom management must be the standard and uncivil behavior must not be tolerated. It does not mean that the classroom should become a stifled, rule-bound environment, but there must be a climate of respect, and teaching faculty and attending students deserve a classroom where learning is optimized, no matter the generation of students. Uncivil behavior may also be a sign of more serious underlying problems with the offending student, and we have witnessed (with some unease) loud and unusual student mutterings over bad grades or short-tempered students in the clinical environment who indeed became even more problematic.

The tragic Tucson incident indicates that any student who has caused that many disruptions on campus certainly should have been identified as meriting an institutional response and that it is important for all faculty to confront incivility early. Students should be referred to counseling if the institution has access to mental health services. Last, incivility can infest and ruin a classroom and course quickly if it is not dealt with expeditiously, and faculty should never feel as though they cannot address a valid student issue for fear of receiving negative teaching evaluations.

Educational institutions must have published policies or regulations that govern student behavior and conduct while they are either on campus or engaged in educational activities. Indeed, many universities' student conduct regulations also apply to off-campus misconduct. These policies will also establish procedures by which campus authorities can enforce the rules and regulations against the offending student.

Faculty members at public institutions can safely assume that these institutional policies and procedures have been vetted by legal counsel to ensure that they meet the minimum legal requirements for procedural due process required under federal and state law. At private institutions, courts will expect that the institution substantially comply with any procedures or processes they have established for the disciplining of students. See *Boehm v. University of Pennsylvania School of Veterinary Medicine*, 573 A.2d. 575 (Pa. Super. Ct., 1990)

Sanctions for violators can range from the most serious, expulsion or suspension from school, to lesser penalties such as requiring medical clearance or mandatory counseling as conditions of returning to or remaining in school. Therefore, these student codes offer powerful and effective tools for faculty and administrators to respond to situations of uncivil or misconduct by students in the classroom, on campus, or at the off-campus clinical training site. It is time for the faculty member to consider using institutional student behavior and conduct regulations when the faculty member's individual effort to modify unacceptable student behavior is unsuccessful.

Of course, in the most serious situations, where a criminal act has been committed or an imminent threat of harm exists, law enforcement authorities should be immediately contacted. At that point, it is no longer a matter of "academic freedom" or of the "rights" of the one—it is the health and safety of the community.

CRITICAL ELEMENTS TO CONSIDER

- Establish your classroom management rules and expected classroom conduct at the beginning. These guidelines are best placed on the syllabus (e.g., no cell phones in class, no texting during lecture, no distractive sidebar conversations).
- Always document any acts of student incivility.
- Keep your course coordinator/course chair up to date with out-of-the-ordinary events that, although innocuous, may portend future negative behaviors.
- Ignore the first minor uncivil act in the classroom but try to communicate nonverbally that you do not appreciate the behavior or comment.
- If it persists, confront the student outside the classroom setting—perhaps in your office. Do not be afraid to have a fellow faculty member witness with you if necessary.
- Make sure your department chair is aware of significant behaviors that occur that disturb you. She or he may be aware of other issues with the student that you are not aware of, and thus the chair may be more able to intervene.
- Your institution may have other resources available to manage the most serious cases. Other institutional offices, such as Student Conduct or Judicial Affairs, Student Life, Student Counseling Services, or Campus Police or Security, will have specialized expertise to assist. In addition, many colleges and universities have developed response plans and a special team or group to handle situations involving distressed, suicidal, or threatening students.
- It is important to stay focused on the problematic behavior or conduct, even if it is suspected that the behavior or misconduct is due to a psychological or medical condition. Be vigilant if you ever feel threatened by a student or feel your safety is at risk. Do not hesitate to call local or campus law enforcement authorities if necessary.

(**HELPFUL RESOURCES**

- "Student Incivility: Teaching and Learning Center"
  http://www.tlc.eku.edu/tips/student_incivility/
- "Classroom Incivility: What Can We Do?"
  http://ctlincivility.project.mnscu.edu/
- Nursing Law & Order
  http://advocatefornurses.typepad.com/my2cents/2008/12/nursing-student-incivility-in-the-classroom-clinical-setting-and-online.html

References

Alsop, R. (2008). *The trophy kids grow up: How the millennial generation is shaking up the workplace.* San Francisco: Jossey-Bass.

American Association of Colleges of Nursing. (2008). *Accelerated nursing programs: The fast-track to careers in nursing.* Retrieved January 15, 2011, from http://www.aacn.nche.edu/publications/issues/aug02.htm

American Association of Colleges of Nursing. (2010). AACN data confirm that nurses with bachelor's degrees are more likely to secure jobs sooner after graduation than other professionals. Retrieved March 5, 2011, from http://www.aacn.nche.edu/Media/NewsReleases/2010/bsngrad.html

Blozen, B. B. (2010). *Accelerated baccalaureate nursing students: Perceptions of success.* Unpublished doctoral dissertation, Seton Hall University. Retrieved January 15, 2011, from http://domapp01.shu.edu/depts/uc/apps/libraryrepository.nsf/resourceid/DC0F5A977FE2694A8525770E0061BEC0/$File/Blozen-Barbara-B_Doctorate.PDF?Open

Boehm v. University of Pennsylvania School of Veterinary Medicine, 573 A.2d. 575 (Pa. Super. Ct., 1990).

Clark, C. M., & Springer, P. J. (2007). Thoughts on incivility: Student and faculty perceptions of uncivil behavior in nursing education. *Nursing Education Perspectives, 28*(2), 93–97.

Criminal charges filed against Jared Loughner. (2011, January 9). cbsnews.com. Retrieved January 15, 2011, from http://www.cbsnews.com/stories/2011/01/09/national/ main7228149.shtml

Dahnke, M. D. (2009). The role of the American Nurses Association code in ethical decision making. *Holistic Nursing Practice, 23*(20), 112–119.

Delorey, R. (2010, December). Evidence based millennials. *Workplace Review,* 37–46. Retrieved January 15, 2011, from http://www.smu.ca/academic/sobey/workplace/documents/delorey_001.pdf

Donovan, L. (2011, January 10). Suspected Ariz. gunman Jared Loughner's five run-ins with college campus police. dailycaller.com. Retrieved January 15, 2011, from http://dailycaller.com/2011/01/10/suspected-ariz-gunman-jared-loughers-five-run-ins-with-college-campus-police/print/

Fahrenholt, D. (2011, January 9). Jared Loughner's college instructor: I was worried he might have a gun in class. Washingtonpost.com. Retrieved January 15, 2011, from http://voices.washingtonpost.com/44/2011/01/loughners-college-instructor-i.html

Frand, J. (2000). The information age mindset: Changes in students and implications for higher education. *EDUCAUSE Review, 35*(5), 15–24.

Johnson, S. A., & Romanello, M. L. (2005). Generational diversity: Teaching and learning approaches. *Nurse Educator, 30*(5), 212–216.

Keating, M. B. (2008). Incivility: More courts are treating rudeness as a reason for sanctions. abajournal.com. Retrieved January 13, 2011, from http://www.abajournal.com/magazine/article/making_the_case_for_change/

Kupperschmidt, B. R. (1998). Understanding generation X employees. *Journal of Nursing Administration, 28*(12), 36–43.

Santos, M. (2011, January 15). In four-minute YouTube video, Loughner calls college "genocide school." Examiner.com. Retrieved January 15, 2011, from http://www.examiner.com/technology-in-national/in-four-minute-youtube-video-loughner-calls-college-genocide-school

Sherman, R. O. (2006). Leading a multigenerational nursing workforce: The generational cohorts. *Online Journal of Issues in Nursing, 11*(2), manuscript 2. Retrieved March 5, 2011, from http://www.nursingworld.org/MainMenuCategories/ANAMarketplace/ANAPeriodicals/OJIN/TableofContents/Volume112006/No2May06/tpc30_216074.aspx

Smith Glasgow, M. E., & Dreher, H. M. (2010). The future of oncology nursing science: Who will generate the knowledge? *Oncology Nursing Forum, 37*(4), 393–396.

Suplee, P. D., Lachman, V. D., Siebert, B., et al. (2008). Managing nursing student incivility in the classroom, clinical setting, and on-line. *Journal of Nursing Law, 12*(2), 68–77.

Swearingen, S. (2004). *Nursing leadership characteristics: Effect on nursing job satisfaction and retention of baby boomer and generation X nurses.* Unpublished doctoral dissertation, College of Health and Public Affairs, University of Central Florida. Retrieved March 5, 2011, from http://etd.fcla.edu/CF/CFE0000205/Swearingen_Sandra_L_200412_PhD.pdf

U.S. Bureau of Labor Statistics. (2009). The employment situation—November 2009. bls.gov Retrieved March 5, 2011, from http://www.bls.gov/news.release/archives/empsit_12042009.pdf

Waite, R., & Nardi, D. (2011). Seeking lifelong mentorship and menteeship in the doctoral advanced practice role. In H. M. Dreher & M. E. Smith Glasgow (Eds.), *Role development for doctoral advanced nursing practice* (pp. 323–340). New York: Springer.

Youssef, F. A., & Goodrich, N. (1996). Accelerated versus traditional nursing students: A comparison of stress, critical thinking ability and performance. *International Journal of Nursing Studies, 33* (1), 76–82.

CHAPTER 20

Managing Faculty Incivility

CASE STUDY

When Faculty Flout Normal Procedures

Your role: You are Dr. Fowler, the associate dean for the division of nursing at State University.

There has been much discussion among your faculty concerning a proposal to offer more teaching credit for undergraduate courses that typically average 53.2 students; the typical graduate course averages only 18.6 students. This disparity has long existed, and faculty members who primarily teach graduate students have enjoyed teaching significantly fewer students in each annual review over the past five years. The undergraduate faculty members feel as if they are carrying a heavier and unfair teaching load compared with members who teach in the master's or doctoral program. The Curriculum Committee At-Large, which represents faculty members who sit on the baccalaureate, master's, and doctoral curriculum committees, has decided to use a blog for faculty members to express their viewpoints on a proposal to give more credit for classes of more than 50 students and also to reduce credit (except a doctoral seminar or doctoral advisement) for any course with fewer than 10 students. Blogs have been used for faculty voting for years, but no specific instructions for using the blog have been established.

The blog has been up now for 10 days, and although many undergraduate faculty members have posted their views, which are largely supportive of the change, very few of the graduate faculty members have posted on the blog. In a previous full nursing faculty meeting, one of the tenured faculty members, Dr. Isherwood, stood up and declared it took more preparation to teach graduate students and she was loudly booed. One of the undergraduate faculty members, Dr. Alami, asked her to prove her statement and to back it up with hard data. Since this confrontation in the full nursing faculty meeting took place, the graduate nursing faculty members have been very defensive but have never put forth the data to support Dr. Isherwood's statement.

After 10 days of the open blog being posted, a full nursing faculty meeting is scheduled for final discussion and a vote taken on the new credit system. One hour before Dr. Fowler is to convene the meeting, open the discussion, and conduct a vote, he receives a letter signed (scanned and sent by e-mail) by six of the eight tenured faculty members, stating their vehement opposition to the proposal. They also write that because they are tenured, their views should carry extra consideration. The dean is copied on the letter to Dr. Fowler. Dr. Fowler is flabbergasted by this last-minute ploy and is furious at what he perceives to be an unprofessional and uncivil act. He knows he has a faculty meeting in only an hour, and he ponders what his best course of action should be.[1]

Questions

- Are the six tenured nursing faculty members being uncivil in their submission of this last-minute letter?
- How should Dr. Fowler first respond?
- What should Dr. Fowler say at the full nursing faculty meeting?
- Should graduate faculty members receive *more* credit for their courses (as some institutions practice) than for teaching undergraduate courses, or should they receive the same or less credit (as this proposal suggests) for teaching small graduate courses on average?
- Should tenured faculty members have a larger or more influential voice than the nontenured or nontenure–track faculty?
- How can the contribution of every faculty member, regardless of position and rank, be valued in any respective nursing division or college?

Managing Faculty Incivility: Legal Principles and Review of the Literature

Although the incivility of students appears to have garnered the most attention in the literature, the problem with faculty incivility cannot be ignored or minimized. The deterioration of student incivility has real parallels to what is happening among faculty in general and nursing faculty in particular. Everyone has likely experienced excessive gossip; faculty members who are very egocentric and overly focused on their own careers or teaching schedules at the expense of the teaching mission of the department, college, or university; too much passive-aggressive behavior and avoidance of real conflict resolution; and disparaging comments made about administrators, even though few nursing faculty members have any desire to become a department chair or an academic nursing administrator (Smith Glasgow, Dreher, et al., 2009). In other words, all too often, there are many critics but few faculty members who want to serve in the very demanding job of an academic nursing executive at any level.

The literature is growing on what is termed *academic incivility* (which encompasses both students and faculty). Clark and Springer (2010) define *academic incivility* as "disruptive behavior that substantially or repeatedly interferes with teaching

---

[1] If there is no faculty governance model, then these changes may be made by fiat or decree by a dean. But when faculty governance is important (or specified in faculty bylaws), these issues (as proposals) generally work their way up through normal internal administrative channels, as they did in this case.

and learning. Incivility on college campuses jeopardizes the welfare of all members of the academy" (p. 319).

Clark and Springer further write that "the challenge of demanding workloads [for nursing faculty], maintaining clinical competence, advancement issues, and a perceived lack of administrative support, contribute to faculty stress" (2010, p. 322), which is characterized by problematic students; long-standing salary inequities; and faculty-to-faculty incivility, bullying, and hazing. Faculty incivility does not occur only between individual faculty members. Clark (2008) earlier noted that student perceptions of faculty incivility toward themselves included faculty members (1) behaving in demeaning and belittling ways, (2) treating students unfairly and subjectively, and (3) pressuring students to conform and comply to unreasonable faculty demands.

Twale and De Luca (2008), in *Faculty Incivility: The Rise of the Academic Bully Culture and What to Do About It* (2008), write of incivility:

> That is what makes the behavior so insidious, because the meaning behind the interaction could be anything from complete sincerity to sarcasm to flagrant manipulation. It could also be harassment, incivility, passive aggression, or bullying as translated by the receiver. (p. 3)

In other words, the parameters of incivility are in the eye of the receiver and not simply in the eye of the beholder. It is not sufficient if the perpetrator did not mean to be uncivil; if the conduct, speech or behavior is perceived as such, then it is damaging in its own right. Imber (2010) vehemently disagrees with this approach in his review of Twale and De Luca's book for the journal *Review of Higher Education*. Twale and De Luca (2010) also conclude that "the only way to eliminate, or at least minimize the impact of, the bully is to recognize the behavior and the perpetrator and address it" (p. 191), and they indicate by doing this the institution is more poised to redirect valuable time and energy to what should occur in higher education: excellent teaching and research.

Also of concern is the ability of nursing faculty to resolve issues of incivility through constructive confrontation or dispute resolution, something we see all too rarely in the nursing profession and in the faculty role. Thomas (2004) wonders whether the "horizontal hostility" in the nursing profession (her phrase for incivility) exists because nurses are predominately women and "trained from birth to be passive-aggressive" (p. 117). Thomas further indicates these behaviors are engrained in nursing students during their nursing education, and it is incumbent on nursing educators to resist this. Role modeling more constructive, assertive behaviors by teaching *and* clinical faculty may be one solution. Chesler (2009), although not a nurse, writes extensively about women's inhumanity to women, and there may be particular parallels to the common acknowledgment that "nurses eat their young"[2] (Brown, 2010).

---

[2] There is a case for ceasing to use the phrase "nurses eat their young" because by using it, it may be itself perpetuated as truth. Maybe the issue should be instead "the incivility of seasoned nurses to novice nurses."

Faculty-to-faculty incivility can technically be both legal (e.g., rudeness, passive-aggressive behaviors, belittling) and illegal (e.g., defamation, libel, harassment). For example, Chapter 2 states that a defamatory statement is a written or verbal publication of a statement or information that is false and has a tendency to injure a person's reputation. Because defamation is a matter of state law, the elements of a defamatory claim can vary slightly from state to state. In general, to succeed in a defamation case, the plaintiff must prove that a false statement of fact (not a mere opinion) was made that is defamatory in nature and was published to a third party who is not the defendant or plaintiff.

The definition of *harassment* is covered in chapters 13 and 14, and although some faculty harassment may not be illegal, if the behavior violates a human resources department policy, then the faculty member could be disciplined or even terminated.

Only a minority of schools have an actual specific faculty code of conduct (see the policy at UC Davis in the "Helpful Resources" section of this chapter). Although faculty code of conduct is often covered by general university code of conduct policies, it is actually innovative for specific guidelines to be developed that address directly faculty-to-faculty incivility and faculty-to-student incivility—something that is written about less but that remains prevalent even in nursing education (Marchiondo K, Marchiondo L, and Lasiter, 2010).

Discussion of Case

Recall the first question from this chapter's case study: Are the six tenured nursing faculty members being uncivil in their submission of this last-minute letter? In this case Associate Dean Fowler was certainly taken aback by the last-minute nature of the approach by these tenured nursing faculty members. Even while acknowledging that there were some valid points in the letter, the complete rejection of the normal procedures for faculty input and voice on matters of curriculum were apparently abandoned with this strategy. Were they really being uncivil or were they simply expressing their opinion on the issue? If he sanctioned them for this uncivil behavior, would he be violating the faculty members' rights of academic freedom or First Amendment free speech rights as this was a public university?

Concerned that any precipitous action on his part might get the university into legal trouble, he put in a quick call to his attorney friend in the general counsel's office. The lawyer explained that whereas the university, as a public state university, could not take disciplinary action for free speech that was protected under the First Amendment, the particular speech in question was not protected. She explained that under a 2006 U.S. Supreme Court case, *Garcetti v. Ceballos*, 126 S.Ct. 1951 (2006), public employees do not have any First Amendment rights when making statements pursuant to their official duties. The attorney felt that because the faculty members were speaking on a matter of internal university operations concerning their own workloads, a court would consider these to be statements pursuant to their official duties. However, the attorney also advised Dr. Fowler that even though he could legally discipline the faculty member, she did not think it was the most prudent course of action given the lack of rules about posting on the blog and its sporadic use for faculty voting. She asked him what he would do if they had posted the letter on the blog just one hour before the meeting? Also, wasn't one of the purposes of the meeting to give the faculty member a last chance to debate the proposal before it was voted on?

Further, as tenured faculty members, do they have a greater voice in decision-making as is apparent by the written statement they subsequently submitted: "As tenured faculty we have a responsibility to be leaders in the development of nursing academic policies that affect the whole. We are concerned that as the non-tenured ranks outnumber us, our views, which we contend are indeed valid, may simply be ignored by voting blocks that do not have the best interest of the graduate faculty or particularly the graduate student (master's and doctoral)." Dr. Fowler was immediately reminded of the PhD tenured faculty member who once suggested to him that she should have first selection over class times for her undergraduate course (over another master's prepared faculty member) and that she should therefore not have to teach an 8 a.m. class. To Dr. Fowler, this was elitist and he simply responded to the tenured faculty member that this was not how faculty course times were scheduled—taking into consideration doctoral preparation or tenure status—and that he did not view that approach as egalitarian or even fair. Dr. Fowler thought it was irresponsible for these six tenured faculty members to allow 10 days to pass without posting any of their concerns on the blog. He thought they should have posted their concerns and perhaps followed up with a letter; then at least the appearance of being constructive would have been helpful.

The second and third questions in this chapter's case study are: How should Dr. Fowler first respond? What should Dr. Fowler say at the full nursing faculty meeting? Within 10 minutes of receiving the e-mail and complaint, the dean responded to Dr. Fowler that she thought the last-minute nature of the letter was simply outrageous. The dean had been following the blog discussion herself but as usual had decided not to post as she did not want to unduly influence the discussion or make other faculty members feel as though they needed to agree with her as dean. As she was a great believer in faculty governance, she was equally adamant that with faculty governance came great accountability and great responsibility. She knew in the end she herself would have to approve any final proposal, but viewing the posts anonymously at least gave her much insight into the issues surrounding the proposal. She also noted to Dr. Fowler that she had not seen any of the tenured faculty posting on the blog, and asked whether they really were proposing that the tenured faculty members should be the "deciders," as the letter actually seemed to indicate. Dr. Fowler decided not to respond to the protest e-mail (which was probably a good thing—quickly written, terse e-mails can sometimes cause more harm) and thought the best strategy was to take a deep breath and figure out how best to approach this at the faculty meeting. He, however, reassured the dean by phone that he would handle it professionally and that he would report to her what took place.

At the full nursing faculty meeting Dr. Fowler made sure every faculty member who entered the room got a copy of the agenda, the previous month's minutes, *and* a copy of the signed letter by the six tenured faculty members. When it was time for that agenda item to be discussed, Dr. Fowler said that some of the tenured faculty members had expressed concerns about the procedures that were being used to vote on the credit allotment for undergraduate and graduate courses and stated to the full congregants that six tenured faculty members had coauthored a letter stating their points. Dr. Fowler had decided that the best strategy was not to be overly confrontational with the four tenured faculty members who attended the mandatory meeting, but that he would calmly ask about the nature of the letter and why they chose not to post these same concerns on the blog. Over the next 45 minutes the four attending tenured faculty members really did not forcefully and publically defend the letter but one did state it seemed like a foregone conclusion that the change was going to be made. She reiterated that six of them decided to put their view in a more formal letter than in a blog post. Dr. Fowler then asked them to help the rest of the faculty members to better understand their position on the proposal. However, they floundered when trying to defend the letter. One undergraduate faculty member asked one of the tenured faculty members, "What is your solution then to this inequity or do you firmly believe there is no inequity with us teaching almost twice the number of students you do annually?" The tenured faculty in attendance really had no responses, and the room became very silent, but overall there was little discussion because it was apparent it was such a volatile issue.

One of the two tenured faculty members who did not sign this letter (she was uncomfortable signing it and told the six others so) sensed this and decided to intervene as she thought there might be a compromise acceptable to all. She rose up and said, "Although I would have preferred that the issues in the letter had been posted on the blog so we could at least debate them according to our normal procedures, I do agree that there are some valid points in the letter. I said 'some'. I would like to recommend that we table a vote for now, go back to the blog for another 10 days, and that any vote be sent to Faculty Affairs [which had elected members from both tenured or tenure-track and clinical faculty members] for their response because this decision ultimately does affect faculty course load and faculty life. The faculty can then vote up or down the recommendations (however modified) from Faculty Affairs. And of course we all know the dean ultimately has to sign off on any of this."

Dr. Fowler immediately stated he thought that was a good idea, and so a vote was taken to follow the new proposed procedures. The vote was 65 in favor, 8 opposed, and 4 abstentions.

WHEN TO CONTACT THE UNIVERSITY COUNSEL

Similar to student violations, a faculty member's contact with the university attorney will generally be through the department chair or other administrator or by a university attorney through human resources. Remember, the job of the university counsel is to represent the institution (this is also her professional and ethical duty as well). The university counsel will not be able to represent an individual faculty member or a group of faculty members who may have a disagreement with institutional policy. If one is from a protected class, then a complaint with the office of equality may be filed if there is bullying, harassment, or discrimination by another faculty member or staff. In extreme circumstances, it may be prudent to consult with a personal attorney if redress within the university is not satisfactory.

Findings and Disposition

After the conclusion of the meeting, one of the department chairs in attendance informed Dr. Fowler that she thought he handled it well. She said it was definitely a very volatile issue but that he did not let the discussion get out of hand, albeit there was apparent hesitancy by many to speak up. Dr. Fowler hoped his tone was tempered and affirmed that the alternative proposal was fine as this policy was actually both a curriculum and faculty affairs issue and that the dean's signature on any change was required regardless of the proposed course load procedures the faculty wanted to follow. Dr. Fowler did express displeasure with the tenured faculty letter authors, not so much because they wrote the letter (he was quite accustomed to turf battles in academia), but because only four out of six showed up to defend the letter. He affirmed they did have some valid points, but was still perplexed about why they became so quiet upon public questioning by their own peers.[3]

The fourth question is: Should graduate faculty members receive more credit for their courses (as some institutions practice) than for teaching undergraduate courses, or should they receive the same or less credit (as this proposal suggests)

---

[3] Or did they consider them "true peers?"

for teaching small graduate courses on average? This is a difficult question. It is rather common, although not universal, that faculty members in some colleges and universities receive more credit for teaching graduate courses.[4] More common[5] are faculty expectations that all faculty members will teach both undergraduate and graduate courses and thus there is no need to give graduate courses more credit. Although some traditionalists may say it takes more effort to teach a graduate course or the faculty in graduate courses must have exceptional scholarly credentials, we attest that these perceptions are unproven, however traditional and extremely unegalitarian. It is more common that faculty members who have a specific graduate appointment may have their credentials reviewed by a graduate council[6] to supervise doctoral students, and this is a sound practice. There is nothing more difficult in nursing education than teaching didactic undergraduate clinical content, especially to a large class and particularly to second-degree/accelerated nursing students. Even doctoral seminars, which we have also taught, are not as difficult to teach.

The fifth question is: Should tenured faculty members have a larger or more influential voice than the nontenured or nontenure-track faculty? Our answer, as two tenured nursing faculty members, is a firm no. Again, this is a very traditional practice and, we think, largely outdated. Tenured faculty members already receive a host of benefits from being tenured, including a lifetime appointment and almost always a lower teaching load than nontenure track (clinical or teaching faculty), and other benefits. Every full-time faculty member has a valuable role to play, and every individual faculty member has made certain choices about his or her career and has chosen to either emphasize teaching (clinical or classroom) or research or administration. This, therefore, essentially answers the sixth question: How can the contribution of every faculty member, regardless of position and rank, be valued in any respective nursing division or college? It is by constructing effective workload policies in which individuals can excel, whether in teaching, research, or administration, without each becoming victim of a strangulating tripartite mission (teaching, scholarship/research, and practice or service) that forces every faculty member to accomplish each equally (including service) and with excellence (Anderson, 2000; Burman, Hart, and McCabe, 2005; Potempa, Redman, and Anderson, 2008).

---

[4] See workload policies at Prairie View A&M University, Prairie View, Texas, where graduate courses receive more credit: http://www.pvamu.edu/pages/1392.asp, or UMASS–Boston, where more credit is given to both graduate courses and large undergraduate class sizes: http://www.umb.edu/academics/provost/documents/FacultyWorkloadGuidelines.pdf

[5] See the University of Minnesota Web site: http://cla.umn.edu/intranet/undergrad/workload.php

[6] See policy at LSU: http://gradlsu.gs.lsu.edu/Graduate%20Faculty/Requirements%20for%20Graduate%20Faculty%20Status/item11939.html

Relevant Legal Case

Ginn v. Stephen F. Austin State University, No. 03-02-00443-CV, 2003 WL
1882264 (Tex. Ct. App. 2003)

In *Ginn v. Stephen F. Austin State University,* Stephen F. Austin State University hired
Mr. Gregory Ginn as an associate professor of management in 1989. At the time
the university did not have a college-wide smoking policy, and Mr. Ginn determined through his own research that the college was in violation of federal Occupational Safety and Health Administration (OSHA) guidelines for not having a
no-smoking policy. On bringing this situation to the attention of university officials, Mr. Ginn was informed that they were technically not in violation of this
policy but that they would provide him some access to a smoke-free environment,
including moving his office. Over the next 2 years Mr. Ginn continued to complain
about the policy. Despite these complaints his contract was renewed in both 1990
and 1991. In 1992 his contract was not renewed. He responded by suing the university for violation of the Texas Whistleblower Protection Act, claiming that he
was fired because he continued his complaints about the smoking policy, including to the university president.

After hearing the evidence, the state court found that he (1) cursed at a student using profane language; (2) referred to a fellow professor by use of an
obscene name in one of his classes; (3) engaged in a heated conversation with
the same professor when she confronted Mr. Ginn about the name-calling;
(4) banged his head against the wall many times in order to stretch his calf while
his students were taking exams; and finally, and what the court of appeals ultimately
ruled led to his dismissal (5) was charged with assault against his department
chair, Mr. Warren Fisher, by shoving him several times while blocking his exit, and
finally grabbing Mr. Fisher by the wrists to prevent him from leaving Mr. Ginn's
office (Texas Ct. of Appeals, Document, Third District, at Austin, 2003). The court
held that these were sufficient to demonstrate that the university had good reasons for not renewing his contract, and ruled against the plaintiff.

Summary

Is incivility on the rise? It is hard to say, but if there is agreement that there is a
rise in incivility in society in general, then it is likely to be happening in academia
too. It is very likely that Representative Joe Wilson's yelling out "You lie!" to President Obama during a 2009 speech on the floor of the House of Representatives
is at least anecdotal evidence that it is on the rise (Parker, 2009). It is very important that a climate of civility be restored to our institutions of higher learning and
that our classrooms actually be places in which safe and civil instruction can take
place. Too often faculty members are adverse to enforcing even modest classroom

management strategies for fear of reprisal from students and even negative teaching evaluations. Strong administrative support is essential so faculty members know they are supported. Clark and Springer (2007) describe the following scenario: Connie seems to challenge everything her nursing professor says. During small-group work, Connie text messages her friends and rarely pays attention. *The professor is impatient and uses harsh language with Connie in front of the other students.* (p. 93; italics added) We have italicized the last part of the quote because it is our belief that one cannot expect civility from students if the faculty members do not accord them professional, civil behavior themselves. Further, the concept of collegiality needs to be revisited so that faculty members indeed treat each other with respect. Didn't Rodney King (n.d.) famously say, "Can't we all just get along?" or words to that effect. It may just be that simple.

CRITICAL ELEMENTS TO CONSIDER

- Victims of bullying or of academic incivility must document these events.
- If attempts to resolve these issues with the offender fail, notify the department chair in writing.
- If the offender is in violation of human resource policies, consider reporting him or her.
- If the normal chain of command is not working, go to the dean and put a complaint and actions taken in writing.
- For faculty disputes that cannot be resolved at the departmental level, we also suggest making use of the campus ombudsman or human resources.
- A faculty witness to bullying behavior by faculty toward students should make every effort possible to speak to that individual directly. If the violation observed is severe or unethical, then report the activity through normal administrative channels.
- Some universities have anonymous ethics hotlines that one can call anonymously.
- Be aware that simply because an activity is reported to a department chair or other administrator, it does not perpetually guarantee the anonymity of the one who reports it.

HELPFUL RESOURCES

- The Academic Ladder, "Getting Help With the Climb Blog—Mean and Nasty Academics: Bullying, Hazing, and Mobbing" http://gblog2.academicladder.com/2008/02/mean-and-nasty-academics-bullying.htm
- "UCSF Code of Conduct" http://chancellor.ucsf.edu/UCSFCOC.pdf
- "UC Davis Administrative Policy: General University Policy for Academic Appointees Section UCD-015, Procedures for Faculty Misconduct Allegations" http://manuals.ucdavis.edu/apm/015.htm

References

Anderson, C. A. (2000). Current strengths and limitations of doctoral education in nursing: Are we prepared for the future? *Journal of Professional Nursing, 16*(4), 191–200.

Brown, T. (2010, February 11). When the nurse is a bully. newyorktimes.com. Retrieved January 18, 2011, from http://well.blogs.nytimes.com/2010/02/11/when-the-nurse-is-a-bully/

Burman, M. E., Hart, A. M., & McCabe, S. M. (2005). Doctor of nursing practice: Opportunity amidst chaos. *American Journal of Critical Care, 14,* 463–464.

Chesler, P. (2009). *Women's inhumanity to women.* Chicago: Lawrence Hill Books.

Clark, C. (2008). Student perspectives on faculty incivility in nursing education: An application of the concept of rankism. *Nursing Outlook, 56*(1), 4–8.

Clark, C., & Springer, P. J. (2007). Thoughts on incivility and faculty perceptions of uncivil behavior in nursing education. *Nursing Education Perspectives, 28*(2), 93–97.

Clark, C. M., & Springer, P. J. (2010). Academic nurse leaders' role in fostering a culture of civility in nursing education. *Journal of Nursing Education, 49*(6), 319–325.

Defamation. (2011). legal-diction.thefreedictionary.com. Retrieved March 6, 2011, from http://legal-dictionary.thefreedictionary.com/defamation

Garcetti v. Ceballos, 126 S.Ct. 1951 (2006).Ginn v. Stephen F. Austin State University, No. 03-02-00443-CV, 2003 WL 1882264 (Tex. Ct. App. 2003).

Imber, M. (2010). Faculty incivility: The rise of the academic bully culture and what to do about it (Review). *Review of Higher Education, 33*(2), 293–294.

King. R. (n.d.) Reconstructing Rodney King. YouTube [video]. Retrieved January 18, 2011, from http://www.youtube.com/watch?v=2Pbyi0JwNug

Marchiondo, K., Marchiondo, L. A., & Lasiter, S. (2010). Faculty incivility: Effects on program satisfaction of BSN students. *Journal of Nursing Education, 49*(11), 608–614.

Parker, K. (2009). Rise in incivility a threat to concept of civilization. Chron.com. Retrieved January 18, 2011, from http://www.chron.com/disp/story.mpl/editorial/outlook/6620712.html

Potempa, K. M., Redman, R. W., & Anderson, C. A. (2008). Capacity for the advancement of nursing science: Issues and challenges. *Journal of Professional Nursing, 24*(6), 329–336.

Smith Glasgow, M. E., Dreher, H. M., Cornelius et al. (2009, November). *A final report on the 2009 National Survey of Doctoral Nursing Faculty (both PhD and DNP) in the United States.* Paper presented at the International Conference on Professional Doctorates (ICPD), UK Council for Graduate Education, London, UK.

Thomas, S. (2004). *Transforming nurses' stress and anger: Steps towards healing* (2nd ed.). New York: Springer.

Twale, D. J., & De Luca, B. M. (2008). *Faculty incivility: The rise of the academic bully culture and what to do about it.* Hoboken, NJ: Jossey-Bass.

CHAPTER 21

Disability Issues for the Student

CASE STUDY

Physical and Learning Disabilities

Your role: You are Dr. Clinton, the BSN program coordinator in a college's nursing department.

This chapter offers analyses of several scenarios regarding undergraduate nursing students with disabilities who make requests for academic accommodations to faculty and academic program administrators. Although these cases initially appear unique, close examination of the underlying principles and related case law reveals common themes that emerge as a basis for discussion of programmatic issues and considerations related to the education of nursing students with disabilities.

Case 1: During the first clinical rotation in a fundamentals nursing course, Lilly Brown informs her clinical instructor, Professor Lindy, that she (Lilly) is unable to participate in physical care activities of adults because of a previously undisclosed physical limitation that does not allow her to lift more than 10 pounds. Ms. Brown declares that she is protected from discrimination in her student role and states that she has a qualified disability. She further states that her intent is to work in a neonatal intensive care unit after graduation and threatens legal action if prevented from continued progression in the nursing program.

Case 2: Donna Glee, a nursing student midway through the nursing program, was denied employment as a nurse's aide for a cooperative education experience in a telemetry unit at a local hospital because of her disclosure of a hearing deficit. Hospital officials cite concerns related to patient safety because Ms. Glee will not be able to hear cardiac monitor alarms. The student wears bilateral hearing aids and is able to converse reasonably well in face-to-face situations. Ms. Glee has been approved for accommodations from the university's office of disability services. The accommodations consist of note-taking support in class and use of an amplified stethoscope in the clinical setting. She has met all academic and clinical requirements to date. However, Ms. Glee acknowledges significant auditory processing problems in large groups or with multidirectional auditory stimuli. The prognosis is that her auditory capacity will continue to decline and she will become totally deaf within an unspecified time frame. Ms. Glee approaches the BSN program coordinator, Dr. Clinton, and questions how the recent denial of employment and associated functional limitations will influence both her continued progression in the nursing program and her career aspirations of becoming a registered nurse.

Case 3: The director of clinical education, Professor Whiting, informs Dr. Clinton that nursing student Jamilla Wyeth, who has a chronic illness, is insisting her clinical assignments be limited to the immediate geographic area, because of her need for ongoing medical treatment. Although Professor Whiting is concerned for the student's welfare, she also feels strongly that granting this request without careful review will have significant negative ramifications for program policies related to student clinical assignments. She predicts that there will be student challenges of preferential treatment, corresponding inequities in student access to a variety of clinical sites, and associated transportation challenges for fellow students (some of whom have significant physical impairments but have not requested special considerations). Professor Whiting asks Dr. Clinton how they are going to resolve the conflict between providing the student's access to needed medical care and program policies regarding to the assignment of clinical sites.

Case 4: Darrell Iseminger, a student with attention-deficit hyperactivity disorder (ADHD) who was previously unsuccessful in a fast-paced, second-degree accelerated nursing curriculum, was granted admission to your 4-year BSN program on the premise that he would be able to meet program outcome standards given that course work would be spread over a longer time period. However, Mr. Iseminger did not initiate the request for academic accommodations with the office of disabilities services until the academic difficulties began to recur. Mr. Iseminger attributes his academic difficulties to ADHD and requests that he be afforded extra time and reduced distraction environment for testing. Because of the urgency of the request, Mr. Iseminger was granted temporary (one term) academic accommodations of extended time and reduced distraction environment by the office of disability services. Doing so gives him time to complete the necessary processes and procedures needed for assessment and evaluation of the nature and extent of formal academic accommodations on an ongoing basis.

Questions

- In each of these cases, do you believe there is a valid disability claim by the student?
- How would you resolve each case individually if you were the academic nursing administrator charged with making a final determination?

Disability Issues for the Student: Legal Principles and Review of the Literature

As the majority of disability issues in higher education pertain to students, the impact of disability law on students will be thoroughly addressed in this chapter.

Legal protection for students with disabilities was initially established by section 504 of the Rehabilitation Act of 1973 but was limited in its applicability to institutions that received federal funds. This protection was extended to all educational institutions by Title II and Title III of the Americans With Disabilities Act (ADA) of 1990. These acts require universities to make reasonable and necessary modifications to rules, policies, and practices to prevent discrimination against students on the basis of disability (Cope, 2005).

As a result of these legislative mandates, advances in technology, and educational supports, the number of students with disabilities who are seeking higher education has tripled in the past 25 years. Data from the National Center for Educational Statistics (NCES) (2003–2004) reveal that 11.3% of all students who pursue secondary education have a disability (NCES, 2011). The NCES report indicates that the most common disabilities in higher education are psychiatric disorders, learning disabilities, and attention-deficit hyperactivity disorder (ADHD).

This trend is also evident in educational programs for health professionals, but the proportion of students enrolled in these programs who report some type of disability is significantly lower than it is in the general undergraduate population. It is unclear whether this disparity is a result of selective admission policies, technical standards, or educational requirements characteristic of health-related disciplines (Newsham, 2008). In a recent study of nursing faculty knowledge and expertise in dealing with disabled nursing students, responses to the types of student disabilities encountered in classroom/clinical settings revealed that 63 of 88 (72%) respondents currently or previously taught students with disabilities. Further breakdown of faculty experiences with students presenting with varied types of disabilities revealed that 60% had encountered students with learning disabilities; 28% had encountered students with ADHD; 25% had encountered students with physical disabilities; 18% had encountered students with significant hearing impairment; and 13% had encountered students with visual impairment (Sowers and Smith, 2004).

Learning disabilities and attention deficit disorders are a heterogeneous group of maladies manifested by significant difficulties in acquisition and use of listening, speaking, reading, reasoning, or mathematical skills. They often present as comorbidities with similar clinical presentations. These disorders are intrinsic to the individual and presumed to be caused by central nervous system dysfunction (Rosenbraugh, 2000). Although physical disabilities are more distinct in etiology and varied in presenting symptoms, there are often similarities in the categories of accommodations needed in the educational setting. Consequently, for purposes of discussion, this chapter focuses on addressing the needs of students with physical disabilities generically.

Nursing, as a profession, maintains a strong advocacy role for individuals with special needs; however, the education of nursing students with disabilities poses unique challenges. Nursing faculty, similar to their counterparts in other professional health disciplines, often exhibit personal bias related to student capabilities, a lack of information, and a lack of confidence in dealing with student disabilities. Clinically focused professional education programs such as nursing are faced with the challenges of simultaneously supporting student learning within the context of public safety, meeting mandated program outcome standards, and ensuring student competency to pass licensure requirements.

Nursing educators have a vested interest in student success, and tend to respond favorably to student requests for assistance in meeting learning objectives. However, granting informal student requests for special considerations related to performance assessments, assignments, or clinical rotations on an ad hoc basis may inadvertently create inequities for other students, delay student access to needed formal academic intervention/supports, and pose legal challenges of discrimination. Limited knowledge about disability issues often contributes to indecision and inconsistency on the part of faculty when approached by students requesting special considerations related to assignments/examinations and/or formal academic accommodations. There is general consensus that educators and administrators alike need to develop a better understanding of the rights of and responsibilities of students and programs within the context of quality in educational curricula and the provision of high-quality health-care services to the public (Stacey and Carroll, 2000; Newsham, 2008; Sowers and Smith, 2004).

Legal protection for students with disabilities in higher education is addressed in federal laws specifically in section 504 of the 1973 Rehabilitation Act (29 U.S.C. § 794) and Title II of the 1990 Americans With Disabilities Act (42 U.S.C. § 12132). These somewhat overlapping laws aim to protect the rights of disabled individuals, those individuals who have a physical or mental disability that "substantially limits" one or more of their major life activities. In academic settings, learning is viewed as a major life activity (Helms, Jorgensen, and Anderson, 2006). These laws require universities to make reasonable and necessary modifications to rules, policies, or practices to prevent discrimination against qualified students based on disability. The ADA also requires that institutions designate a compliance officer (and disability staff as needed) to address ADA compliance issues, qualify students with disabilities, and identify appropriate academic adjustments as indicated (Cope, 2005).

Although these two federal regulations do not specifically address higher education, subsequent administrative rules and case law provide insight and guidance related to a nursing program's obligation to the student, its educational mission, preparation for licensure, and eventual employment of the student as a registered nurse. Courts are understandably particularly interested in cases involving the health professions because of the direct effect on the health and safety of patients. Initially, few suits from students came forward. However, legal experts in this area suspect that more cases will arise given the dramatic increase in accommodation given in the high schools making more students with disabilities eligible, the increase in activity from disability advocacy groups, and the interest from policy makers to expand those eligible for accommodations (Rothstein, 2000).

Three foundational terms must be defined to understand these laws. A *qualified disability* is a physical or mental impairment that substantially limits one or more major life activities of an individual compared to the conditions, manner, or duration under which these activities can be performed by the general public or comparable student group. *Otherwise qualified* in postsecondary educational settings means that a student with a disability is one who is able to meet a program's admission, academic, and technical standards either with or without accommodation *in spite of* the limitations imposed by the disability. *Reasonable accommodations* are the program/activity adjustments that enable an otherwise qualified individual fair opportunity to achieve outcome standards. Adjustments are not intended to create unfair advantage or require significant adjustments to program/activity—do not result in lowering program/activity standards—and are not intended to cause undue burden to the sponsoring entity.

Several principles guide the fair and reasonable implementation of accommodating students during the continuum of their enrollment to graduation in an academic nursing program. These include the following:

1. Formal notification by student of perceived or qualified disability
2. Disability verification/qualification by designated disability personnel
3. Integrity of educational program and academic standards
4. Determination of reasonable accommodations
5. Notification and implementation of accommodation
6. Established procedures for complaints and appeals[1]

It is the student's responsibility to formally notify an institution, either through the program administrators or the office of disability services, to self-identify the existence of disability (perceived or qualified), and to request consideration of formal academic accommodations. If the student fails to make such notification to an institution, program administrators and faculty cannot be held responsible for untoward student outcomes, requests for retroactive accommodations, or related allegations of disability discrimination. Once the student requests disability status, the case should be handled in a confidential, expeditious, and comprehensive manner.

---

[1] Just a reminder that due process for *private* universities is not required. What private universities follow is something close to due process but is technically not called *due process.*

Assuming a student appropriately reports a disability, he or she must then provide supporting documentation from appropriate/qualified medical or educational professionals to establish a qualified disability. However, the existence of documentation of physical or learning limitations, in and of itself, may not be sufficient to qualify the student for academic accommodations because the associated impairment must substantially limit major life activities. In addition, disabling conditions that can be mitigated or ameliorated with medications or corrective devices may negate requests for disability accommodation. In instances in which supporting documentation is not available (or deemed inadequate) to support a claim of disability, the cost of all related testing and professional evaluative measures to document the existence of a qualified disability are the responsibility of the student. The institution and its representatives bear no accountability for the provision or procurement of these services. Qualified disability status (and related accommodations) cannot be granted unless all verification requirements are met in accordance with the law.

Accommodations/academic supports are intended to minimize the impact of a qualified disability and enable the student to participate fully in the educational process. These adjustments are not intended to fundamentally alter the education and training program in an academic setting, create excessive burden to the sponsoring organization, or create an unfair advantage with regard to other students in learning experiences and evaluative measures. However, courts have asked that institutions bear the higher burden than the individual because they are better situated to do so (Rothstein, 2000).

Once reasonable accommodations are determined by the office of disability services, the student is given an academic verification letter (AVL), or equivalent documentation, outlining the specific nature of the accommodation and related considerations. It is extremely important that faculty do not grant any academic adjustments in any way without the AVL letter. Granting accommodations in the absence of this documentation establishes precedence that the academic unit acknowledges the student as disabled. As a result, the individual is automatically qualified to receive similar academic supports/considerations in the future, thereby circumventing the evaluation/verification processes inherent in disability legislation. Once established, institutions have limited recourse for cessation of academic accommodations, even if it is felt that they are no longer warranted (Newsham, 2008). It is the institution's responsibility to ensure that accommodations are implemented in a consistent and equitable manner and that equivalent backup supports are available in the event that usual accommodation mechanisms fail. Both students and faculty (who are charged with implementing accommodations) should also have access to formal appeal mechanisms should the designated accommodations be viewed as inadequate or unreasonable.

Academic accommodations are not intended to lower program outcome standards in any way. It is important for both faculty and students to understand the important distinction that all students, even those with qualified disabilities and academic accommodations, are held to the same academic standards and program outcome requirements. Correspondingly, technical standards/essential functions are established for the continuum of students' participation in the nursing program from admission, to graduation and practice as a registered nurse. These standards typically range from the very general, such as sense functioning and locomotion, to motor ability, observational ability, communication ability, conceptual and quantitative ability, sociobehavioral ability, and ability to handle stress (Evans, 2005). Individuals who are unable to meet such technical standards, with or without reasonable accommodations, are not permitted to complete the nursing program and will be counseled to pursue alternative careers. In circumstances in which achievement of technical standards or course/program outcomes is deemed unsatisfactory, the student should be afforded access to formalized appeal procedures.

Discussion of Cases, Findings and Disposition, and Relevant Legal Cases

Unlike previous chapters, this one explores four different cases and therefore the discussion of each case, the resulting findings and disposition, and relevant legal citation will be integrated in one section.

In Case 1, Lilly Brown, a fundamentals nursing student, stated that she was unable to lift more than 10 pounds. Despite Ms. Brown's claim of protection under ADA legislation, she did not disclose her physical limitation, nor did she proactively seek the office of disability services with request for accommodation on admission to the nursing program or in advance of her clinical rotations. She, like many others, assumed that the mere existence of a severe physical limitation would place her in a protected class and afford special consideration with regard to meeting clinical requirements and technical standards inherent to the nursing curriculum.

Ms. Brown's case was referred to the office of disabilities services for evaluation and recommendation. Although the medical documentation of her physical limitations met the criteria of substantially limiting her performance of manual tasks, the nature of her disability made it impossible for her to meet programmatic technical standards associated with motor ability and patient care activities for individuals across the life span. In addition, it was determined that her physical condition would place her at significant risk for personal harm and she did not have the physical stamina to meet the demands of physical exertion required for safe performance in the clinical setting. There were also no medications or ameliorating devices that would permit her to meet these requirements. It was noted that students who have disabilities for which there are no reasonable accommodations do not meet the criteria of being reasonably qualified for admission to or continued progression in a nursing education program. In addition, internships and clinical requirements are considered essential components of nursing curricula. Dismissal from the nursing program was upheld on the basis that Ms. Brown's requested accommodations would necessitate significant alteration to the undergraduate nursing curriculum and related program requirements and necessitate significant alterations/limitations in student clinical learning activities beyond the scope of available resources.

Doherty v. Southern College of Optometry, 862 F.2d 570, 575 (6th Cir. 1988), cert. denied, 493 U.S. 810, 110 S.Ct. 53, 107 L.Ed.2d 22 (1989)

Courts have been clear that health professions education programs can require the full complement of standards and practice. For example, in *Doherty v. Southern College of Optometry*, an optometric student was not otherwise qualified because his neurological disorder inhibited him from using necessary clinical tools of the profession. The court also ruled that reasonable accommodation does not include waiving an essential component of the educational program.

Shin v. University of Maryland Medical System Corp., 369 F. App'x. 472 (4th Cir. 2010)

In the case of *Shin v. University of Maryland Medical System Corp.*, a medical intern with mental and behavioral disabilities associated with attention-deficit disorder (a low working memory and impairment in visual-spatial reasoning) was not deemed an otherwise qualified person under the ADA because he was unable to meet program requirements. The courts upheld that the nature and extent of needed accommodations would require extensive restructuring of the academic program and modifications in academic/clinical standards resulting in undue burden for the academic entity.

Southeastern Community College v. Davis, 442 U.S. 397 (1979)

In Case 2, Donna Glee was a nursing student midway through her nursing program but with significant hearing impairment. The seminal case of a student with disabilities in the nursing context is the U.S. Supreme Court case of *Southeastern Community College v. Davis*. The court determined that a nursing college's denial of enrollment to a deaf applicant was not a violation of section 504 of the Rehabilitation Act of 1973, in which accommodation to perform essential functions of work would require major accommodations by, and lowering the standards of, the nursing program (e.g., taking only academic classes and not participating in the clinical portion of the nursing program). However, subsequent cases have clarified the original ruling explaining that programs could be expected to make reasonable accommodations such as those made available to this student to date.

In this case, Ms. Glee continued to meet all academic and clinical requirements of the nursing program, but there was ongoing concern that her academic performance on examinations was negatively affected by the continued progression of her hearing deficits. She had been provided a stenographer to take notes during class sessions as an auxiliary aid to enhance learning. It is well established that students with sensory impairments may require an intermediary to facilitate communication in areas and activities outside the classroom. However, the use of these intermediaries is highly controversial in the clinical health-care arena. Privacy concerns related to patient confidentiality and potential violation of the Health Information Portability Accountability Act of 1996 are inherent to inclusion of an independent third party in the client-caregiver relationship. It is also difficult to determine to what degree the intermediary simply transfers information or influences the nature of the communication and student judgment (Hafferty and Gibson, 2003). Cost and availability of providing such services outside the classroom raise considerations of undue burden on the part of the program; however, the burden of proof in this situation rests largely with the academic entity (Newsham, 2008).

The denial of Ms. Glee for employment for a university and program-sponsored cooperative education requirement highlights the fact that while on clinical rotations and cooperative work-related activities, students are invited guests of the host facility and subject to their decisions regarding patient care delivery in their respective institutions. The nursing program maintained that it would continue to assist Ms. Glee in finding quality clinical educational experiences and alternative clinical sites that would provide opportunities for her to increase knowledge and skills in fulfillment of her degree requirements. However, it was beyond the academic program's purview to demand that health-care facilities honor the range of accommodations provided to students in the academic environment. If Ms. Glee's disability worsens to the extent that her academic/clinical performance is significantly compromised, safety issues emerge, or reasonable accommodations are no longer feasible, her continued progression in the nursing program would need to be reevaluated. Ms. Glee was also advised that, although there is established precedent that individuals with significant hearing impairment have successfully transitioned to clinical practice roles as registered nurses, there is no guarantee that the extent of accommodations available in postsecondary education programs will be deemed reasonable by potential employers. Consequently, she was counseled that her employment options in the future, although available, may be limited by the nature of her disability.

In Case 3, Jamilla Wyeth had a chronic illness. She subsequently voluntarily disclosed that she had a genetic disorder resulting in anemia, the need for close medical follow-up, and frequent blood transfusions. However, Ms. Wyeth did not reveal the associated degree of disability or details regarding her ongoing plan of treatment. The director of clinical education, Professor Whiting, identified several concerns related to the request for exemption to program policies related to the student's assignments for clinical rotations: (1) safety concerns for both patients and the student; (2) the request for special consideration in the assignment of clinical rotations would create inequity in the application of related policies for other students (some of whom also had certification of qualified physical limitations); and (3) late notification (after clinical assignments had been finalized) left no reasonable alternative clinical assignment due to agency-specific clinical compliance requirements associated with student placements.

Consistent with program policies, Ms. Wyeth was asked to provide a note from her health-care provider that she could participate fully in clinical activities without posing undue risk to herself or others. She was also informed that special consideration could not be provided without formal verification of disability and related academic accommodations from the office of disability services.

Ms. Wyeth subsequently provided documentation from her health-care provider that she was not able to participate fully in course-related clinical activities without limitation and chose to pursue her request for special consideration in the assignment of current and future clinical placements to avoid the need to utilize public transportation or seek alternative means of transportation to distant clinical sites. After review of the case, the office of disability services requested that the nursing program grant the student's request and provide priority consideration for clinical placement sites in this instance and for future clinical rotations.

Professor Whiting remained adamant that such accommodation was unreasonable, limited the student's exposure to varied clinical settings, and created inequity for other students in the application of program policies related to assignment of clinical rotations. It was also noted that Ms. Wyeth had previously completed a prior clinical rotation in a suburban hospital without any discussion of undue burden or negative impact on her medical condition or treatment regimen.

Further discussion with the student revealed that her appointments for recurring blood transfusions and medical follow-up always occurred on the same day of the week. Therefore, Professor Whiting (with the consultation of Dr. Clinton) was able to move the student's clinical assignment to a different day within the same clinical facility, permitting the student access to needed medical treatment within the clinical guidelines and expectations set for all students in the nursing program. The office of disability services agreed that the academic accommodation for Ms. Wyeth should be amended to encompass only the scheduling of the student's future clinical rotations to accommodate ongoing medical treatment and follow-up. It would be Ms. Wyeth's responsibility to notify Professor Whiting of any adjustments to her scheduled treatment regimen, allowing ample time for clinical assignments associated with future nursing courses to be adjusted accordingly.

In this case, the student qualified as disabled because of her chronic medical condition and the need for blood transfusions on a regular basis. However, the initial recommendations for accommodation, subsequent negotiations, and the evolution of revised, mutually agreed upon accommodations highlight the need for close collaboration between the nursing program and the office of disability services. Although disability professionals are well versed in processes related to certification of disability status and generic academic supports, they do not have knowledge of discipline-specific standards, technical standards, and operational complexities associated with clinically oriented health-care disciplines.

In Case 4, nursing student Darrell Iseminger had ADHD. He successfully completed all academic and clinical requirements during the semester with temporary accommodations (extended time and reduced distraction environment for testing) in place. However, he did not complete the qualifications process within the initially agreed-on time line and did not contact the office of disability services for an extension of academic supports. Mr. Iseminger verbally notified course faculty of his diagnosis of ADHD, but did not follow through with faculty recommendations to contact the disability services despite being reminded of academic policies prohibiting special considerations in the absence of official verification of qualification for academic accommodation. Mr. Iseminger elected to take exams without the accommodations of extended time or a distraction-free environment that were in place previously, citing that he did not want to take advantage of the system. Mr. Iseminger subsequently failed both exams and was in jeopardy of failing out of the nursing program, consistent with academic policies, for a second time. He appealed both failing grades and demanded the opportunity to retake the failed exams citing that his previous accommodations served as an acknowledgment of disability by the nursing program and that prior accommodations should have automatically been extended.

Mr. Iseminger then contacted the office of disability services and requested additional time to complete the disability certification process. He was granted an additional 3-month extension of temporary accommodations, but was notified that retroactive application of academic supports was not possible and that he had no basis for appeal in that regard. Correspondingly the nursing program permitted Mr. Iseminger to continue in the nursing program, but with the clear stipulation that (with or without academic accommodations in place) he must meet all established academic and clinical requirements or face dismissal from the nursing program for a final time.

This case highlights several important considerations associated with students who request disability accommodations. Although the diagnosis of ADHD was medically documented, the diagnosis alone is insufficient to qualify the student as disabled. In addition, responsibility to complete the certification process or request extension of time to do so rests solely with the student.

The faculty member's response to the student's verbal notification of a diagnosis of ADHD and denial of accommodations in the absence of an official academic verification letter, consistent with program and university policies, was appropriate. A faculty member is technically an agent of the university. Consequently, had he or she granted academic accommodations without formal documentation of same, it would have resulted in the student being regarded as disabled. In this instance, it would be virtually impossible to discontinue related accommodations, whether or not they were justified, in the future (Thomas, 2000).

The case of Mr. Iseminger also exemplifies the requirement that student disability (perceived or qualified) does not exempt an individual from academic policies and technical standards. It is well established in case law that students with disabilities (with or without related accommodations) must demonstrate that they are otherwise qualified to meet all programmatic requirements or are subject to denial of continued academic progression and dismissal (*Rosenberger v. Rector and Visitors of the Univ. of Virginia*, 145 Fed. Appx. 7 [4th Cir. 2005]; *Hash v. University of Kentucky*, 138 S.W. 3d 123 [Ky.Ct. App. 2004]).

Powell v. National Board of Medical Examiners, 34 F.3d 79 (2nd Cir. 2004)

Another case from the University of Connecticut *(Powell v. National Board of Medical Examiners)* describes a situation in which a student diagnosed with dyslexia, attentions-deficit disorder, anxiety, and depression was dismissed from medical school after failing to meet academic standards despite being afforded multiple opportunities to do so. The court held that she never proved that she was a qualified individual with a disability. As a result, the court found that the university did not discriminate against the student in any way. The court further acknowledged that by granting the student multiple opportunities to meet academic standards, the university went above and beyond usual standards to support her educational endeavors. The temporary academic accommodations granted to the nursing student in this case scenario (in support of the student completing the necessary verifying processes to qualify her ADHD as a disability) would likely be viewed in a similar manner.

⚖ WHEN TO CONTACT THE UNIVERSITY COUNSEL

As mentioned earlier in this chapter, the need to support students with disabilities has intensified in both its nature and extent, and university officials should expect that students will seek legal representation.

WHEN TO CONTACT THE UNIVERSITY COUNSEL—cont'd

Therefore, it is important for the academic administrators in the nursing programs to first be familiar with the representative from the general counsel office who will handle such cases; know how to access this individual for a consult; and be proactive in the educational process and information exchange. In most universities, the director of the office of disability services will have more frequent contact in handling students with disability concerns than will the academic administrators. However, as we emphasize in this chapter, the nursing program administrators need to ensure that legal counsel is briefed on how a clinical education program differs from other academic programs in handling student progression and overall clearance for licensure examination. It would be important to meet with general counsel staff prior to the rise of a problem to explain the types of issues anticipated. Updated student handbooks should be on file in the general counsel office with more in-depth discussion about competencies and technical standards. General counsel should also periodically review admission standards as they relate to students' ability to *fully participate* in didactic and clinical components of the program.

General counsel should be able to review correspondence sent to these students, especially if there may not be agreement between the office of disability services director and the nursing program administrators. Dismissal letters should, without a doubt, be reviewed by counsel. Communiqués that significantly alter the student's degree plan or time to degree completion should be reviewed by counsel. Rulings and decisions on official complaints (not necessarily grievances) are worth reviews by counsel. Decisions on rulings that the student may believe his/her disability confounded the less than expected score or grade on an assessment is worth a review by general counsel. Nursing program administrators should not be hesitant about contacting general counsel on these matters.

Considerations of Students With Disabilities in Nursing Education

Sharby and Roush (2009) suggest that the process of supporting students with disabilities begins long before the student submits an accommodation verification letter endorsed by the office of disability services to a faculty member. It is important that academic administrators and nursing faculty develop a systematic process to anticipate, review, and respond to student requests for accommodation. A discussion of considerations in nursing education must address the specific needs and challenges of students with disabilities from both a legal and conceptual viewpoint.

Clear Articulation of Admission Policies, Pedagogical Requirements, Academic Policies, and Technical Standards

The first step in addressing the needs of nursing students with disabilities involves a detailed review of existing university/program admission criteria for compliance with current legal mandates. Preadmission inquiry concerning whether a prospective applicant has a disability is not permissible under the law. However, questions related to substance abuse and criminal convictions are permissible because of the direct relationship with clinical nursing practice, professional licensure requirements, and the student interface with vulnerable patient populations during clinical rotations (Thomas, 2000).

The use of testing, evaluation of preexisting course work, or other criteria that may influence the admission decision is permissible only if applied equitably to prospective students and if the criteria have been deemed valid and reliable predictors of student success in the nursing program. It is also important to note that when the use of standardized testing is used as major criterion in the admission decision process, these tests must reflect the applicant's aptitude or achievement level rather than sensory, manual, or verbal skills (Thomas, 2000). It is common for third-party testing administrators to note if the tests were taken in nonconforming conditions (testing accommodations provided). Preadmission test scores with such a notation should not be relied on as a sole predictor for admission or rejection of a candidate's application, and should be viewed within the context of other universally applied admission criteria, including prior academic performance, background, and life experiences.

Technical standards deemed fundamental for admission and successful student progression/graduation in the nursing program must also be clearly defined and must be defensible as essential elements of the curriculum. These essential requirements are generally classified in terms of (1) the ability to observe and communicate; (2) physical capacity and motor skills; (3) cognitive skills and intellectual capacity; (4) decision-making skills; and (5) behavioral, social, and professional attributes (Helms, Jorgensen, and Andersen, 2010). Once established, the technical standards should be included in student recruitment and application materials, posted in program Web sites, and published in student handbooks. This information should also be readily available to both theory and clinical faculty so that the standards are applied in a consistent manner. Refer to the *Drexel University Technical Standard Policy* located on http://davisplus.fadavis.com for a detailed example.

Courts have consistently demonstrated great respect for faculty professional judgment and expertise with regard to establishment and implementation of technical standards in professional education programs when reviewing disability discrimination cases. However, it is also necessary for program administrators to ensure timely and ongoing review of these standards to verify conformance with current standards of practice, fair and equitable application of principles, and ongoing compliance with disability law. It is essential that academic administrators take a systematic, disciplined approach to these reviews and seek consultation from legal counsel as needed.

Centralized/Integrated Student Disability Services Functions

The Americans With Disability Act also requires institutions to designate a compliance officer to oversee compliance issues, student disability qualification processes, and accommodation determinations and to serve as a subject matter expert for consultation with faculty and program administrators. This function can be operationalized in a variety of ways. Small, stand-alone nursing programs may choose to designate a faculty member and committee supported by outside consultants and legal counsel. Nursing programs associated with most colleges and universities have the benefit of institutional legal counsel and a formal department dedicated to disability services.

Academic adjustments in nursing and other health-care education programs may be similar to other academic programs in many instances, but often differ substantially in clinical education activities. As noted previously, the office of disability, legal counsel, and their respective staffs are content experts in disability law and generally accepted academic accommodations, but they often lack the professional insight and expertise to adapt generic academic adjustments to clinical course work and related clinical experiences. Close collaboration among nursing program administrators, faculty, university academic support services, and office of disability is needed to address the specific nuances and challenges of addressing discipline-specific nuances and clinical agency requirements for the development and implementation of accommodations in the clinical setting.

Consideration of accommodations in the clinical setting must take into consideration policies and procedures of the host clinical facility and availability of associated resources that may present associated challenges of feasibility or undue burden. Until now, it has not been uncommon for nursing programs to establish policy that academic accommodations do not transfer to the clinical arena because of patient safety concerns and the inability of the university to mandate policies and procedures of clinical affiliates. However, ongoing advances in technology and the availability of sophisticated assistive devices for students with disabilities continue to stretch the limits of possibility in developing creative, unobtrusive, and economically feasible support for students with disabilities in clinical settings. Consequently, it is imperative that the office of disability, program administrators, nursing faculty, and representatives from clinical affiliate sites work together in consideration of student requests for accommodation and evaluation of program standards and related organizational policies/procedures.

Support From Key Stakeholders

Although the law and institution-specific policies serve as the foundation for the determination of applicable accommodations, inherent complexities in nursing education necessitate active involvement and support from key stakeholders.

Nursing Faculty

Nurse educators have the responsibility of ensuring that disabled students have equal access to the nursing profession. The most significant factors affecting disabled student access and academic success in nursing education programs are the perceptions and attitudes of faculty (Ashcroft, Cheronomas, Davis et al., 2008; Sowers and Smith, 2004). Unfortunately for nursing students with disabilities, there is often a disproportionate preoccupation with safety concerns compared to the general nursing student population. However, there is no documented evidence to support those concerns. There have also been no reported instances of students or nurses with qualified disabilities causing harm or substandard care.

Another misconception often voiced by faculty is concern that accommodating students with disabilities will have a negative impact on program outcome standards. These concerns reveal a misunderstanding of intent and requirements of the law, which is to an otherwise qualified individual fair opportunity to achieve outcome standards. Accommodations are not intended to create unfair advantage or require significant adjustments that would substantially alter the nature of the activity.

A study by Sowers and Smith (2004) focusing on faculty perceptions about nursing students with disabilities revealed that nursing faculty viewed students with learning disabilities less favorably than those with physical disabilities. The researchers were also surprised to find that given the emphasis on technical standards in nursing education, respondents were less negative than expected regarding the ability of wheelchair-bound individuals to complete a nursing program and practice as nurses. They suggest that possible contributing factors to these findings include prior experience with wheelchair-bound professional colleagues; minimal faculty effort associated with accommodations associated with physical infirmities that can be implemented with minimum disruption to faculty routines; a lack of understanding of the need for accommodations associated with hidden disabilities; and the need to exert substantial effort in modifying teaching practices to meet the needs of students with learning disabilities (Sowers and Smith, 2004). There is general agreement regarding a significant need for faculty orientation and ongoing education related to potential for students with disabilities to complete an academic nursing program; strategies to promote student success; implementation of needed accommodations; and associated legal mandates (Ashcroft et al., 2008; Konur, 2002; Sowers and Smith, 2004).

Clinical Affiliates

Agencies contracted as clinical sites for nursing student experiences with direct patient care have the dual responsibility of fulfilling these contractual obligations to nursing education programs and the provision of quality health care. These entities are faced with several regulatory requirements (e.g., accreditation standards, licensure requirements, health information privacy laws, patient-quality benchmarks) and liability concerns. Although they may be philosophically supportive of nursing education, their primary focus is the "business" of health care. Nevertheless, they are also subject to compliance with disability statutes.

Understandably, perceived potential liability issues and patient perceptions become important considerations in granting access to a disabled student (who is essentially a guest in the host facility). It is incumbent on nursing faculty and academic administrators to provide education and needed supports to alleviate affiliate clinical agency concerns. It may also be beneficial for the program administrator to take advantage of established relationships with key individuals in clinical agencies when soliciting cooperation and support for student accommodations in the clinical setting such as introducing the use of adaptive devices and suggesting possible modifications to policies/procedures that will enhance student learning and the provision of safe, effective nursing care. Once the feasibility of such accommodations is established, it is likely that other clinical affiliates will be more receptive to requests for needed clinical accommodations in their respective organizations.

Students

For those who have had little exposure to individuals with disabilities, it may be difficult to understand the associated challenges faced by peers with physical or learning disabilities. Students may sense faculty concern about the ability of disabled students to meet clinical and academic standards. Nondisabled students may have apprehensions that sharing the learning environment with individuals who need extra support may negatively affect their own personal learning objectives and outcomes. Open dialogue, experiential learning, and faculty support will provide opportunity for students to reframe paradigms, work collaboratively with individuals with disabilities (in both personal and professional roles), and provide nursing care from a more holistic framework that will enhance the learning experience for all.

Embrace the Use of Technology and Evolving Pedagogy

Rapid advances in technology and assistive devices and evolving pedagogy continue to open new worlds of possibilities for assimilation and achievement for individuals with disabilities thought impossible not long ago (Dorman, 1998; Leigh, 2008; Smith Glasgow, Dunphy et al., 2010). In addition to increased sophistication of adaptive and assistive devices, these technological supports are also becoming more affordable and accessible to the general public.

Corresponding advances in special education and the move from teacher-dominated to learner-focused pedagogies, which enable students with diverse learning needs to process information more efficiently and effectively, enhance student acquisition of knowledge and skills. Simulated patient-care experiences and virtual learning environments enable nursing students to practice clinical skills, develop clinical judgment, and demonstrate mastery of essential professional competencies (Leigh, 2008; Smith Glasgow, Dunphy et al., 2010). Although the advances in technology have benefited the entire nursing student population, these scientific and technological breakthroughs have had a profound effect on minimizing or eliminating barriers for nursing students with physical and learning disabilities in both the classroom and clinical arena (Ashcraft et al., 2008; Broadbent, Dorow, and Fisch, 2006; Busby, Gammel, and Jeffcoat, 2002; Coombs, 2002; Evans, 2005; Preece et al., 2007; Sowers and Smith, 2004; Tee et al., 2010; Tincani, 2004) Consultation with colleagues in other nursing programs and other health-related disciplines will provide insight into innovative teaching strategies, evaluative measures, physical adaptation devices, learning aids, and technological supports that would enable disabled nursing students to meet program outcome standards both in the classroom and at the point of care.

Create a Supportive Environment

It is generally accepted that a supportive educational environment is conducive to learning and achieving program outcomes for all students. Information for the range of academic and clinical support services available, including the office of disability services, should be made available to students in advance of matriculation into the nursing program, at general orientation sessions, and on an ongoing basis. Because students with disabilities may be hesitant to disclose limitations for fear of negative consequences, it is essential that an attitude of acceptance and support permeate all aspects of the educational experience. There are many and varied strategies and accommodations that provide students with learning and other disabilities an equal opportunity to be successful in didactic and clinical settings. An open, supportive environment will encourage students with disabilities to feel more comfortable in openly discussing their learning needs and accessing available supports. Some examples of how this can be accomplished include the following:

1. Inclusion of an introductory course (or equivalent) focusing on the transition to college which includes information related to time management, organizational skills, study strategies, stress management and personalized introductions of staff from student support services available through the university
2. Inclusion of the office of disability services in course syllabi
3. Implementation of a nonfaculty adviser role that serves as a student advocate and liaison for addressing student issues and concerns in a nonjudgmental manner
4. Ongoing monitoring of student progress in course work with established early warning mechanisms to facilitate recognition and activation of needed support systems
5. Development of nursing-specific academic and clinical support functions that complement course content (practice labs, content review, remediation activities, test-taking skills, etc.) that accommodate the need for additional time and practice associated with mastery of course content and proficiency in clinical skills
6. Education of administrators, faculty, and staff regarding disability law, and information regarding accommodation and access
7. Provision of sensitivity training workshops and understanding of disability as a cultural competency throughout all aspects of the nursing curriculum
8. Encouragement of student input and maintenance of ongoing dialogue regarding needed educational supports
9. Provision of timely responses and comprehensive ongoing follow-ups for inquiries and issues associated with disability services
10. Development of case-by-case evaluation, complaint, and appeal procedures for student disability issues
11. Establishment of ongoing review, update, and widespread dissemination of practices and policies associated with student disability services

Evolving Trends

As a result of greater acceptance of individuals with disabilities in society, some nursing educators are questioning the longstanding emphasis on physical attributes associated with technical standards for admission and progression in nursing programs. Marks (2007) asserts that nursing students with disabilities will foster a new set of knowledge, skills, and abilities in the nursing profession and challenges that technical standards and essential standards in nursing curricula need to be redefined accordingly. She also suggests that students with disabilities have the potential to improve nursing care and advance culturally relevant care as a result of their unique understanding of disability issues. There is also a growing number of nursing faculty and professionals who argue that relying exclusively on a list of physical attributes and technical skills that tend to dominate the nursing profession undermines the profession's desire to move beyond the perception of nurses as skilled laborers (Sowers and Smith, 2004).

Carroll (2004) suggests that the technical standards model in nursing should be replaced by a creative access model that is outcomes based and acknowledges that more than one process can be used to achieve desired outcomes. This model focuses on the availability of accommodations, not the type and severity of the associated disability. Arndt (2004) proposes that because delegation, direction, and supervision of certain tasks are essential components of professional nursing practice, it should also be considered as a possible accommodation for nursing students with physical disabilities in the clinical setting. She further asserts that "every nurse needs to be caring, deliver that care with integrity, effectively interact with others and able to think critically. Not every nurse needs to be able to lift 25 lbs., climb stairs, or be able to start an intravenous solution" (Arndt, 2004, p. 205).

Evans (2005) presents a compelling example of a paraplegic student who successfully completed a baccalaureate nursing program and successfully transitioned to practice as a registered nurse. She outlines curricular and procedural adaptations that permitted the student to meet both academic and clinical program standards and enabled faculty to think in new ways about clinical competencies and innovative teaching strategies. Faculty deemed that when the student learned the concepts underlying a psychomotor skill and demonstrated her knowledge through verbalization, simulation using a manikin, and theoretical testing, she had fulfilled her academic obligations similar to nondisabled students who learn the same concepts but never had the opportunity to practice on a live patient in the clinical setting (Evans, 2005).

In revisiting these important concepts, nursing educators are challenged to move away from a task-oriented perspective and the mindset that disabled students need special treatment, and focus instead on the range of strategies and technologies that will enable these students to exercise their full range of abilities in meeting essential functions inherent in professional nursing practice. The dialogue and debate will undoubtedly continue; however, ongoing communication and collaboration will serve as a foundation curricular innovation now and in the future.

Summary

Federal laws require universities to make reasonable and necessary modifications to rules, policies, and practices to prevent discrimination against students on the basis of disability. As a result of these legislative mandates, advances in technology, educational supports at all levels of schooling, and the work of advocacy groups for students with disabilities, more and more students with disabilities are seeking postsecondary degrees. Nursing, as a profession, maintains a strong advocacy role for individuals with special needs; however, the education of nursing students with disabilities poses unique challenges. Clinically focused professional education programs such as nursing are faced with the dichotomous challenge of supporting student learning within the context of public safety, mandated program outcome standards, and licensure requirements. Despite the significant body of literature on postsecondary students with disabilities, there is a paucity of literature related to students with disabilities in nursing and the health professions compared with other disciplines (Sharby and Roush, 2009). There is also no definitive agreement regarding the nature and extent of accommodations and related academic supports in meeting the needs of nursing students with disabilities with regard to program outcome standards at this time. Courts are, understandably, particularly interested in cases involving the health professions because of the direct effect on the health and safety of patients.

In your role as an academic nursing administrator to support faculty and students in the teaching and learning process, you also have a legal and moral responsibility to protect your school from claims of discrimination on the basis of disability. However, the complex and varied roles of the nurse educator and academic administrator also necessitate that you transcend legal mandates and embrace the associated ethical and professional responsibilities to students, faculty, clinical affiliates, and the public for the education of nursing professionals who provide high-quality, culturally sensitive nursing care. This chapter offered analyses of several scenarios regarding undergraduate nursing students who present requests for academic accommodations (perceived or officially verified) to faculty and academic program administrators and pointed out significant considerations in the management of these issues.

Bohne (2004) suggests consideration of two essential questions that provide the foundation for personal reflection and academic leadership in policy development, curricular evolution, and programmatic accommodations/supports for nursing students with disabilities: (1) "If people with disabilities can use their skills to execute the nursing process to achieve desired nursing outcomes in a nursing role, do these individuals have a right to pursue a career in nursing?" *and* (2) "...beyond the letter of the law, does the nursing profession have a professional responsibility to support them to doing so?" (Bohne, 2004, p. 202)

As an academic administrator of a nursing program, you are positioned in a key leadership role to challenge traditional paradigms and proactively assist faculty in exploring curricular innovation and academic/clinical supports which will support disabled nursing students in achieving program outcome standards as they transition to professional nursing roles.

The disposition of cases in this chapter is based on the technical standards model prevalent in nursing education today. As a result of ongoing advances in technology, changing societal perceptions, new conceptual models of nursing education, and the evolution of increasingly diverse professional opportunities, similar cases may have very different outcomes in the future. The principles and practices presented in this chapter also provide a framework for compliance with legal mandates, evaluating and implementing academic accommodations, and understanding the needs of students with physical and learning disabilities in contemporary nursing education programs.

Qualified individuals with physical and learning disabilities have the potential to improve nursing care and advance culturally relevant care with their unique understanding of related obstacles and challenges. Consequently, it is also critical that academic administrators in nursing education build upon the status quo and assume a proactive role in reexamining existing admission criteria; redefining technical standards and essential competencies; exploring creative teaching and evaluation strategies; and participating in the ongoing evolution of best practices and professional standards for individuals with disabilities in nursing education and practice, now and in the future.

CRITICAL ELEMENTS TO CONSIDER

- Examine admission and progression policies for conformance with disability laws; consult legal counsel as needed.
- Maintain working knowledge of regulatory changes, case law, and professional standards, and licensure regulations affecting nursing education and practice.
- Provide early and ongoing student access to comprehensive disability services and individualized case analysis and disposition.
- Review technical standards and essential competencies with regard to trends in nursing education and professional practice.
- Expand conceptualization of disability beyond the focus of physical limitations and disorders.
- Provide education sessions for faculty related to evolving trends and advancements in addressing students with physical and learning disabilities.
- Develop collaborative relationships for determination and implementation of student academic and clinical accommodations; ensure that accommodations are not made without formal verification.
- Keep abreast of evolving advances in technology and educational practices that will assist disabled individuals in achieving programmatic outcomes.

CRITICAL ELEMENTS TO CONSIDER—cont'd

- Participate in ongoing dialogue regarding evolving trends and best practices in addressing the needs of nursing students with disabilities within the context of quality in educational curricula and the provision of high-quality health-care services to the public.

HELPFUL RESOURCES

- US Department of Education, "Students With Disabilities Preparing for Postsecondary Education: Know Your Rights and Responsibilities" http://www2.ed.gov/about/offices/list/ocr/transition.html
- "10 Tips for College Students With Disabilities" http://www.npr.org/templates/story/story.php?
- College Funding for Students With Disabilities http://www.washington.edu/doit/Brochures/Academics/financial
- Colleges With Programs for Learning Disabled Students http://www.college-scholarships.com/learning_disabilities.htm

References

Arndt, M. E. (2004). Educating nursing students with disabilities: One nurse educator's journey from questions to clarity. *Journal of Nursing Education, 43*(50), 204.

Ashcroft, T., Cheronomas, W., Davis, P., et al. (2008). Nursing students with disabilities: One faculty's journey. *International Journal of Nursing Education Scholarship, 5*(1), 1–26.

Bohne, J. J. (2004). Valuing differences among nursing students. *Journal of Nursing Education, 43*(5), 202–203.

Broadbent, G., Dorow, L. G., & Fisch, L. A. (2006). College syllabi: Providing support for students with disabilities. *Educational Forum, 71*, 71–80.

Busby, R. R., Gammel, H. L., & Jeffcoat, N. K. (2002). Grades, graduation and orientation: A longitudinal study of how new student programs relate to grade point averages and graduation. *Journal of College Orientation and Transition, 10*(1), 45–50.

Carroll, S.M. (2004). Inclusion of people with physical disabilities in nursing education. *Journal of Nursing Education, 43*(5), 207-212.

Center for Education and Employment Law. (2010). *Higher education law in America.* Malvern, PA: Author.

Coombs, N. (2002). FIPSE: Empowering students with disabilities. *Change, 34*(5), 42–48.

Cope, D. (2005). The courts, the ADA, and the academy. *Academic Questions, 19*(1), 37–47.

Doherty v. Southern College of Optometry, 862 F.2d 570, 575 (6th Cir.1988), cert. denied, 493 U.S. 810, 110 S.Ct. 53, 107 L.Ed.2d 22 (1989).

Dorman, S. M. (1998). Assistive technology benefits for students with disabilities. *Journal of School Health, 68*(3), 120–123.

Drexel University. (2010, September). *Student handbook: Bachelor of science in nursing co-operative education program* (pp. 23–25). Philadelphia: Drexel University, College of Nursing and Health Professions.

Evans, B. C. (2005). Chapter 1: Nursing education for students with disabilities: Our students, our teachers. *Annual Review of Nursing Education, 3,* 3–22.

Hafferty, F. W., & Gibson, G. G. (2003). Learning disabilities, professionalism, and the practice of medical education. *Academic Medicine, 78,* 189–201.

Hash v. University of Kentucky, 138 S.W.3d 123 (Ky.Ct. App. 2004).

Helms, L., Jorgensen, J., & Anderson, M. A. (2006). Disability law and nursing education: An update. *Journal of Professional Nursing, 22*(30), 190–196.

Konur, O. (2002). Access to nursing education by disabled students: Rights and duties of nursing programs. *Nurse Education Today, 22,* 364–374.

Leigh, G. T. (2008). High-fidelity patient simulation and nursing student's self-efficacy: A review of the literature. *International Journal of Nursing Education Scholarship, 5*(1), article 37. doi:10.2202/1548-923X.1613

Marks, B. (2007). Cultural competence revisited: Nursing students with disabilities. *Journal of Nursing Education, 46*(2), 70–74.

National Center for Educational Statistics. Washington, DC: NCES, U.S. Dept of Education. Accessed February 7, 2011, from http://www.ces.ed.gov/fastfacts.

Newsham, K. (2008). Disability law and health care education. *Journal of Allied Health, 37*(2), 110–115.

Powell v. National Board of Medical Examiners, 34 F.3d 79 (2nd Cir. 2004).

Preece, J., Roberts, N., Beecher, M., Rash, P., Shwalb, D., & Martinelli, E. (2007). Academic advisors and students with disabilities: A national survey of advisors' experiences and needs. *NACADA Journal, 27*(1), 57–72.

Rosenberger v. Rector and Visitors of the University of Virginia, 145 Fed. Appx. 7 (4th Cir. 2005).

Ridley, J., Stanley, N., Manthorpe, J., & Harris, J. (2008). Disabled students and staff: Disclosing disability. *Community Care* (1717), 32–33.

Rosenberger v. Rector and Visitors of the Univ. of Va., 515 U.S. 819 (1995).

Rosenbraugh, C. J. (2005). Learning disabilities and medical schools. *Medical Education, 34,* 994–1000.

Rothstein, L. F. (2000). The American With Disabilities Act: A ten-year retrospective: Higher education and the future of disability policy. *Alabama Law Review.* 52 Ala. L. Rev. 241.

Sharby, N., & Roush, S. (2009). Analytical decision-making model for addressing the needs of allied health students with disabilities. *Journal of Allied Health, 38*(1), 54–62.

Shin v. University of Maryland Medical System Corp., 369 F. App'x. 472 (4th Cir. 2010).

Smith Glasgow, M. E., Dunphy, L. M., & Mainous, R. O. (2010). Innovative nursing educational curriculum for the 21st century. *NLN Educational Perspectives, 31*(6), 355–357.

Southeastern Community College v. Davis, 442 U.S. 397 (1979).

Sowers, J., & Smith, M. R. (2004). Nursing faculty members' perceptions, knowledge, and concerns about students with disabilities. *Journal of Nursing Education, 43*(5), 213–218.

Stacey, M., & Carroll, S. M. (2004). Inclusion of people with physical disabilities in nursing education. *Journal of Nursing Education, 43*(5), 207–212.

Tee, T. R., Owens, K., Plowright, S., et al. (2010). Being reasonable: Supporting disabled students in practice. *Nurse Education in Practice, 10,* 216–221.

Thomas, S. B. (2000). College students and disability law. *Journal of Special Education, 33*(4), 248–257.

Tincani, M. (2004). Improving outcomes for college students with disabilities. *College Teaching, 52*(4), 128–132.

CHAPTER 22

Disability Issues for the Faculty

A New Graduate Nursing Faculty Hire Demands to Teach Online From Home Due to Disability

Your role: You are Dr. Lopez, the department chair of the adult health division in the college of nursing.

An extensive search committee has led to the hiring of Dr. Bostridge, an experienced faculty member who has taught in several nursing schools during her 15-year academic career. Although Dr. Bostridge was the leading recommendation of the graduate nursing search committee, you had some reservations about the relative job-hopping that you discerned from her curriculum vitae. As the department chair who had either to agree to the hire or reject the recommendation, at the final interview you had queried Dr. Bostridge about it. She stated she had moved around because of her husband's job; that seemed plausible to you, although you knew there was no way to confirm this. Even by contacting previous employers you knew they would likely indicate only whether Dr. Lopez was eligible for rehire or not. Nevertheless, you always aimed to do more due diligence when making a final hiring decision, particularly at the faculty level. You checked Dr. Bostridge's personal references, did a quick license check, and found that Dr. Bostridge's RN license was active in the state with no pending actions. Finally, you thought you needed at least one confirmation of the applicant from someone whom you know at one of Dr. Bostridge's previous employers. Unfortunately, Dr. Bostridge worked in smaller nursing programs, and the individuals on the faculty whom you do know, you know only remotely and feel uncomfortable calling them for a reference. With some reservation, you made an offer to Dr. Bostridge, who promptly accepted.

Dr. Bostridge's hire date was the first Monday of August for the fall semester. Human resource benefits commenced 30 days after the hire date, and classes commenced in mid-September. Approximately 35 days after Dr. Bostridge was hired and 3 days before classes were to begin, she sent you a letter indicating that she has Huntington's disease and could only teach online from home due to her disability.

Questions

- How should Dr. Lopez first proceed?
- Can Dr. Bostridge legally demand to teach online from home?
- Does Dr. Bostridge have any particular protections under the Americans With Disabilities Act of 1990?
- If there was anything fraudulent in Dr. Bostridge's application, could the university immediately terminate her?

Disability Issues for the Faculty: Legal Principles and Review of the Literature

Any discussion of disabilities in the workplace must begin with the Americans With Disabilities Act (ADA) of 1990 signed into law by President George H. W. Bush (U.S. Dept. of Justice, 2011). Since its enactment in 1990, there have been voluminous court rulings on the exact interpretation of the intent of the ADA law, and various court cases that Congress deemed as having gone beyond the original intent of the act led to a major amendment of this federal law, the ADA Amendment Act, which was signed into law by President George W. Bush on September 25, 2008 (which went into effect January 1, 2009) (Equal Employment Opportunity Commission, 2009).

From the amended act of 2008, the following definitions apply to *disability* and *major life activity.*

(1) Disability

The term "disability" means, with respect to an individual

(A) a physical or mental impairment that substantially limits one or more major life activities of such individual;

(B) a record of such an impairment; or

(C) being regarded as having such an impairment (as described in paragraph (3)).

(2) Major Life Activities

(A) In general

For purposes of paragraph (1),[1] major life activities include, but are not limited to, caring for oneself, performing manual tasks, seeing, hearing, eating, sleeping, walking, standing, lifting, bending, speaking, breathing, learning, reading, concentrating, thinking, communicating, and working.

(B) Major bodily functions

For purposes of paragraph (1), a major life activity also includes the operation of a major bodily function, including but not limited to, functions of the immune system, normal cell growth, digestive, bowel, bladder, neurological, brain, respiratory, circulatory, endocrine, and reproductive functions (Section 12102, 2009).

The law further protects individuals who are merely "regarded as having such an impairment" and states the following:

(A) An individual meets the requirement of "being regarded as having such an impairment" if the individual establishes that he or she has been subjected to an action prohibited under this chapter

---

[1] This refers to the section 1 definition of *disability.*

because of an actual or perceived physical or mental impairment whether or not the impairment limits or is perceived to limit a major life activity.

(B) *Paragraph (1) (C) shall not apply to impairments that are transitory and minor. A transitory impairment is an impairment with an actual or expected duration of 6 months or less.*

The ADA is an incredibly complex law, and it is beyond the scope of this chapter to explain it in great detail, but there are a few important general principles to emphasize. First, the ADA does not apply to all employers; depending on the nature of the organization, it applies to workers employed in companies having 15 to 25 workers. Second, the ADA does not apply to all workers in these organizations, but to "qualified individuals." A "qualified individual" is:

an individual who, with or without reasonable accommodation, can perform the essential functions of the employment position that such individual holds or desires. For the purposes of this subchapter, consideration shall be given to the employer's judgment as to what functions of a job are essential, and if an employer has prepared a written description before advertising or interviewing applicants for the job, this description shall be considered evidence of the essential functions of the job. (Section 12111, 2009)

Last, although "qualified individuals" working in organizations/companies covered by the ADA are by law entitled to "reasonable accommodation," employers are not required to bear "undue hardship" (meaning requiring significant difficulty or expenses) to accommodate employees claiming disability. The definition of *reasonable accommodation* is the following:

(A) *making existing facilities used by employees readily accessible to and usable by individuals with disabilities; and*

(B) *job restructuring, part-time or modified work schedules, reassignment to a vacant position, acquisition or modification of equipment or devices, appropriate adjustment or modifications of examinations, training materials or policies, the provision of qualified readers or interpreters, and other similar accommodations for individuals with disabilities. (section 12111, 2009)*

This is where the crux of the debate between employers and employees lies: Is the employee legitimately disabled and is the accommodation requested or needed by the employee reasonable? Indeed, Kirkland has written in *Fat Rights: Dilemmas of Difference and Personhood* (2008) that "disability studies scholars and activists hoped the social model of disability [rather than its medicalization] would dominate discussion of what would need to change to provide real opportunity for persons with disabilities" (p. 128)[2] In other words, many believe the ADA has not led to broad acceptance and integration of individuals with disabilities into the vast spectrum of contemporary modern society, but instead a mindset has evolved in which society meets only the technical requirements of accommodation.

Kirkland indicates the case for justice for individuals with disability lies within the challenge of difference (2008). She writes:

A prominent idea in American law is that similarly situated people ought to be treated similarly. Equality, in this view, is not about treating each and every person in exactly the same way. Instead, it is about knowing which differences among persons really matter. (p. 1)

---

[2] For the record, except in rare circumstances (e.g., morbid, incapacitating obesity), obesity is not considered a disabling impairment under the ADA (Adamitis, 2000).

Kirkland indicates that if individuals are different and not similarly situated, they can be legally treated differently, and she uses children as a case example. In this case, children are not adults and therefore not held to the same standards. They may be treated differently and very often should be treated differently from the way in which adults are treated.

In the case of the difference characterized by a medical illness such as Huntington's disease, Miller (2007) indicates that it can be difficult to claim disability with this disease (especially in its early stages) because there are numerous problems that may lead to one's inability to work and because in the early stages the individual affected may look and act perfectly normal.[3] A great deal of leeway is granted, however, to employers who often deal with employees with cancer who are undergoing chemotherapy or who face other serious medical issues. Our experience is that employers, particularly when the employee has created good will, are often willing to accommodate employees as they seek treatment and begin either a transition back to full-time employment in the organization/company or who are transitioning out of the workplace because of the severity and perhaps permanence of the illness. Employees who have created substantial bad good will in the organization may find themselves treated to the letter of the ADA law, and even these individuals are rarely in a position to push forth with accusations that they are being treated unfairly. These are, for better or worse, some of the realities of the U.S. workforce, especially because there is no national health insurance program in full operation as of the writing of this text.[4]

Discussion of Case

Recall from this chapter's case study that you are Dr. Lopez and have just received a letter from Dr. Bostridge, telling you that she has Huntington's disease. How would you first proceed? Dr. Lopez was initially shocked by the suddenness of the letter and the demands made by Dr. Bostridge. She was also very remorseful about her own sloppiness with her due diligence of this faculty hire. Her intuition told her that there was something awry with the applicant, but she had failed to do the second level of reference checks that had been her usual practice. Nevertheless, she thought it preposterous that Dr. Bostridge would be making this request for accommodation with class to begin in only a few days. She was already determined that Dr. Bostridge's request was not reasonable, but she knew she would have to do more fact-finding and first meet with Dr. Bostridge. Dr. Lopez e-mailed Dr. Bostridge to schedule a meeting for the next day, but Dr. Bostridge e-mailed back stating that she was sick and unable to come in, and that she wasn't sure if she would be well by the first day of class. She reiterated that she was certain she

---

[3] The issues of disability caused by the early stages of multiple sclerosis are similar to those of Huntington's disease (Perkins & Perkins, 2008.).

[4] President Obama's health-care reform bill, if not repealed, will not be in full operation and covering all U.S. citizens until 2015 (Jackson & Nolan, 2010).

would be able to teach online, but because her condition had suddenly worsened, it was very unlikely she would be able to make it in to class and stand all day.

Bewildered by what she perceived as outright stalling tactics, Dr. Lopez called her associate dean, Dr. Vizny, and informed her of what had transpired. Dr. Lopez told Dr. Vizny that she planned on calling university counsel for guidance. Dr. Vizny endorsed the strategy, and said she would inform the dean and get back to her if she had any further advice. Upon calling the university counsel, Mr. Callas, Dr. Lopez asked him, "Can she legally demand to teach online from home?" Mr. Callas was concerned about how to proceed, especially with a diagnosis of Huntington's disease, if it could be confirmed. Having previously dealt with a similar case with an employee with longstanding multiple sclerosis who had worked many, many years at the university until his behavior became so bizarre his employment had to be terminated, Mr. Callas suspected that many individuals in the early stages of Huntington's disease would likely not need any kind of accommodation. He drafted a letter to Dr. Bostridge stating that (1) Dr. Bostridge had to provide certified documentation of a disabling condition; and (2) indicate what major life activity Dr. Bostridge could not fulfill. He also stated in his letter that because the college had no faculty who teach 100% online, Dr. Bostridge's request for such an accommodation appears unreasonable at first glance and recommended that she revise her accommodation request to one that is more reasonable.

WHEN TO CONTACT THE UNIVERSITY COUNSEL

As happened in this case, the department chair contacted university counsel when she had a question arising out of a new employee's demands that her working conditions be immediately modified. Dr. Lopez also followed the chain of command by keeping her superiors well informed about the incident and her likely actions. This was a very prudent course to take, and in cases in which a faculty member (possibly the chair of a search committee) faces any of these issues, consultation first with the department chair is highly recommended. It is also recommended that nursing administrators develop a strong relationship with their human resources department so policies and procedures are being interpreted and can be strictly enforced. Familiarity with appropriate and legal diversity strategies and affirmative action policies in recruitment and hiring is also essential.

Findings and Disposition

The third question in this chapter's case study is: Does Dr. Bostridge have any particular protections under the Americans With Disabilities Act of 1990? The simplest answer is that it is very likely that she does, especially if Dr. Bostridge is able to provide the certified documentation of the disability that interferes with at least one major life activity. But in this case, the resolution is not so clear-cut. Dr. Lopez was certain that she had discussed (and documented in at least one e-mail) the prospective teaching load for Dr. Bostridge and indicated that most faculty teach one online course per year. She also discussed with Dr. Bostridge (when queried) that most graduate students take classes in the evenings, so classes are scheduled sometime between 5 and 8 p.m. She therefore thought that Dr. Bostridge had been dishonest in her intentions when she agreed to the teaching assignment and did not raise any issues at that time. The fourth question in this chapter's case study is: If there was anything fraudulent in Dr. Bostridge's application, could the university immediately terminate her? Although the answer to this question is yes, there was nothing immediately identifiable that was false—only that Dr. Bostridge had agreed orally and in writing to her teaching assignment and was suddenly stating she could not meet her obligations without her requested accommodation.

Dr. Bostridge subsequently replied to Mr. Callas's request but failed to produce the certified documentation. In her letter, Dr. Bostridge raised the fact that the building, where her assigned classes and office are located is not wheelchair-accessible on any floor. Dr. Bostridge then went on to state that if she is not allowed to teach online, as she has requested, she may be forced to file a complaint with state or federal authorities.

A subsequent investigation discovered that indeed Dr. Bostridge had incorrectly cited her previous length of employment at two previous colleges, thereby providing a justifiable and nondiscriminatory basis for termination. Regarding the accessibility of the building to which Dr. Bostridge was assigned, the college was prepared to reassign Dr. Bostridge's office and her classes to a different building on campus, which was completely accessible, thus negating Dr. Bostridge's threats of filing a complaint. After communicating to Dr. Bostridge these facts, it was decided that the best course of action was to offer Dr. Bostridge a very small settlement to resign with an accompanying release, or else they would terminate her for falsifying her application. Dr. Bostridge accepted the settlement, her employment was terminated, and the case was closed.

Relevant Legal Case

Mingo v. Oakland Unified School District, No. 104055 (105 LRP 7028)
(Cal. Ct. App. 2005)

This case rested on the principle that knowledge of depression does not equate with knowledge of a depression-related disability. The plaintiff in this case, Mr. Mingo, was a typing teacher in an Oakland, California, school district. Although he had a longstanding history of depression and was undergoing treatment for it, he had never notified his employer that his depression was a disabling condition. Upon being accused of sexual harassment and making threats against other district employees, he was terminated. He immediately filed a federal lawsuit, claiming disability discrimination under the California Fair Employment and Housing Act (Pima Community College, n.d.).

At trial it was revealed that before he was terminated, Mr. Mingo's neurologist had notified the school district of his patient's threats[5] and dangerous behavior and the school district promptly issued a restraining order. Mr. Mingo's therapist testified at a hearing, and his psychiatrist and psychologist wrote letters to the school district urging that the restraining order be lifted, on the basis that Mr. Mingo suffered from depression. The courts ruled against Mr. Mingo, indicating that although it was evident he had depression, it was never reported as a disability nor in any of the court correspondence by the psychologist or psychiatrist did they refer to the depression as a disability. Further, Mr. Mingo never claimed to the court that his sexual harassment or threats were due to his depression, and the case was dismissed. The conclusion to this case is that in order for a court to rule that an individual was fired due to a disabling condition, the employer must have first been formally notified that the employee had a disabling condition, and not after the fact (Pima Community College, n.d.).

Summary

It will be increasingly common that universities will employ new faculty or whose own current faculty will suffer from disabling conditions such as those noted above, including chronic fatigue syndrome, chronic back pain, and other medical conditions (De Souza and Frank, 2011; Jason et al., 2011). The issues of disability are becoming even more prevalent in contemporary society with some estimates that 40 million or more Americans (roughly one in seven) have some form of disability (Lander, 2007) and that number is expected to rise with an aging population. We are also seeing thousands of veterans return from wars in Iraq and Afghanistan who are disabled, and some so severely with amputations of limbs and traumatic brain injuries (Schneiderman, Braver, and Kang, 2008). The challenge for the future will be for society to find ways to better integrate many of these disabled individuals into the mainstream of working life so that they can remain productive citizens and also contribute to the federal and state tax base.

Individuals with disabilities are protected by the ADA, but in the context of employment, the individual must be qualified, meaning able with or without an accommodation to perform the essential functions of a job. Although there are legal protections for qualified individuals who seek employment, matching the best individual for any given position often may leave a disabled individual at a

---

[5] The court record is not clear what precise threats were made. The inference is that the neurologist was walking a fine line between both disclosing confidential health information and withholding other information discerned from the physician–patient relationship.

disadvantage. It is important for employers to put the time and effort into writing job descriptions, defining very carefully what are essential functions and what are not, so that when employment decisions need to be made involving individuals with disabilities and reasonable accommodations need to be discussed, the ultimate decisions will be less fraught with claims of actual as well as perceived discrimination on the basis of disability.

In the context of a university or college, figuring out how teaching faculty can be reasonably accommodated in that unique work environment (generally high intellect, low physical requirement), especially with the huge growth of online learning, may give rise to new meanings in academia of what constitutes "reasonable accommodation" (Parry, 2010).

CRITICAL ELEMENTS TO CONSIDER

- Although this chapter is focused on faculty, it should be iterated that for nursing programs (at all levels—BSN, MSN, and PhD/DNP or others) it is important to have technical standards.
- There may also be technical standards that would apply to faculty too—especially if they are being hired for undergraduate or graduate clinical teaching or supervision.
- It is possible that some degrees, the PhD for instance, may have very few real technical requirements and might permit both students and faculty to have higher levels of enrolled or employed individuals with disabilities.
- Employers cannot ask employees if they have a disability, but they can inquire whether employees can meet the technical requirements of the job. Note that it is not a requirement that an applicant or student disclose anything about a medical condition or disability in advance of being hired by or admitted to the university. Therefore, failure to do so should not be viewed as dishonest or misrepresentation.
- If applicants indicate that they would need reasonable accommodation to perform the job, one cannot simply not hire them because they are requesting an accommodation. The employer can assess whether the accommodation would necessitate an undue hardship that the employer is not required to accommodate.
- These issues are very delicate and are ripe for litigation, and it is always wise to consult a human resources representative for any clarifications before any job offers are made or job offers are denied. Any decisions, made following disclosure by an applicant of any medical condition or disability during the hiring process, should be reviewed in advance with a human resources representative or university counsel.

CRITICAL ELEMENTS TO CONSIDER—cont'd

- Individuals involved in the hiring process (e.g., chairs and members of search committees) *must* be trained in proper methods of the recruitment and hiring process, and they must follow federal, state, and local laws in their procedures. For instance, someone on a search committee cannot ask an applicant if she is pregnant or what the applicant plans to do for child care once the baby arrives. Although the applicant is free to disclose the fact that she is pregnant and discuss child care herself, those conducting the interviews should be careful and direct the conversation back to the qualifications and essential functions of the job. A disclosure of pregnancy may not disqualify an applicant from a respective job search.

HELPFUL RESOURCES

- Americans With Disabilities Amendments Act of 2008
  http://www.access-board.gov/about/laws/ada-amendments.htm
- Top Disability Web Sites
  http://www.topdisabilitywebsites.com/
- "Understanding Disabilities When Designing a Web Site"
  http://www.digital-web.com/articles/understanding_disabilities_when_designing_a_website/
- United States Equal Employment Opportunity Commission
  http://www.eeoc.gov/

References

Adamitis, E. M. (2000). Appearance matters: A proposal to prohibit appearance discrimination in employment. *Washington Law Review, 75,* 195.

De Souza, L., & Frank, A. O. (2011). Patients' experiences of the impact of chronic back pain on family life and work. *Disability and Rehabilitation, 33*(4), 310–318.

Jackson, J., & Nolan, J. (2010, March 21). Health care reform bill summary: A look at what's in the bill. cbsnews.com. Retrieved February 7, 2011, from http://www.cbsnews.com/8301-503544_162-20000846-503544.html

Jason, L., Evans, J. M., Brown, M., Porter, N., Brown, A., Hunnell, J., et al. (2011). Fatigue scales and chronic fatigue syndrome: Issues of sensitivity and specificity. *Disability Studies Quarterly, 31*(1). Retrieved February 8, 2011, from http://www.dsq-sds.org/article/view/1375/1540

Kirkland, A. (2008). *Fat rights: Dilemmas of difference and personhood.* New York: New York University Press.

Lander, S. J. (2007, May 21). Number of disabled expected to rise; More research urged. Americanmedicalnew.com. Retrieved February 8, 2011, from http://www.ama-assn.org/amednews/2007/05/21/hlsb0521.htm

Miller, M. L. (2007). Self-advocacy, part two: Documenting disability. *Huntington's Disease Advocacy Center.* Retrieved February 7, 2011, from http://www.hdac.org/features/article.php?p_articleNumber=278

Mingo v. Oakland Unified School District, No. 104055 (105 LRP 7028) (Cal. Ct. App. 2005).

Parry, M. (2010, January 26). Colleges see 17 percent increase in online learning. *Chronicle.com.* Retrieved February 8, 2011, from http://chronicle.com/blogs/wiredcampus/colleges-see-17-percent-increase-in-online-enrollment/20820

Perkins, L. E., & Perkins, S. (2008). *Multiple sclerosis: Your legal rights.* New York: Demos Medical Publishing.

Pima Community College. (n.d.). Recent case information: Disability. Retrieved February 8, 2011, from http://www.pima.edu/employee/eeoaa/Recent_Case_Info.shtml

Schneiderman, A. I., Braver, E. R., & Kang, H. K. (2008). Understanding sequelae of injury mechanisms and mild traumatic brain injury incurred during the conflicts in Iraq and Afghanistan: Persistent postconcussive symptoms and posttraumatic stress disorder. *American Journal of Epidemiology, 167*(12), 1446–1452.

U.S. Department of Justice. (2011). U.S. Department of Justice Americans With Disabilities Act ADA home page. ada.gov. Retrieved February 7, 2011, from http://www.ada.gov/

U.S. Equal Employment Opportunity Commission. (2009). Notice concerning the Americans With Disabilities Act (ADA) Amendments Act of 2008. www.eeoc.gov. Retrieved February 7, 2011, from http://www.eeoc.gov/laws/statutes/adaaa_notice.cfm

CHAPTER 23

Dealing With Mental Health Issues Among Students

CASE STUDY

Mental Health Issues

Your role: You are a clinical faculty member on a medical-surgical unit.

Sarah Brown is a 48-year-old nursing student in her final semester of the BSN accelerated nursing program. She had taken a leave of absence last year after receiving a failing theory grade in her last medical-surgical course and returned to the accelerated BSN program to complete this course and another course. You are the clinical faculty member for the last medical-surgical course. In your opinion, Ms. Brown is extremely anxious and is having a great deal of difficulty meeting the clinical objectives. She cannot answer questions about her patients' diagnoses and medication regime; therefore, you have placed her on clinical warning because of her poor clinical performance. You have also developed a detailed learning contract with Ms. Brown. Given your concerns, you ask the course coordinator, Joan Horowitz, to also evaluate/observe Ms. Brown because she is in her final semester. Professor Horowitz agrees with your observations that Ms. Brown does not have adequate knowledge about her patients' diagnoses or medication regimes.

At the end of the clinical day, you and Professor Horowitz invite Ms. Brown to your office. When you describe your concerns to Ms. Brown, she begins to cry uncontrollably, shake, and yell, "I can't take this course again, I can't do it; I can't do it!" She also bangs her head on the wall and says, "I might as well kill myself," as she continues to cry.

Questions

- Whom should you consult?
- Would you allow this student to leave your office?
- What is your best course of action?

Legal Principles and Review of the Literature

There is no doubt that higher education in general, and course work in clinical care in particular, is stressful. Students have always had difficulty in responding to the stress, and faculty have dealt with that issue for years. But mental health crises appear to have exploded on college and university campuses around the country. Meunier and Wolf (2006) report that more than 90% of college counseling center directors describe the problems presented by students with significant psychological problems as a growing concern. Research indicates that the number of students with mental health issues arriving on college campuses will continue to rise (Lake and Tribbensee, 2002).

One likely cause of this is the evolution of our culture. The 1960s and 1970s exposed a generation to the right to express themselves as individuals and to act out, and those students are today's administrators and faculty. Another likely cause is the law: lawsuits and lawyers (and the fear of both) and the ease with which claims can be asserted (and costs imposed) have caused college administrators to accept and retain students longer than they had been willing to do so in years past. These forces have combined in two landmark federal laws—the Rehabilitation Act of 1973 and the Americans With Disabilities Act (ADA) of 1990—which together afford students a better chance of entering and remaining in college by protecting their rights as persons with psychiatric (or physical) disabilities (Bowe, 1992). Section 504 of the Rehabilitation Act was the first to require all postsecondary institutions receiving federal aid (i.e., virtually all colleges and universities) to make their programs accessible to students with mental health issues (Meunier and Wolf, 2006).

A third likely cause is pharmaceuticals. The numbers of students who are able to function in an academic setting despite anxiety disorders, mood disorders, depression, psychiatric illness, and other such issues have grown as more effective treatments and medications have been developed and made available (Kaplan and Reed, 2004). More and more students have been diagnosed and treated successfully in high school, leading to greater opportunity for students with mental health issues to enter college. These issues may or may not be disclosed to the university.

Practice pointer: A university may or may not want to know about a student's mental or physical health issues. Unlike high school, a university is not obligated to take care of students. Conversely, if the college knows about a student's problems (and medications), it can react appropriately when the student begins to demonstrate those problems. Such knowledge may become problematic, however. If the college asks for and has this knowledge, it might be considered to have created a "special relationship" with the student, and might be held liable for failing to step in and act to prevent harm to the student or others. This is often called *parens patriae.* Many universities do not want to assume this responsibility voluntarily, and have disclaimed such responsibility. See, for example, Drexel University's disclaimer : http://www.drexel.edu/univrel/health_disability

An additional factor contributing to students' dealing with mental illness on campus involves the timing of psychiatric illness presentation. Psychiatric illnesses are most often diagnosed in young adulthood and may very well be triggered by stressful situations germane to college life. Some of the stressors that contribute to the development of mental health problems in college students include living in a new place, sharing a confined space, peer pressure, greater academic demands, and less structure (Cook, 2007). College students are faced with these multiple changes during this transition, not to mention the physical absence of parents and decreased structure in their lives in general. Nursing majors not only must cope with the general pressure associated with college life, but they also have additional stress associated with clinical education and the hospital environment. Although policies may exist for students in crisis on academic campuses, there is a shortage of literature related to the undergraduate nursing student in the clinical area with severe exacerbation of his or her mental illness.

Although many students with a disability will register with the office of disability services, there are still others who choose not to disclose a disability, especially students with a mental illness or psychiatric disability who are concerned about stigma and believe that they will not be treated confidentially or fairly. When any of these nursing students starts to experience psychiatric symptoms and exhibits distress in the classroom and/or the clinical area, a different type of problem solving is required, one that takes on a more complex set of stakeholder considerations. In these cases, faculty may not be clear about how to manage a student emergency situation. It is useful for a university to have an emergency student protocol in place to assist faculty in supporting students when they begin to act out seemingly unreasonably or suggest that they may be acting in imminent danger to themselves. It is important that faculty members are aware of distress signals, methods of immediate intervention, and sources for help for students. However, there are very few instances of the existence of such protocol (Cook, 2007).

The situation is made more complex by the rights that adults have to privacy. The Family Education Rights and Privacy Act (20 U.S.C. § 1232g; 34 CFR Part 99) is a federal law that protects the privacy of student education records. The law applies to all schools that receive funds under an applicable program of the U.S. Department of Education. In essence, it requires schools to keep confidential—from anyone at the college unless they have a need to know, and even from parents—the student's academic record, including complaints about behavior, allegations of misconduct, and event punishments imposed by student judicial bodies. For this reason, it is not easy for a member of the faculty or administration to decide

whom they can talk to or what they can say. Talking to a university attorney, however, is always permissible.

Discussion of Case

Recall this chapter's case study, in which student Sarah Brown is having difficulties. Faculty can surely understand this student's distress, and they will want to be
supportive. What makes the situation reach a higher level of concern is the student's physical symptoms and voiced reference to suicide. (The more difficult situation might well be when the student does not express the thought of suicide.)
Uncontrollable crying and shaking as well as statements such as "I can't take this
course again" and "I might as well kill myself" are very serious, have implications
well beyond the classroom, and require immediate evaluation by qualified professionals. Thus the response is clear: faculty must immediately refer the student to
a professional provider of psychiatric services (for the student's good) and also to
the university's office of student life (for the good of all students and the health
of the academic community). All campus personnel who play a part in this student's campus experience should be notified of the student's self-initiated descriptions of problems. The faculty member needs to stay with the student in crisis and escort her to the emergency room or to a consultation with a psychiatric
mental health professional immediately. The student should not be left alone
given the suicidal statement and general emotional condition. The situation can
likely be successfully addressed with in-patient or out-patient treatment and medication and then with a combination of medication and counseling. However, as
long as the student is exhibiting these behaviors, the faculty member needs to ensure the safety of the student and patients. The student's clinical experiences
should be suspended until such time as a mental health professional confirms
that the student can safely return to the clinical arena and assume patient care
responsibilities.

WHEN TO CONTACT THE UNIVERSITY COUNSEL

Consult the university counsel related to policy development and
implementation.

Findings and Disposition

The faculty member escorted Ms. Brown to the emergency room (ER) for an evaluation. Dr. O'Brien, director of the BSN accelerated nursing program, was also
notified. The student's behavior at the office visit and her referral to the ER were
also documented in her academic file.

Ms. Brown was hospitalized, released, and successfully treated. She was allowed to reenter the nursing program after a period of time, with a note from her treating health-care providers, and successfully graduated from the program.

PREVENTION TIPS

- Offer faculty development sessions on signs of psychological distress, and appropriate support resources for students.
- Educate faculty about the emergency protocol for students exhibiting severe psychological distress.
- Remind students on a routine basis to consult university counseling services during high-stress periods (midterm and final exams, etc.).

Relevant Legal Cases

Schieszler v. Ferrum College, No. 7:02CV00131 (W.D. Va. 2002)

Shin v. Massachusetts Institute of Technology, No. 020403, 2005 WL 1869101 (Mass. Super. Ct. June 27, 2005)

The law clearly shapes university policies that are related to students with mental illness. For centuries, common law held that suicide was a criminal act on the part of the individual and not the responsibility of universities (Gray, 2007). However, the recent increase in the number of suicides on campus (and the attendant reporting of them by the media) has fueled litigation that challenges this traditional approach. Universities are usually challenged on one of the following legal theories: duty to protect, duty to prevent, and permitting or allowing the cause (Smith and Fleming, 2007).

In *Schieszler v. Ferrum College* (2002) and *Shin v. Massachusetts Institute of Technology* (MIT) (2005), the parents of students who committed suicide argued that universities have a special relationship with their students that impose a duty on the school to protect the students even from themselves. In *Schieszler v. Ferrum College,* the student, Michael Frentzel, hung himself with a belt. Distraught after a fight with his girlfriend, Mr. Frentzel was seen banging his head against a wall and heard talking about killing himself. This was reported by other students in his dormitory to college officials, but the officials did not do what a jury later decided was required of them. The court held that the college was liable for his death based on the foreseeability of the suicide and the special relationship it had with him (Cohen, 2007).

Elizabeth Shin was a student at MIT who killed herself by setting herself on fire. While a freshman, she had required a week-long hospitalization for suicidal behavior based on an overdose of Tylenol with codeine. Following hospitalization, Ms. Shin gave permission for her parents to be notified. Ms. Shin, her parents, and the MIT medical team decided that the student should receive care from the medical team at MIT. In her sophomore year, Ms. Shin again required hospitalization for mental health issues and recovered at home. Upon her return from spring break, Ms. Shin told her friends that she intended to kill herself—and her friends immediately called the university, who alerted the medical team. The team scheduled an appointment to discuss her case the next day, but Ms. Shin committed suicide that same night. The parents filed a wrongful death suit against the university, the medical team, and others. MIT was granted summary judgment, but the medical team was not. The court based its finding on the duty of care that the medical team owed Ms. Shin and on its conclusion that a special relationship existed between them and Ms. Shin because they had a specific knowledge that she was at high risk for suicide and it was likely that she would hurt herself without proper supervision (Pavela, 2006). The lawsuit was settled out of court for an undisclosed amount (Cohen, 2007).

Stress, anxiety, and depression—either alone or combined with other psychiatric disorders—can lead students to act out in a variety of unfortunate ways, including considering suicide. It will be impossible for faculty or administrators to know whether the student is serious; they must not place themselves in the position of making that kind of judgment. Both of these cases illustrate the need for faculty members to find help *immediately* for a student who has verbally or textually voiced the intention (or the idea) to commit suicide; they should not attempt to help suicidal students themselves because doing so would qualify them as having a special relationship with the student. Nor is it enough just to diagnose the situation properly: immediate action is required. Scheduling an appointment for the student with a specialist for "the next day" is too risky, as shown in *Shin v. Massachusetts Institute of Technology*. Instead, if university faculty members directly or indirectly hear of suicidal intent, then they should immediately report the incident and do whatever they can to get the student help—for example, taking the student to the ER—as soon as possible. If the student commits suicide and the courts rule that the university did not act on their knowledge to protect the student, then the university and the faculty personally will be held liable.

Summary

Nursing faculty members may respond to a student in distress by acting in accordance with their professional nursing training and attempt to help the student. This is the wrong response, because it will impose much higher obligations and duties as a result of the special relationship doing so creates. Nursing faculty should immediately contact the university counseling center, as should faculty members from other academic disciplines. Psychiatric and mental health nursing faculty members are especially cautioned not to establish a special relationship with students. Just as nursing faculty would call 911 as they provided CPR or other lifesaving emergency techniques, in an emergency situation, they should also ensure the safety of the student in a psychological emergency and seek qualified psychiatric care for the student. Case law clearly cautions faculty about switching their role to care provider (establishing a special relationship). It is in the student's and clinical faculty's best interest for the clinical faculty member to refer a student rather than attempt to counsel the student on his or her own, as this could be considered a special relationship. In nonemergency situations, faculty should also refer students to the university counseling center, as would be expected of faculty members from other academic disciplines. Psychiatric and mental health nursing faculty members are especially cautioned not to establish a special relationship with students (Cook, 2007).

In an effort to manage students in crisis effectively, universities need to develop protocols on emergency situations to guide faculty. Protocols serve as a resource in assisting faculty during interventions with students who may be in imminent danger to themselves or others (see the Emergency Student Protocol Guide). Drexel University's resource center provides one such example: http://www.drexel.edu/StudentLife/ch/CC_Info_for_Faculty&Staff.html. The need for management protocols for nursing students in crisis, particularly those with suspected severe mental health issues or psychiatric disabilities, cannot be understated. Academic nursing programs need to be cognizant of the safety of the student and the patients that student might treat, while respecting the student's own rights and the law (e.g., the ADA). Furthermore, faculty encounter problems in the clinical setting when a student has not disclosed a mental health problem; therefore, it is important for the faculty member to consult the counseling center, academic administrator, office of disability, and legal counsel for advice.

An analysis of how colleges and universities have responded in the aftermath of the shootings at Virginia Tech was reported at the 2008 Annual Forum of the Association of Institutional Research (Lederman, 2008). According to a media report published by *insidehighered.com*, data indicate that many colleges have significantly altered their campus safety procedures, especially how students are notified of possible danger and how procedures are implemented to deal with students who display signs of trouble. However, these same reports indicate that "campus leaders generally shunned the sort of wholesale changes to their admissions or other policies that might have been seen as severely restricting the campus culture or trampling on individual rights. While more than half of respondents said they had considered installing metal detectors at entrances to classroom buildings, only about a third said they had contemplated adding questions to their admissions applications that asked would-be students whether they had had previous psychiatric treatment" (p. 1). Finally, and perhaps sadly, one coauthor of the report stated, "It's interesting what they talked about and *didn't* do" (p. 1). Dealing with students exhibiting mental health problems needs to be proactive, professional, and cognizant of both the student's and patient's well-being.

CRITICAL ELEMENTS TO CONSIDER

Faculty should consider these essential recommendations on how to manage a student with a mental health issue effectively:

- Recognize signs of behavioral distress, such as deterioration of clinical performance or attendance, lack of energy, disruptive behavior, confused thoughts or speech, anxiety, mood changes/swings, weight change, and loss of contact with reality. This should be documented in the student's file.
- Speak with the student privately about your concerns, share your observations, and make an assessment of the urgency of the situation. This should be documented in the student's file.
- Determine if the situation requires immediate intervention. The most basic criterion is whether the student is a danger to him- or herself or to others. If the student is perceived to be a danger, then the faculty member must contact security or public safety representatives immediately. It is imperative that the student receive a psychiatric evaluation and subsequent treatment. Do not isolate yourself when dealing with a student with a serious mental health issue: consult with staff at the university's counseling center and legal counsel.
- Universities can support their faculty members—and, more specifically, their nursing faculty members—by making sure that they have the policies and procedures in place to manage emergency situations that involve the rights of the person with a disability, the care and safety of patients, the care and safety of the student at risk, and the safety of other students involved.
- Faculty development sessions should be offered to new faculty members to acquaint them with behaviors that warrant concern as well as the appropriate action to take in these situations, with periodic reinforcement of this information to ensure awareness and accessibility of these possibilities. Written guidelines should be prepared and made easily accessible to all faculty, instructing them what to do, and when.
- The university's interpretation of Family Education Rights Privacy Act (FERPA) and its emergency exceptions should be emphasized (Baker, 2005). FERPA is addressed in detail in Chapter 35.

References

Baker, T. R. (2005). Notifying parents following a college student suicide attempt: A review of case law and FERPA, and recommendations for practice. *National Association of Student Personnel Administrators Journal, 42,* 513–533.

Bowe, F. (1992). *Adults with disabilities: A portrait.* Washington, DC: President's Committee on Employment of People With Disabilities.

Cohen, V. K. (2007). Keeping students alive: Mandating on-campus counseling saves suicidal college students' lives and limits liability. *Fordham Law Review, 75,* 3081.

Cook, L. J. (2007). Striving to help college students with mental health issues. *Journal of Psychosocial Nursing, 45*(4), 40–44.

Drexel University student handbook. (2008). Philadelphia, PA: Drexel University College of Nursing & Health Professions, 2008–2009.

Gray, C. E. (2007). The university-student relationship amidst increasing rates of student suicide. *Law and Psychology Review, 31*(137), 1–7.

Kaplan, B., & Reed, M. (2004). College student mental health: Plan designs, utilization, trends and costs. *Student Health Spectrum.* Retrieved August 5, 2008, from http://www.chickering .com/uploads/documents/spectrum/2004%20Spring%20-%20Mental%20Health%20On%20Campus.pdf

Lake, P., & Tribbensee, N. (2002). The emerging crisis of college student suicide: Law and policy responses to serious forms of self-inflicted injury. *Stetson Law Review, 32,* 125–157.

Lederman, D. (2008). What changed, and didn't, after Virginia Tech. Insidehighered.com. Retrieved August 28, 2009, from http://www.insidehighered.com/news/2008/05/28/vatech

Meunier, L. H., & Wolf, C. R. (2006). Mental health issues on college campuses. *NYSBA Health Law Journal, 11*(2), 42–52.

Pavela, G. (2006). Should colleges withdraw students who threaten or attempt suicide? *Journal of American College Health, 54*(6), 367–370.

Schieszler v. Ferrum College, No. 7:02CV00131 (W.D. Va., 2002).

Shin v. Massachusetts Institute of Technology, No. 020403, 2005 WL 1869101 (Mass. Super. Ct., June 27, 2005).

Smith, R., & Fleming, D. (2007). Student suicide and colleges' liability. *Chronicle of Higher Education, 53,* B24–B26.

CHAPTER 24

Dealing With Mental Health Issues Among Faculty

Mental Health

Your role: You are the dean.

Professor Reilly is a nontenured faculty member in the acute nurse practitioner program. You receive a phone call from the department chair of a local nurse practitioner program, Dr. Wilson, informing you that Professor Reilly was drunk at the National Organization for Nurse Practitioner Faculty (NONPF) meeting, slurring her words and falling asleep at the table. When you ask Dr. Wilson if you can use his name, he tells you that he was not at the meeting but he will ask the faculty members who reported the incident to him if you can use their names. He then calls back and says that the two faculty members do not wish to be involved. You consult with Professor Reilly's department chair, who did not attend this particular meeting; however, she notes that Professor Reilly has been absent many Fridays and Mondays and has multiple excuses. She does not note any unusual behavior.

In consultation with the department chair, you also ask to see the nurse practitioner faculty members who attended the same NONPF meeting about their observations. The faculty members confirm Professor Reilly's behavior at the national meeting. One of the faculty states that Professor Reilly has a serious drinking problem and has been hospitalized in the past. She also reports that she has seen Professor Reilly go to her car to get a drink during the day. You are also concerned because Professor Reilly has a clinical position at a local hospital in the cardiothoracic intensive care unit once a week where she practices as an acute nurse practitioner.

Questions

- How would you proceed?
- Is disciplinary action appropriate?
- Is Professor Reilly protected under the Americans With Disabilities Act?
- Should Professor Reilly be reported to the state board of nursing?

Mental Health: Legal Principles and Review of the Literature

University counsel will tell you that employment law is the single greatest challenge (or risk) that universities face. This is largely because disputes typically present issues of fact, meaning that they will have witnesses on both sides of the dispute, causing disruption on the campus; experts on both sides, causing confusion and expense; decisions being made by juries who are not experts; judges issuing decisions that are often contradictory. All of these factors combine to become very lengthy, complicated, and costly issues to address, even when the decisions made are appropriate and legally defensible.

Employment claims are often difficult to assess in the area of disability. The academy is clearly a place where a person's lack of physical mobility should be irrelevant in determining the quality of the person's mind or ability to create new knowledge. It is also a place where differences are respected, even prized, for adding new perspectives in the search for truth. It is difficult enough when faculty perceive students who are differently abled, but the challenge becomes all the greater when evaluating colleagues. However, all must ensure that decisions are made on a faculty member's or student's merits and not on the basis of stereotypes, assumptions, or prejudices.

To prevent such discrimination, Congress enacted the Americans With Disabilities Act (ADA). It prohibits discrimination on the basis of disability and perceived disability in employment and other areas. To be protected by the ADA, one must have a disability or have a relationship or association with an individual with a disability. An individual with a disability is defined by the ADA as a person who has a physical or mental impairment that substantially limits one or more major life activities, a person who has a history or record of such impairment, or a person who is perceived by others as having such impairment. Title I requires employers with 15 or more employees to provide qualified individuals having disabilities an equal opportunity to benefit from the full range of employment-related opportunities available to others. For example, it prohibits discrimination in recruitment, hiring, promotions, training, pay, social activities, and other privileges of employment. It requires that employers make reasonable accommodation to the known physical or mental limitations of otherwise qualified individuals with disabilities, unless it results in undue hardship. Universities are subject to ADA Title I requirements.

Universities also have responsibilities under section 504 of the Rehabilitation Act of 1973 and ADA Title II to ensure that employees with a disability do not experience discrimination based on their disability (U.S. Department of Justice, 2005). The Rehabilitation Act prohibits discrimination on the basis of disability in programs conducted by federal agencies, in programs receiving federal financial assistance, in federal employment, and in the employment practices of federal contractors. The standards for determining employment discrimination under the Rehabilitation Act are the same as those used in Title I of the ADA. Section 504 states that "no qualified individual with a disability in the United States shall be excluded from, denied the benefits of, or be subjected to discrimination under" any program or activity that either receives federal financial assistance or is conducted by any executive agency (U.S. Department of Justice, 2005).

According to the Equal Employment Opportunity Commission (EEOC), alcoholism is considered an impairment, and people with alcoholism who are substantially limited in a major life activity have a disability under the ADA. However, even if a person with alcoholism meets the definition of disability, an employer may legally discipline or discharge an employee who is an alcoholic whose current use of alcohol adversely affects job performance or conduct to the extent that s/he becomes not "qualified" to perform the work (EEOC, 1992). That being said, the university would initially offer the faculty member paid or unpaid leave for medical treatment, just as they would for any physical illness, because alcoholism is a disease (EEOC, 2000).

An employer may not discipline a faculty member with alcoholism more severely than nonalcoholic faculty for the same conduct. Although employers must provide reasonable accommodations to individuals with alcoholism in certain cases, an employer is never required to provide an accommodation to facilitate employee alcoholism or to tolerate substandard performance resulting from alcoholism. Reasonable accommodation may include allowing an alcoholic employee time off to participate in a rehabilitation program or to attend Alcoholics Anonymous meetings. Employers are not required to provide a reasonable accommodation that creates undue hardship for the employer.

The ADA specifically provides that employers may create reasonable workplace standards, and then enforce them. In particular, employers may take the following measures: prohibit alcohol in the workplace; require employees not to be under the influence of alcohol in the workplace; and require the same job performance and behavior from employees with alcoholism as other employees. For example, a university may enforce a policy against a faculty member with alcoholism, but only if the university enforces the policy in the same manner against other faculty and employees (Workman and Jorgensen, 1997). Private employers are also able to have drug and alcohol tests administered; by contrast, this ability is significantly restricted in public universities because of constitutional prohibitions against a state performing illegal searches and seizures.

Alcoholism, also called alcohol dependence, is a disease that includes four symptoms: craving (a strong need, or compulsion, to drink), loss of control (the inability to limit one's drinking on any given occasion), physical dependence (withdrawal symptoms, e.g., nausea, sweating, shakiness, and anxiety), and tolerance (the need to drink greater amounts of alcohol in order to get high) (National Institutes of Health, National Institute on Alcohol Abuse and Alcoholism, 2008).

It is also important to note that steps to recognize and assist an alcoholic colleague may be more successful in nonuniversity settings than in university settings for several reasons. First, faculty work autonomously, deciding how to divide their time, and they are free to work at home. Second, the high degree of autonomy creates low visibility and a wide range of acceptable behaviors, which might include episodes of drinking heavily at professional meetings away from home. Third, faculty performance is not evaluated by the same methods used in nonuniversity settings. Fourth, key administrative officials find it difficult to evaluate deterioration of job performance in colleagues and are not necessarily trained in recognizing alcohol-related behavior. There is also a desire to protect the privacy of colleagues; therefore, faculty administrators are reluctant to participate in the constructive confrontation needed for a successful assistance program (Spickard and Billings, 1986).

When the faculty member has clinical duties, it is important to remember that a key reason for reporting inappropriate behavior is to protect patients. It is the responsibility of the person who discovers a problem to report it via appropriate channels. A management intercession should then be conducted and include the department chair and/or associate dean, a human resources administrator, and a representative from the university's employee assistance program (EAP) if available. If the faculty member refuses to participate in the intervention or to undergo a physician's evaluation or treatment, then the department chair can properly begin disciplinary procedures that include written warnings, suspensions, and termination with reporting to the state board of nursing if the faculty member is actively engaged in clinical practice (Dunn, 2005).

A department chair or dean's decision to report a nurse faculty member to the state board of nursing is an individual and difficult one. It depends on whether:

- The state has a mandatory reporting law
- The state has diversion legislation (i.e., a rehabilitation option in lieu of discipline) and rehabilitation programs
- A hazard exists that poses a threat to public health and safety
- The nurse is motivated to seek treatment
- There is evidence of satisfactory participation in a treatment program (Fisk and Devoto, 1990)

In addition, university legal counsel would be consulted throughout these proceedings to guide administrators through the reporting process.

Discussion of Case

Recall this chapter's case study, in which there are several problems. First, the members of the faculty need to be reminded of and discuss their obligations to the community, which they violated when they failed to let the department chair and dean know about Professor Reilly's conduct. Now it is no longer a private matter because she has performed poorly at a national conference—and that has the potential to adversely affect the school's reputation.

The department chair and dean promptly address the problem internally. They meet with Professor Reilly about what they have heard from her colleagues and faculty members related to her behavior at the NONPF meeting and about other behaviors that are consistent with alcohol abuse. A human resources representative should also attend the meeting and possibly a representative from the university's EAP. If the faculty member agrees to seek treatment, then human resources would work with the faculty member to construct a remediation plan, which could include a medical leave in accordance with the Family Medical Leave Act (FMLA). If the faculty member refuses to participate or undergo a physician's evaluation or treatment, then the department chair should begin disciplinary procedures and report the faculty member to the state board of nursing.

> ## WHEN TO CONSULT THE UNIVERSITY COUNSEL
> Consult counsel for advice when you suspect or receive reports that a faculty member or staff member is abusing alcohol or other substances.

Findings and Disposition

In this case, Professor Reilly agreed to be examined and to undergo treatment. Given that the university's nursing students had clinical rotations in regional drug and alcohol rehabilitation centers, the university human resource department and Professor Reilly's insurance company permitted Professor Reilly to undergo treatment at an in-patient facility in an out-of-state drug and alcohol rehabilitation center, which allowed the matter to remain private. Professor Reilly returned to the university after a 12-week leave.

Professor Reilly was diagnosed with alcoholism, a disease, and it was determined that this was a disability under the ADA. Before Professor Reilly was allowed to return to her faculty position after a 12-week leave, she was required to discuss the situation with the Office of Disability Services (ODS), and together they came to the following accommodation plan:

- She was allowed use of paid leave for medical treatment and committed to participating in the medical plan her doctors had prescribed.

- She was suspended from her practice as an acute nurse practitioner until such time as her doctors confirmed her fitness to return to duty.
- She was allowed use of paid leave or flexible scheduling for counseling or Alcoholic Anonymous meetings with the department chair's approval.
- She was excused from work events where alcohol was served.
- She signed a copy of the university's drug and alcohol policy and of the university's code of conduct, confirming her understanding of the prohibitions they contained on the consumption of alcohol and the rendering of employment services while under the influence of alcohol.

PREVENTION TIPS

- Educate faculty and administrators about the behaviors consistent with alcohol or substance abuse.
- Develop policies that not only specify and sanction conduct that is unacceptable, but that also treat and support—not ignore and discharge—faculty who are impaired.

Relevant Legal Case

Anthony L. Mayo v. Columbia University, 8 Wage & Hour Cas. 2nd (BNA) 1562 (S.D.N.Y. 2003)

In this case, Anthony Mayo was an administrative coordinator and director of student affairs at Columbia University who was repeatedly absent from work without prior authorization or notification of supervisors. Mr. Mayo claims he left voice messages that he would not be in and that he spoke with administrative staff about his absences, but these conversations were not recorded in any records. He called his supervisor and informed her that he was an alcoholic. He later met with the interim director of the occupational therapy program, a director of the physical therapy program, and the manager of the return-to-work program (part of human resources department), and signed a work agreement, under which he was given a paid leave to enter a treatment program for alcoholism and then committed to workplace performance standards following his return, including documenting his participation in ongoing treatment as required. He took a paid leave of absence from August 16, 2000, to September 18, 2000. When Mr. Mayo failed to submit the required documentation (despite receiving an extension of time to do so), he was terminated. He then filed a lawsuit alleging discrimination on the basis of disability, sexual orientation, and race, in violation of the Americans With Disabilities Act, the Rehabilitation Act, the Family Medical Leave Act, and various other federal and state laws. Reviewing the record on motions for summary judgment, the court determined that the university and its officers had acted appropriately in granting reasonable accommodations to the employee and in terminating him for failure to perform in accordance with the agreement he had made, and therefore granted judgment to the defendants on all claims arising under federal law. (The court declined to exercise jurisdiction over the employee's state law claims.)

Summary

The abuse of alcohol is just one of several possible causes of inadequate performance of duties at a university. People respond differently to stress. There will be times when unique behaviors cross a line and become either worrisome (concern for the person) and/or inappropriate (concern for others). Faculty and administrators may be slow to act because of their respect for the person's right to privacy or right to be different, or because of their worry that they might be violating a legal right (and perhaps subjecting themselves to liability).

Universities should not leave such important matters to individual determination. They should have policies in place that not only specify and sanction conduct that is unacceptable, but that also treat and support—not ignore and discharge—faculty who are impaired. In assisting an impaired faculty member, education and early intervention are critical, as is documentation of the efforts that are made. It is important to educate faculty and staff to do the following:

- Speak to the colleague about the perceived problem and suggest that the colleague visit employee assistance program or other counseling services.
- Bring concerns about a colleague with an apparent alcohol problem to the attention of the relevant administrator, such as the department chair, associate dean, or dean.
- Educate faculty and administrators about the behaviors consistent with alcohol or substance abuse. Universities must follow their own human resources policies related to personnel issues.

CRITICAL ELEMENTS TO CONSIDER

- Consult human resources and the employee assistance program.
- Document employee behaviors and written and verbal communications when you suspect alcohol abuse.
- Consult the alcohol and drug abuse policy at your institution.
- Follow your own policies.
- Maintain the confidentiality of the faculty member or employee.
- Consult the state board of nursing for reporting advice and direction.

Continued

CRITICAL ELEMENTS TO CONSIDER—cont'd

- The office of disability and/or human resources should discuss specific limitations that the faculty member with alcoholism experiences with the faculty member's department chair or supervisor.
- The office of disability and/or human resources should discuss how these limitations affect the faculty's job performance with the faculty member's department chair supervisor.
- In consultation with the office of disability services (ODS), accommodations may be available to reduce or eliminate problems.
- Once accommodations are in place, ODS should meet with the faculty member with alcoholism to evaluate the effectiveness of the accommodations.
- Provide the faculty member with due process if discipline or discharge is warranted.

References

Anthony L. Mayo v. Columbia University, 8 Wage & Hour Cas. 2nd (BNA) 1562 (S.D.N.Y. 2003).

Dunn, D. (2005). Substance abuse among nurses: Intercession and intervention. *AORN Journal, 82*(5), 775–799.

Equal Employment Opportunity Commission. (1992). *A technical assistance manual on the employment provisions (Title I) of the Americans With Disabilities Act.* Retrieved January 25, 2010, from http://www.jan.wvu.edu/links/ADAtam1.html

Equal Employment Opportunity Commission. (2000). *Enforcement guidance on disability-related inquiries and medical examinations of employees under the Americans with Disabilities Act.* Retrieved February 26, 2010, from http://www.eeoc.gov/policy/docs/guidance-inquiries.html

Fisk, N. B., & Devoto, D. A. (1990). The nurse employee who uses alcohol/other drugs. *Nurse Managers Bookshelf, 2,* 110–129.

National Institutes of Health, National Institute on Alcohol Abuse and Alcoholism. (2008). *Alcohol alert: Alcohol and other drugs.* Retrieved February 26, 2010, from http://pubs.niaaa.nih.gov/publications/AA76/AA76.htm

Spickard, W. A., & Billings, F. T. (1986) Alcoholism in an university faculty. *Transactions of the American Clinical & Climatological Association, 97,* 191-199.

U.S. Department of Justice. (2005). *A guide to disability rights laws.* Retrieved February 27, 2010, from http://www.ada.gov/cguide.htm

Workman, M. T., & Jorgensen, J. (1997). Alcoholism is a disability under the ADA. *Triangle Business Journal.* Retrieved February 26, 2010, from http://triangle.bizjournals.com/triangle/stories/1997/02/03/smallb8.html

CHAPTER 25

The Challenge of Online Learning: Discussion Boards and Blogs

CASE STUDY

Online Discussion Board

Your role: You are the department chair of the graduate nursing program.

The office of equality contacts you. Kia Johnson, a graduate student, has filed a complaint that another graduate student, William Wilson, made racist comments during an online class while blogging on the discussion board and that the faculty member in charge, Dr. Lawson, did not address the matter. You review the online discussion board (blog) and note that Wilson had responded to another student's posting to the question "Why Isn't Nursing More Diversified?" with this comment:

I agree that African Americans have been handed a raw deal in the past. But times have changed, or the election that ends tomorrow would not be taking place. In addition, all ethnicities have suffered indignities and genocides. The ghettos that today house the African Americans and Latinos did not just develop. These were the same ghettos that housed the Jews; before the Jews, they housed the Germans and Italians; and before them, they housed the Irish. All of these people pulled themselves up by their bootstraps, and now it is time for the current inhabitants to do the same. Saying that recruiters do not target these communities is audacious. No one came knocking on my door begging for me to be a nurse, and no particular nursing school recruited me. I decided with my own last two brain cells that a career as a paramedic was going nowhere and that my only choice was to switch to nursing.

All cultures have in their past gone through horrors. The pilgrims came from England to escape religious persecution. Americans did their best to annihilate the American Indian. The Armenian genocide was a large part of World War I. Ethnic cleansing in Yugoslavia occurred through most of the twentieth century. Racism in America has caused extreme hardship for blacks. The Nazis killed millions of Jews, Stalin killed even more Russians. Japan killed untold Chinese, and Koreans. Pol Pot devastated Cambodia. Genocide continues in Darfur and other African nations.

People need to get past the victim mentality and develop some inner drive to succeed. If you would rather drive a Lincoln Navigator than live in better housing or pay for your education, so be it.

The student complainant, Johnson, was offended by Wilson's comment, calling it racist. In her view, Dr. Lawson had agreed with the posting when she did not address the issue, condemn the language, or discipline the student. Johnson is refusing to participate in the discussion board until the matter is addressed to her satisfaction. Dr. Lawson has warned her that this will result in her receiving an incomplete or zero (F) on assignments and failing the class, and this has made Johnson even more resolute in her refusal to participate. Dr. Lawson was recently hired at the university. This is her first academic appointment.

Questions

- Whom should you consult?
- What policies should exist related to online discussion boards?
- What is your best course of action?

Legal Principles and Review of the Literature

The National Center for Education Statistics (2008) estimated that 12.2 million people were enrolled in college-level credit-granting distance education courses in 2006 to 2007. Out of this number enrolled, 77% were reported in online courses (U.S. Department of Education, 2008). The 2010 Sloan Survey of Online Learning revealed that enrollment in online courses continues to rise. In a survey of more than 2,500 colleges and universities nationwide, it was found that approximately 5.6 million students were enrolled in at least one online course in fall 2009.

Webopedia (2009) defines *blog* as short for *Web log*; a blog is a Web page that serves as a publicly accessible personal journal for an individual. A blog is an electronic site where an individual, group, or corporation presents a record of activities, thoughts, or beliefs. Some blogs operate mainly as news filters, collecting various online sources and adding short comments and Internet links. Other blogs concentrate on presenting original material. In addition, many blogs provide a forum to allow visitors to leave comments and interact with the publisher (*Encyclopedia Britannica*, 2009). Typically updated very regularly (daily, if not even more frequently), blogs often reflect the personality of the author.

Defamation is an act of communication that causes someone to be shamed, ridiculed, held in contempt, or lowered in the estimation of the community; it refers to the damage done to a person's reputation. Although speech on the Internet (in blogs, on social networking sites, and otherwise) can quickly be communicated to countless people, it is still regarded as individual communication (not mass media) and is still regulated primarily by the common law and its traditional remedies in tort (for invasion of privacy, or defamation). Under the common law, a person who publishes (communicates to another) a defamatory statement by another bears the same liability for the statement as if he or she had initially created or made the statement. Thus a book publisher or a newspaper publisher can be held liable for anything that it prints (Duran, 2004). The premise behind this publisher liability is that a publisher has the knowledge, opportunity, and ability to exercise editorial control over the content of its publications (Ciolli, 2007; Duran, 2004). The Communications Decency Act of 1996 changed this rule for the Internet by granting immunity for defamation to Internet service providers (ISPs), and providing that they could not be held responsible for content (Ciolli, 2007; Duran, 2004).

In terms of higher education, Title VI was enacted as part of the landmark Civil Rights Act of 1964. It prohibits discrimination on the basis of race, color, and national origin in programs and activities receiving federal financial assistance. Section 601 prohibits intentional discrimination based on race, color, or national origin in covered programs and activities (U.S. Department of Justice, 2010). Students have legal relationships not only with the university but also with other students, faculty members, and staff. For student peer relationships, the most relevant internal law is likely to be found in the student code of conduct, housing rules, and student organization bylaws. Because student rules are created and enforced by and in the name of the university, universities are sometimes implicated in the resolution of disputes among students and may become liable for acts of students that injure other students (Kaplin and Lee, 2007).

Neither the law nor academia guarantees freedom from offense by what someone else says or believes. Indeed, the constitutional guarantees we do have— of speech, of belief, and of the press—were enacted precisely because the Founders knew that people often say offensive things and wanted to make sure that the government did not have the power to regulate what people say or believe. Before a lawsuit can be prosecuted, the plaintiff must show that he or she has suffered personal injury or individualized harm. For this reason, maligning a group of people (or an entire race) does not constitute defamation that is actionable under the law. The law does not provide a remedy for every injury. In online learning, discussions are different from those in face-to-face settings, students are less easily controlled, and the faculty member must rely on different skills from those typically used in traditional classroom settings.

Academia imposes additional restrictions on conduct for those who are members of its community. They are typically expressed in student codes of conduct or in policies regarding online academic activity or use of the university's technology. Private universities may more easily regulate what is expressed over their systems or in their classes, because the constitutional protections of free speech only prohibit action by the state, and therefore apply to public universities. You consulted with legal counsel, and did not find this to be the case. If a student is offended and decides not to participate in a class or an activity, then that is the student's choice; but failure to participate can be sanctioned, if participation is required or included in grading.

Students can always choose not to participate in their classes. If participation in class (or online) is evaluated and graded or included in grades, then faculty may properly respond to nonparticipation by assigning incompletes or failures to the student, and reducing grades accordingly. Faculty do not have to concern themselves with deciding which reasons are good reasons and which are not. Students can always appeal the award of a perceived unfair grade through established procedures. A single action in the class can be so excessive, or a number of similar actions can repeat so often, that the environment itself becomes hostile. In such an instance, there is the possibility that rights have been violated (see Chapter 13, Dealing With Student-Student Harassment, for a discussion of this problem).

Discussion of Case

Recall this chapter's Case Study. When Dr. Lawson was made aware of Kia Johnson's complaint, she had a detailed discussion with Mr. Wilson about how his first and last paragraphs could be easily perceived as offensive and racist by others. The student was counseled to be more sensitive to the concerns of others from different racial, cultural, or ethnic backgrounds. He protested that he did not mean to be racist, but did intend to raise issues that had bothered him. He did intend to use hyperbole and criticized himself as well ("my two brain cells"), because he wanted to provoke his classmates to get to "the real issues here" and respond to his ideas so he could learn from them. He admitted that the comments could be construed as racist and, afterward, he apologized to the class by e-mail and by phone to Kia Johnson, at Dr. Lawson's suggestion; however, this was not satisfactory to Ms. Johnson.

Dr. Lawson was new to teaching and this was her first online course. Dr. Lawson, readily admitted that she was uncomfortable with the comments but did not know what to do, so she did not deal with the online posting situation. She felt that Mr. Wilson had the right to express his opinion, and was hoping that his classmates would pounce on what he had written and eviscerate it themselves, without her getting involved, which she thought would be important. Appreciating her logic, you, as department chair, counseled her to seek assistance the next time that she is confronted with a new teaching situation. She was also counseled that she could have injected herself into the discussion, identifying them as offensive and very likely to be interpreted as racist (although surely not meant to be so), restating the points without reference to stereotypes, and directing the discussion to the argument and questions that Mr. Wilson had raised. In the future, the faculty member should also set ground rules for what is and is not appropriate content for online discussions. In these cases, the department chair should consult legal counsel for guidance.

WHEN TO CONSULT THE UNIVERSITY COUNSEL

Faculty should consult with their program directors or department chairs on how to handle conduct in a class (online or otherwise) that is offensive in ways that they think could violate the law, but which may also be protected free speech. Often the best response is to educate the author as well as the class about the conflicting interests, and instruct all on the importance of civil debate; but legal counsel should be consulted when the conduct is so outrageous or when it happens more often than irregularly.

Findings and Disposition

You (the department chair) call Dr. Lawson immediately and tell her about the complaint. You ask her why she did not bring this matter to your attention when it occurred, telling her that it is always better for a department chair to learn of these issues from the faculty directly instead of from a university official doing an investigation.

After a review of the online discussion board by both you and the university's equality officer, Dr. Lawson was counseled on how to manage difficult online situations of this nature. Dr. Lawson was also counseled to intervene immediately when she felt online discussions "crossed the line" and were so offensive as to impair the academic experience; and to seek the department chair's assistance if she is unsure how to respond to or manage such situations. At that time, Dr. Lawson agreed to apologize to the student who issued the complaint, Kia Johnson, which she did in the context of an e-mail sent to the entire class in which she established guidelines for blogging. The formal complaint was resolved by a three-way phone conversation among the student, you, and the equality officer. Ms. Johnson, received an incomplete in the course and was given additional time to submit her assignments and complete the course.

PREVENTION TIPS

- Post Web etiquette policies on student blogs and online discussion boards.
- Reinforce the school's professional code of conduct policies and the consequences of not following those policies to students at the beginning of each term.

Relevant Legal Cases

Yoder v. University of Louisville, No. 32009cv00205 (W.D. Ky. 2009)

Bryant v. Independent Schools District of No. I-38 of Gavin County,
334 F.3d 928 (10th Cir. 2003)

Byrnes v. University Johnson County Community College (D. Kan. 2010)

Nina Yoder was a nursing student at the University of Louisville. She was expelled after the university became aware that she had been blogging about her experience as a nursing student on her MySpace page. In her blog, Ms. Yoder detailed events related to her clinical day, evaluated her experiences and offered her opinions, and identified herself as a University of Louisville nursing student. On March 2, 2009, Ms. Yoder was dismissed from the University of Louisville's School of Nursing (SON) because of the nature of her Internet postings. One week later, her appeal to the university for reinstatement was denied; and three days after that, she filed suit in federal court. Ms. Yoder alleged that she did not violate the University of Louisville's student code of conduct, that what she did was "private" and that her First Amendment rights of freedom of speech had been violated. The federal court ruled in her favor and ordered her reinstated.

The School of Nursing had expelled Ms. Yoder on the basis of its student honor code, which referred to each student as a "representative of the School of Nursing" and imposed on them the obligation to act with "professionalism." The court noted that Ms. Yoder's blog was purely personal, and was not created or used in any professional context. For that reason, her postings did not violate the honor code. The court wrote that if the SON wanted the professionalism requirements in the honor code to apply to every act of a SON student in all places, at all times, and in all contexts, it had failed to give any notice of that expectation and intention, nor had it explained such obligation clearly. Because the case was decided on a notice issue, the court did not issue any decision on the merits about whether the code would have survived constitutional challenge had it been explicit.

A federal appellate court has held that students have a private cause of action against their school if the school "intentionally allowed or nurtured a racially hostile educational environment...by being deliberately indifferent to incidents of peer harassment of which it was aware." In the case of *Bryant v. Independent Schools*, the students claimed that the school had allowed the presence of offensive racial slurs, epithets, swastikas, and the letters KKK inscribed in school furniture and in notes placed in African American students' lockers and notebooks. They claimed that white males were allowed to wear T-shirts adorned with the Confederate flag in violation of the dress code prohibiting offensive and disruptive clothing. They also claimed that parents and students had complained about this and that the school's principal was personally aware of the hostile environment, but did nothing to remedy the situation, which led to a fight among students. Although all of the students had been involved in the fight, only African American students were expelled (because it was their second fight).

At the trial level, the district court held that the school had not acted against the students on the basis of their race, and concluded that the students were properly dismissed. On appeal, however, the circuit court held that a school can be held liable under the law where its administrators are deliberately indifferent to "[racial] harassment, of which they have actual knowledge, that is so severe, pervasive, and objectively offensive that it can be said to deprive the victims of access to the educational opportunities or benefits provided by the school." It described the duties owed by the school's administrators as follows: "We are not necessarily holding that school administrators have a duty to seek out and discover instances of discrimination or risk being held liable for intentional discrimination under [Title VI of the Civil Rights Act of 1964]. However, we are holding that when administrators who have a duty to provide a non-discriminatory educational environment for their charges are made aware of egregious forms of intentional discrimination and make the intentional choice to sit by and do nothing, they can be held liable under [that law]." It therefore remanded the case to the district court for trial.

In the case of *Byrnes v. University Johnson County Community College,* four nursing students were dismissed from the college after one of them posted a picture of them on Facebook, taken in a laboratory with a human placenta. The student who posted the picture, Doyles Byrnes, sued, claiming that her instructor had given her implicit permission to post the picture, that she suffered a "temporary lapse in judgment," and that the college had violated her right to due process in dismissing her. Further, Byrnes's attorney claimed that nothing in the college's code of conduct addresses photos or social media. A college official issued a letter that stated, "Your demeanor and lack of professional behavior surrounding this event was considered a disruption to the learning environment and did not exemplify the professional behavior that we expect in the nursing program" (Campbell, 2010). At the time of this writing, the suit has just been filed and a verdict has not been reached.

Summary

Academia promises the free flowing of ideas. The Web allows individuals to express their opinions to the world without the kinds of checks that exist in face-to-face or classroom discussions. For academic institutions to contend with the excesses that can so easily occur on online discussion boards or blogs, institutions need to educate their students on academic etiquette and make sure that students understand that it applies not just in the physical classroom but online as well, in any school-related activity. Web etiquette policies should be readily accessible (e.g., posted on university Web sites and addressed in student handbooks); universities should provide instruction and warnings from the start (admission and orientation); and faculty should be sure to remind their students of those obligations repeatedly throughout their university experience. Consequences for breaching academic etiquette—whether on the Web, in class, or otherwise—must be clearly outlined and enforced, with sensitivity to the core mission of academia of allowing freedom of thought and expression and the exploration of ideas, regardless of how offensive some might find them to be. Because cyberspace allows hyperbole and excess to go viral, personal intentions are irrelevant, and the best remedy for misuse is education and prevention. Web etiquette policies may go a long way in curbing inappropriate postings. In the case of professional programs, such as nursing, academic and clinical policies need to be developed in relation to the student's expectations of professional conduct as outlined in the American Nurses Association (ANA) Code of Ethics. Such policies should include professional Web etiquette or expectations. In any situation in which a student is alleged to have violated academic etiquette, the university must be sure to afford the student due process, for both the student's sake and the university's.

CRITICAL ELEMENTS TO CONSIDER

- Develop Web etiquette policies related to in-course discussion boards and university blogs.
- Develop a code of professional conduct for nursing majors to include conduct concerning blogs and Internet postings that is congruent with the ANA Code of Ethics.
- Include Web etiquette policies and professional code of conduct policies in new student orientation.
- If you are an experienced faculty member or academic administrator, educate new faculty about students' due process rights.
- Educate nursing students about the importance of following hospital policies related to protected health information derived from the Health Insurance Portability and Accountability Act (HIPPA) and the sharing of protected health information to include information shared on Web sites and discussion boards. All information on electronic devices should be password as well as fingerprint protected.
- *Note:* The HIPAA privacy rule regulates the use and disclosure of certain information held by covered entities (generally, health-care clearinghouses, employer-sponsored health plans, health insurers, and medical service providers). It establishes regulations for the use and disclosure of protected health information (PHI). PHI is any information held by a covered entity that concerns health status, provision of health care, or payment for health care that can be linked to an individual. This is interpreted rather broadly and includes any part of an individual's medical record (Terry, 2009).

References

Bryant v. Independent Schools District of No. I-38 of Gavin County, 334 F.3d 928 (10th Cir. 2003).

Byrnes v. University Johnson County Community College, No. 10-2690 (D. Kan. 2010).

Campbell, M. (2010, December 31). Nursing students dismissed for Facebook photo. *The Kansas City Star.* Retrieved January 6, 2011, from http://www.kansascity.com

Ciolli, A. (2007). Bloggers as public figures. *Boston University Public Interest Law Journal, 16,* 255.

Duran, S. (2004). Hear no evil, see no evil, spread no evil: Creating a unified legislative approach to internet service provider immunity. *University of Baltimore Intellectual Property Law Journal, 12,* 115.

Encyclopædia Britannica. Blog. Encyclopædia Britannica Online. Retrieved September 14, 2009, from http://www.britannica.com/EBchecked/topic/869092/blog

Kaplin, W. A., & Lee, B. A. (2007). *The law of higher education* (4th ed.). San Francisco: Jossey-Bass.

Sloan Foundation. (2010). Class differences: Online education in the United States, 2010. Retrieved December 26, 2010, from http://sloanconsortium.org/publications/survey/class_differences

Terry, K. (2009). Patient privacy—the new threats. *Physicians Practice Journal.* Retrieved September 14, 2009, from http://www.physicianspractice.com/index/fuseaction/articles.details/articleID/1299/page/1.htm

U.S. Department of Education. (2008). *Distance education at degree-granting postsecondary institutions: 2006–2007.* Retrieved December 26, 2010, from http://www.distancelearning.com/distance-learning-statistics/

U.S. Department of Justice. (2010). *Overview of Title VI of the Civil Rights Act of 1964.* Retrieved December 26, 2010, from http://www.justice.gov/crt/cor/coord/titlevi.php

Webopedia. (2009). Definition of *blog.* Retrieved September 14, 2009, from http://www.webopedia.com/ TERM/B/blog.html

Yoder v. University of Louisville, No. 32009cv00205 (W.D. Ky. 2009). (NOTE: Yoder v. University of Louisville, 2011 WL 1345051 [6th Cir. April 8, 2011]. The 6th Circuit overturned Yoder v. University of Louisville on procedural grounds and remanded to the district court to try again.)

CHAPTER 26

Issues Surrounding Drug Testing and Monitoring of Students

CASE STUDY

Drug Monitoring

Your role: You are the chair of the nurse anesthesia program.

Robin Jones is a second-year student in the nurse anesthesia program. You receive reports from several students that Ms. Jones is abusing prescription drugs. One student, Elise Markowitz, tells you that Ms. Jones is "really out of it" when she speaks to her on the phone at night and even asked her to give her some Percocet, a prescription that Ms. Markowitz had from a previous surgery. Two other students, Marisol Rodriguez and Tanya Brown, have also contacted you about Ms. Jones, expressing worry about her and giving you similar reports about her conduct. You note that Ms. Jones was on leave last year because of chronic back pain related to a car accident. She is currently on her pediatric rotation. Quickly scanning Ms. Jones's clinical file, you see that her clinical coordinator has noted that "Robin sometimes appears tired and down."

Questions
- How would you proceed?
- Do you have enough evidence to support a drug test?
- Do you need to report Ms. Jones to the state board of nursing?

Drug Testing: Legal Principles and Review of the Literature

Drugs are everywhere today. Television advertisements for them appear all the time. Even children are able to procure them. The problem has escalated to such an extent that Congress enacted the Safe School and Drug Free Communities Act in 2002. In addition, the distribution and consumption of alcohol is a matter of state criminal law, making the off-campus use by students and faculty a matter of concern for universities (Drexel University, 2009).

Noting the corrosive effects that drugs and alcohol have on both academic and social life, many institutions of higher learning have adopted policies that prohibit student or staff possession and/or use of narcotics or drugs other than those prescribed for that person by a doctor. Professional organizations have also responded to these issues by offering best practices on policies as well as confidential assistance to individual members. For example, the American Association of Nurse Anesthetists (AANA) Peer Assistance Advisors provides an important resource to serve certified registered nurse anesthetists (CRNAs); nurse anesthesia students; and institutions in their formulation of guidelines for intervention, treatment, aftercare, and reentry into the workplace (AANA Peer Assistance, 2010).

It is often difficult to identify an impaired student or colleague. The challenge is even greater in the university setting, where we encourage the acceptance of differences; allow (even encourage) individualism and self-discovery; and are accustomed to people following the beat of a different drummer, even to the point of neglecting sleep, food, and hygiene. However, faculty, clinical supervisors, and RN student peers may have certain legal responsibilities in identifying and reporting the chemically dependent nurse or student nurse. Many states have mandatory reporting laws that may hold colleagues responsible for harm to patients if they fail to report a coworker in whom substance abuse is suspected. In those states having alternative programs (a rehabilitation option in lieu of discipline), confidential reporting to the programs absolves the colleague from reporting to the nursing regulatory board (AANA, 2010).

Aside from seriously affecting the physical and psychological integrity of the user, substance abuse may significantly affect the ability of students to administer safe care to the patients who are entrusted to them in a clinical health-care setting. For these reasons, it is important that academic nursing programs have policies and procedures related to the detection of drug and alcohol use and that they authorize the testing and monitoring of students. This is particularly important for those who hold an RN license or who are otherwise involved in patient-care activities. Such policies should inform students who are enrolled in a major that includes a clinical health-care component.

Drug and alcohol testing and monitoring policies should be explicit. They should prohibit use that is illegal or that impairs conduct. They should state when students are required to submit to drug testing, whether randomized or for cause. For example, a student may be required to undergo drug or alcohol testing when the administrator of the program, or designee, determines through direct observation or reports from faculty or clinical supervisors that there is reasonable suspicion that the student is impaired due to illegal drug or alcohol use, or the use or misuse of prescribed over-the-counter medications (Drexel University, 2009). Once there is a written policy and procedure, faculty and administrators must be sure to act in accordance with it: going beyond what's written will likely be viewed as an invasion of the student's privacy.

The problems caused by an impaired health-care practitioner are so significant that the consequences of drug or alcohol misuse go beyond the academy and may implicate professional licensure when the problem might pose a risk to the public. A department chair or dean is sometimes called on to decide whether to report a student who is an RN to the state board of nursing. That will always be a difficult decision and will depend on the circumstances of that particular case, but will involve considering whether:

- The state has a mandatory reporting law
- The state has diversion legislation (e.g., a rehabilitation option in lieu of discipline) and rehabilitation programs
- A hazard exists that poses a threat to public health and safety
- The nurse is motivated to seek treatment
- There is evidence of satisfactory participation in a treatment program (Dunn, 2005; Fisk & Devoto, 1990)

If the school's state has a mandatory reporting law, then the dean has no choice but to report the student to the state board of nursing. However, even that is not necessarily an easy decision: because the report may forever damage the nurse, the requirements of the law must be carefully read against the actual facts known, and the report must be made only if the facts fit the law's requirements. If the state does not have a mandatory reporting law (or if its requirements are not strictly satisfied), then the dean must consider the options listed above and decide whether a report is warranted or if another response (e.g., rehabilitation) is satisfactory.

Discussion of Case

Given the serious allegations and the fact that they are made separately by three people, you consult with the assistant dean for clinical compliance, who is responsible for clinical health clearance and safety. Concurring in the concern, the assistant dean calls Ms. Jones to a meeting in her office and from there escorts her to the office for student and employee health for a drug test. A urine and hair analysis is obtained in accordance with the college's substance abuse policy for student majors that include a clinical component in the curriculum. You also suspend Ms. Jones from her clinical rotation pending an investigation and drug screen results.

WHEN TO CONSULT THE UNIVERSITY COUNSEL

Consult the university counsel when you need:

- To seek advice related to verbal/written communication with student
- To interpret the state board of nursing reporting law(s)
- To seek advice related to temporary suspension
- To review documentation

Findings and Disposition

Ms. Jones's drug test is positive for OxyContin. You and the assistant dean for clinical compliance meet with Ms. Jones to discuss your findings and concerns. You learn from Ms. Jones that she has a prescription for tramadol for chronic back pain. She does not have a prescription for OxyContin.

At the meeting, Ms. Jones denies having a problem and states that she took one of her mother's pills (OxyContin) because she was out of tramadol. You encourage her to seek treatment and she becomes angry and denies that she has a problem. You say to her, "Robin, I am trying to save your life." She continues to deny that she has a problem. You inform her that you will be reporting the incident to the state board of nursing for further investigation and that she is suspended from clinical courses for the time being. You will also report the matter to the nursing student conduct committee for review. You refer Ms. Jones to the student counseling center.

Ms. Jones is dismissed from the program in accordance with the university's drug policy. She does not return to the nurse anesthesia program. However, a student who has been dismissed, suspended, withdrawn, or taken an approved leave of absence from the program because of substance abuse may be eligible to reenter the program in certain circumstances if he or she can demonstrate satisfactory evidence of successful completion of treatment and documentation of 24 months of sustained recovery. Factors that have been identified as helpful for reentry into practice include 12-step program participation, random drug screens, and sponsorship in a peer-assisted support group. The student must also provide medical clearance from the appropriate individual coordinating the therapeutic intervention and evidence of current, active nursing licensure if required by the program.

Relevant Legal Cases

Mississippi State Board of Nursing v. John Wilson, No. 91-CA-0054, 624 So. 2d 485 (Miss. 1993)

Woodis v. Westark Community College, 160 F.3d 435 (8th Cir. 1998)

In the case of *Mississippi State Board of Nursing v. John Wilson*, John Wilson was a registered nurse who was employed as a nursing supervisor in the chemical dependency unit at the Mississippi State Hospital. Following the introduction of considerable evidence at hearings, the state board concluded that he was guilty of three violations of using habit-forming drugs—primarily cocaine—and issued a final order revoking his license. Mr. Wilson appealed this decision to the local court (the Hinds County Chancery Court). After a trial, the court found that Mr. Wilson did have a history of drug use, but that the incidents were isolated, being separated by periods of three to eight years. Because this did not constitute continuous use of habit-forming drugs, the court reversed the finding of the board that Wilson was addicted to or dependent on habit-forming drugs. For that reason, the court held that his license should not have been revoked and reversed the decision of the state board. The state board then filed an appeal, and the Mississippi Supreme Court upheld its original decision, reversing the trial court and sending the case back to the state board to implement its original decision.

In *Woodis v. Westark Community College,* Rosia Woodis was enrolled as a nursing student and pursuing a degree as an LPN. In her third semester in the program, the police arrested Ms. Woodis for attempting to obtain a controlled substance using a fraudulent prescription. Upon receiving notice of the arrest and the charges against the student, Dr. Sandi Sanders, the community college's vice president of student affairs, promptly suspended Ms. Woodis pending the outcome of the police investigation. Dr. Sanders sent a letter to Ms. Woodis advising her of this decision and of her due process rights as set forth in the Westark student handbook. Ms. Woodis appealed the decision to a five-member disciplinary appeals committee, which not only upheld the suspension but, hearing the evidence behind the arrest, concluded that Ms. Woodis had violated the school's code of conduct and imposed the sanction of expulsion. Ms. Woodis appealed those decisions to the court. In upholding the expulsion decision, the court held that the disciplinary committee had properly found that the student had violated the school's code of conduct and that the student's rights to due process had not been violated.

Although the courts ruled differently in each of these cases, both *Woodis v. Westark Community College* and *Mississippi State Board of Nursing v. John Wilson* reveal that specific policies regarding drug use and abuse are invaluable when acting on suspicion or reports of student substance abuse. For example, the Westark student handbook's specific descriptions of the conduct that was not allowed and the process that would be followed during a drug and police investigation left the courts satisfied that the student's interests were protected while the university was conducting its investigation. The problem for the Mississippi State Board of Nursing's substance abuse policy was that it was not entirely clear: had it been specific in stating that the board could revoke a nurse's license solely based on illegal drug use (as opposed to addiction or regular use), then there probably would not have been a disagreement between the trial court and the supreme court, and the trial court would have been more likely to affirm the decision of the board based on clear warning given in the policy. In other words, the question of whether the appellee was addicted to the drug would not have made a difference in their decision. These cases illustrate the need for colleges and universities to have a policy for drug use, testing, and monitoring that is clear, and a process for investigating allegations of violations that moves quickly toward a resolution while protecting the rights of all involved. Refer to the *Drexel University Substance Abuse Policy* located on http://davisplus.fadavis.com for a detailed example.

PREVENTION TIPS

To help prevent substance abuse in students, educate students about the risk of chemical dependency among health-care providers and the risk that it causes not just to patients, but also to society at large. Enhance their ability to recognize impaired health-care professionals, and reinforce the importance of reporting and the significance of appropriate intervention. Make sure that students have the contact information for people who can help them or their colleagues if substance abuse becomes an issue. It is also important to remind students of the school's substance abuse policy and to show them where they can locate a copy of it.

Summary

When a student or nurse is suspected of substance abuse, it is suggested that faculty or fellow nurses and peers confront the student or nurse by taking the individual aside and privately addressing their concern about the behavior. The faculty member should also consult an administrator to receive assistance and support (Banerjee, 2006). Except in extreme situations, it is likely that an appropriate response is for the individual and the university to enter an agreement by which the individual agrees immediately to cease the improper conduct and begin addictions treatment with the goal to return to work/school and maintain client safety (O'Hagan, 2005). The academic institution will have to render a decision regarding the student's eligibility to continue in the program—at the time, after a suspension, or never. The student should be allowed to continue in school based on conditions consistent with the institution's drug and alcohol policy. Although a report of the transgression may be required at the time of the conduct, the state board of nursing will not become involved until the student graduates and a decision is needed about whether to issue an initial registered professional nursing license. What is certain is that faculty and students require education about this very important issue. Academic institutions need drug and alcohol use and screening and monitoring policies firmly in place to deal effectively with this persistent social problem.

CRITICAL ELEMENTS TO CONSIDER

- Assess students for signs of substance abuse.
- Offer faculty development programs on substance abuse.
- Maintain student confidentiality.
- Follow your institution's substance abuse policy.

CRITICAL ELEMENTS TO CONSIDER—cont'd

- Consult legal counsel for advice.
- Consult the dean of students for assistance and support.
- Document faculty report of suspicion of drug/alcohol use.

Please include the following information in documentation:

- Date, time, and location of incident
- Behavioral, visual, olfactory, or auditory observations
- Whether the student admitted to use of drugs/alcohol
- Whether drugs/alcohol were discovered on the student
- Witnesses to the student's behavior
- Whether the student agreed to drug/alcohol testing
- Results of drug/alcohol test (if completed)
- Consult the state board of nursing for reporting advice.

References

American Association of Nurse Anesthetists Peer Assistance. (2010). Signs and behaviors of impaired colleagues. Retrieved April 21, 2010, from http://www.aana.com/peerassist.aspx

Banerjee, L. (2006). Ask a practice advisor: Substance abuse and chemical dependency by nurse. *SRNA Bulletin.* Retrieved April 15, 2010, from http://www.srna.org/nurse_resources/pa/2006_pa_substance.pdf

Dunn, D. (2005). Substance abuse among nurses: Intercession and intervention. *AORN Journal, 82*(5), 775–799.

Drexel University. (2009). *Official student handbook 2009–2010.* Retrieved April 21, 2010, from http://www.drexel.edu/studentlife/studenthandbook/Handbook.html#code

Fisk, N. B., & Devoto, D. A. (1990). The nurse employee who uses alcohol/other drugs. *Nurse Managers Bookshelf, 2,* 110–129.

Mississippi State Board of Nursing v. John Wilson, No. 91-CA-0054, 624 So. 2d 485 (Miss. 1993).

O'Hagan, R. (2005). Consensual complaint resolution agreement: Dealing with an addiction/chemical dependency. *SRNA Bulletin.* Retrieved March 24, 2010, from http://www.srna.org/communications/newsbulletin/bulletin_oct_05.pdf

Woodis v. Westark Community College, 160 F.3d 435 (8th Cir. 1998).

CHAPTER 27

Issues Surrounding the Tenure Process

CASE STUDY

Issues Surrounding the Tenure Process

Your role: You are the new dean in the college of nursing.

You are the new dean in the college of nursing. The University Tenure Appeals Committee voted unanimously to sustain the appeal of Professor Sally Saks, a member of your college's faculty, who was denied tenure last year. By unanimous vote (9 to 0), the University Tenure Appeals Committee recommends the case be returned to the college of nursing as the result of a serious failure that occurred during the tenure process.

The problem identified by the University Tenure Appeals Committee is that there was no formal midterm review of Professor Saks, as required by the tenure policy. Instead, there had only been a meeting between the former dean of the college of nursing and Professor Saks addressing Professor Saks's progress toward tenure. The former dean then sent a letter via e-mail to Dr. Saks in which she summarized the key points of their meeting (in which many deficiencies were discussed); however, no formal midterm review committee was ever formed to evaluate the candidate's tenure dossier, and there was no formal review of that dossier by such a committee, thus violating the tenure policy. The committee identified a second failure as well: Professor Saks was never provided with an official mentor from the department, which the tenure policy also required. The University Tenure Appeals Committee was unanimous in concluding that these two failings were fundamentally unfair to the candidate.

You also learn that the college of nursing's tenure committee had unanimously voted to deny tenure to Professor Saks last year. As the process proceeded, her department chair and the former dean of the college also voted to deny her tenure. She received no letters of support from her colleagues. In addition, her former direct reports were on her Department Tenure Review Committee.

The former dean, department chair, and tenure committee all focused on Dr. Saks's lack of collegiality and failure to meet her service obligations. They found her quality of teaching and publication record to be adequate.

Questions

- What are the major violations in this case?
- Is Professor Saks receiving a fair review?
- Is lack of collegiality a justifiable reason to deny tenure?

Tenure Process: Legal Principles and Review of the Literature

The notion of tenure has been in place since the 12th century. It is intended to protect faculty members by safeguarding academic freedom, ensuring a fair process prior to dismissal, and providing job security (Adams, 2006). The process of being awarded academic tenure typically requires review of three key areas of participation within the academy: publishing, research, and program funding; service to the institution and community; and teaching. The emphasis and relative weight placed on each of these categories vary by academic institution.

The decision to award or deny tenure is perhaps the single most important decision in the career of a member of the faculty. Negative tenure decisions can cause extreme stress for tenure candidates, ill will in departments, and costly lawsuits for universities. Because careers can be broken by denials, challenges to denials are to be anticipated; and because fairness is both promised and demanded, all involved in the process (including judges who are often called in to review it at the end) are very sensitive to how fairly the candidate was treated. The tension arises when everyone agrees that on the merits the candidate does not deserve tenure, but also agrees that the college did not do what it should to hold up its end of the bargain. In a field such as nursing in which the faculty have spent their careers rendering aid and assistance to people, there may perhaps be even greater empathy and emphasis on protecting the candidate.

Most colleges and universities have well-articulated tenure policies. Tenured faculty and administrators have collaborated on developing standards and procedures that match their unique institutional circumstances. However, some aspects of a tenure policy may be unclear or incomplete, creating the potential for ambiguity or conflict. If a step is missed in the process, or if the tenure denial is based on a criterion that does not specifically appear in the written policy, or if the criteria changed after the candidate was initially hired on the tenure track, then the unsuccessful candidate may argue that the decision was unfair or improper.

Some courts are sympathetic to these claims. Other courts give universities latitude in interpreting, for example, research as including the ability to attract external funding, or teaching as including social skills in relating to students. The safest course for colleges and universities is to articulate written standards that reflect the major criteria that are actually used. The evaluators at all stages in the tenure process should know—and apply—the criteria (American Association of

University Professors, American Council of Education, & United Educators Insurance Risk Retention Group [AAUP, ACE, and United Educators], 2000).

The American Association of University Professors, the American Council on Education, and the United Educators Insurance Risk Retention Group (2000) issued a report that provides guidance on conducting tenure evaluations. The report, *Good Practice in Tenure Evaluation: Advice for Tenured Faculty, Department Chairs, and Academic Administrators*, recommends that tenure decisions be guided by four principles:

- Clarity in standards and procedures. Institutions should ensure that both the criteria and the process for tenure decisions are clearly delineated in writing, that they are communicated to candidates, and that they are followed in practice.
- Consistency in decisions. Tenure criteria should be applied consistently to all candidates regardless of personal characteristics—such as race, gender, disability, or national origin—that are protected by law or by university policy. It is also important that individual candidates be given consistent information and feedback during the probationary period.
- Candor in evaluations. Senior faculty should not back away from offering constructive criticism and a realistic assessment of how well a tenure candidate is meeting tenure requirements.
- Caring for unsuccessful candidates. Faculty and academic administrators should treat unsuccessful tenure candidates in a respectful and professional manner, making sure that they do not become isolated during the terminal year and providing whatever assistance possible to assist them in finding a new position.

The report stresses that faculty and administrators must collaborate to clarify tenure guidelines and adhere to tenure processes. In addition to following these principles, faculty and academic administrators should review their past tenure evaluations and ask the following questions: Have candidates who have been denied tenure been surprised by the decisions? Have lawsuits or disputes over tenure arisen? If so, what was learned as a result, and how can the policy or procedures be changed to reduce those risks in the future? It should also be made clear to candidates at the beginning of their appointment that annual evaluations may not be the same as tenure evaluations: the criteria for receiving a lifetime appointment are not the same as for receiving an annual pay increase. Negative tenure decisions that are preceded by positive evaluations and optimistic departmental promises are particularly problematic.

Faculty committees that hold tenure-granting rank are also considering collegiality when they make their tenure decisions. *Collegiality*—the spirit of collaboration and cooperation—recognizes important aspects of a faculty member's overall performance (American Association of University Professors

[AAUP], 1999). According to the AAUP (1999), collegiality does not have a distinct capacity to be assessed independently of the established three-part tenure test but is a quality whose worth is expressed in the successful implementation of three criteria—teaching, scholarship, and service. The AAUP (1999) also reminds members that collegiality is not simply enthusiasm, dedication, or a display of deference for the sake of harmony; rather, "such expectations are flatly contrary to elementary principles of academic freedom, which protect a faculty member's right to dissent from the judgments of colleagues and administrators" (p. 2).

That said, faculty members do have a duty of collegiality in the fulfillment of their job responsibilities and in satisfying their dual role as employees and managers in self-governance (Adams, 2006). As noted by Pertnoy (2004), "Each of us decides, depending on our individual interpretive mechanisms, whether being collegial means having a personality trait that suits ours, being able to disagree without being disagreeable, or having to forfeit one's contrary opinion to another's for the sake of keeping peace" (p. 202). With that said, universities are not insisting on congeniality but rather collegiality, which is generally viewed as promoting and participating in supportive interactions among colleagues. Despite concerns that collegiality is counter to a culture of thoughtful debate and a lively exchange of ideas and opinions in the academy, faculty exchanges should be conducted in a culture of mutual respect (Tacha, 1995). Collegiality plays an essential role in maintaining a respectful, supportive climate that supports the teaching, research, and service mission of the university.

The point is that if universities do want to use collegiality as a criterion in the consideration of tenure candidate, it is only fair (and smart) to include it in the list of essential factors, so that candidates have notice in advance of what will be on the test, so to say. When it is included as a factor, the decisions that are made will be left alone. Courts recognize that the tenure decision is among the most personal decisions that a university can make, and therefore give significant deference to universities' tenure decisions, recognizing the subjective and evaluative nature of the decision. This applies to interpreting what is meant by the word *collegiality*. In fact, Connell and Savage (2001) state that "there is no case in which a court rejected consideration of collegiality unless there was evidence of discrimination or a violation of free speech or academic freedom" (p. 833).

Discussion of Case

Convening a tenure midpoint review committee is a specific step in the tenure review process, and the failure to do so is a violation of the tenure policy. This is more than just a checklist item. The midpoint review provides an opportunity for the tenure candidate to obtain feedback on how well he or she is meeting the tenure requirements, and for the college to articulate its standards of performance for its permanent faculty and provide instruction to candidates on how they can do a better job fulfilling the college's expectations and needs. Without such review, the college cannot get the most out of its tenure-track faculty, and the candidate is at a significant disadvantage concerning what he or she needs to do to be successful for tenure. Although it could be argued that the former dean provided such a review, Professor Saks did not receive the full benefit of a full review of her work by senior tenured faculty. She also did not receive a formal written notification of the committee's assessment of her progress toward tenure. The college did not follow its own tenure policy.

Conversely, tenure policies are not designed to be tests that the administration must pass at the end of the tenure review process or a game by which candidates can avoid harsh decisions by finding missteps. The tenure track is intended to be a pathway to learning as well as evaluation, and tenure candidates have duties as well as rights. If a step is missed, the tenure candidate should be expected to point it out and request the benefit. The failure to do so could be argued to be a waiver by the candidate of that right.

As per AAUP, ACE, & United Educators (2000) in *Good Practice in Tenure Evaluation: Advice for Tenured Faculty, Department Chairs, and Academic Administrators*, tenure criteria should be applied consistently to all candidates regardless of personal characteristics—and certainly without regard to such factors as race, gender, disability, sexual preference, national origin, or other factors that the law defines as illegal. It is also important that individual candidates be given consistent information and feedback during the probationary period. In this case, the university's tenure criteria were not applied consistently because other tenure candidates had the benefit of a midpoint review whereas Professor Saks did not.

Because Professor Saks did not receive a formal midpoint review, the senior tenured faculty did not have an opportunity to address Professor Saks's faculty and peer relationships and lack of collegiality. Professor Saks did not have an opportunity to respond to the feedback, receive mentoring and advice from more senior faculty, and adjust her behavior.

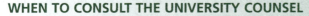

WHEN TO CONSULT THE UNIVERSITY COUNSEL
- Consult counsel with tenure policy changes and implementation.
- Consult counsel if violations in the tenure policy occur.

Findings and Disposition

In this particular case, the dean accepted the findings and recommendations of the University Tenure Appeals Committee, and decided to add two years to Professor Saks's tenure clock. The dean requested that Professor Saks be provided with a development plan that would cover the ensuing 2-year period, similar to what she could have expected to receive at the intended midpoint review. Professor Saks was also assigned a faculty mentor. During her additional 2-year probationary period, Professor Saks continued to have difficulty with her faculty and peer relationships. At its end, Professor Saks was reevaluated for tenure in a new process. Once again, she received poor evaluations by her department and by a new tenure committee, and was denied tenure.

Relevant Legal Case

University of Baltimore v. Iz, 716 A.2d 1107 (Md. Ct. Spec. App. 1998)

University of Baltimore v. Iz was a lawsuit against the University of Baltimore for sex and national origin discrimination under Title VII, violation of equal protection and breach of contract, which Dr. Iz filed following the denial of her tenure candidacy. The steps in the tenure review process were as follows:

- In 1989, the University of Baltimore hired Dr. Iz as a visiting assistant professor under a 1-year contract. Her appointment was in the Department of Information and Qualitative Sciences in the Merrick School of Business.

- In 1990, Dr. Iz accepted the university's offer of a tenure-track position. Based on credit for a prior faculty appointment at Miami University, her initial tenure review date was the 1994–1995 academic year, but the applicable policy permitted early tenure review. Against the advice of senior departmental colleagues, Dr. Iz decided to undergo tenure review one year early, in 1993–1994. Although the policy on early review does not require a vote, the tenured members of her department voted (5 to 1, with one abstention) to recommend against early tenure review. Dr. Iz appealed to the university's central administration, and the president informed her that she could seek early review but, if she were denied tenure, then she would not receive another review. She decided to proceed with the early review, and the provost instructed the Merrick faculty to consider her for tenure with promotion to the rank of associate professor.

- At the first stage of review, Dr. Iz's tenured colleagues in the department voted 3 to 2 against tenure, with one abstention. Relying on a recent review of her teaching, research, and service, which had been required at the end of her third year, her colleagues noted in a written report that Dr. Iz "has been showing progress and would have a stronger case next year." In addition, the former department chair, who had held the position for 17 years and had hired Dr. Iz, e-mailed his vote while he was away on sabbatical; providing one of the three recommendations against tenure, he stated that she was a good teacher, had publications, and was involved in professional service activities, but he expressed concern about "her attitude and collegiality."

- The current department chair, however, recommended in favor of tenure and promotion, judging her as meeting or exceeding the necessary qualifications for teaching, research, and service.
- Next, the school's Tenure and Promotion Committee voted 6 to 4 in favor of awarding tenure to Dr. Iz.
- After receiving these three recommendations, the dean voted against tenure and promotion. In his opinion, Dr. Iz met or exceeded the qualifications for research and service but not for teaching. He also observed that she was reluctant to accept "peer evaluation" and that her colleagues had "strongly recommended that she not apply early for tenure and promotion."
- Before making his final determination, the provost met separately with Dr. Iz and the department chair to give them an opportunity to be heard on the points where Dr. Iz's performance had been found inadequate in the process. In a follow-up letter, the department chair confirmed that Dr. Iz was inflexible, defensive, and unwilling to take constructive advice, including peer evaluation. Further, he explained that he had not included this information in his recommendation because he had not regarded it as a pertinent criterion in the tenure and promotion process.
- Subsequently, the provost recommended against tenure and promotion. Although acknowledging Dr. Iz's strengths in research and service, he found significance in her difficulties with her departmental colleagues.
- Dr. Iz filed an internal appeal. The Tenure Appeals Committee was split and could not reach an agreement on whether or not to uphold the provost's tenure denial.
- The president accepted the provost's recommendation against tenure.
- Dr. Iz sued the university on the basis of sex and national origin discrimination under Title VII, violation of equal protection and breach of contract. The breach of contract claim was based on Dr. Iz's assertion that the university could only use criteria that were specifically listed in the university tenure policy, and that collegiality was not one of those factors.
- The jury determined that the university had breached Dr. Iz's contract and awarded $425,000 in compensatory damages.
- The university filed an appeal.

The only issue before the appellate court was whether the university had the right to use collegiality as a criterion for tenure, even though it was not specifically referenced. "We are persuaded that collegiality plays an essential role in both teaching and service" (716 A.2d at 1122). The court held that the trial court should have ruled, as a matter of law, that the university could use collegiality as a tenure criterion.

Among other things, it is worth noting that the appellate court's decision was rendered 4 years after the tenure process had occurred. The amount of time, expense, and disruption this process caused cannot be underestimated. Simply including collegiality among the factors that would be considered for tenure would have prevented it all.

Summary

Consideration for tenure is a fundamental moment in an academic's career. Therefore, it is imperative that tenured faculty and administrators use best practices discussed in this chapter as well as the advice outlined in *Good Practice in Tenure Evaluation: Advice for Tenured Faculty, Department Chairs, and Academic Administrators* (AAUP, ACE, and United Educators, 2000). A consistent, fair, and transparent process is in the best interest of the tenure candidate, faculty, administrators, and the university.

PREVENTION TIPS

- Institutions should ensure that both the criteria and the process for tenure decisions are clearly delineated in writing, that they are communicated to candidates, and that they are followed in practice (AAUP, ACE, 2000).
- Offer development sessions to department chairs and academic administrators on offering constructive feedback during the annual faculty review process.
- If universities wish to use collegiality as a criterion in the consideration of tenure candidates, it is only fair (and smart) to include it in the list of essential factors, so that candidates have notice in advance what will be used as a criterion for tenure.

CRITICAL ELEMENTS TO CONSIDER

- The tenure policy should comprehensively list all the major criteria used for evaluation.
- The policy and procedures should be reviewed by the university attorney to determine areas in which they are unclear or might not fully express the university's expectations for tenured faculty.
- The evaluators at all stages in the tenure process should know—and apply—the criteria.
- The tenure policy should address whether tenure evaluators will consider positive events occurring after the tenure application has been submitted.

CRITICAL ELEMENTS TO CONSIDER—cont'd

- The tenure policy should indicate what steps the institution will take if a faculty member under consideration for tenure is charged with misconduct or if other negative events emerge.
- The tenure policy should indicate times when the "clock" will stop, slow, or otherwise be adjusted (e.g., leave for disability or pregnancy, maternity, military service).
- The tenure policy should address the voting protocol when an evaluator serves at more than one level of review (e.g., department chair in the same discipline).
- Individual faculty members may wish to express their own opinions about a tenure candidate to members of the campus-wide promotion and tenure committee or to the administration. The tenure policy should address how the recipients should treat these individual opinions.
- All reviewers should meticulously follow tenure procedures. The probationary faculty members should also be instructed as to their obligation to be a full participant in the process, and their duty to call errors to the attention of the dean (or other appropriate official).
- Conduct workshops for department chairs on the appointment and evaluation of tenure-track faculty.
- Conduct workshops on tenure procedures for faculty serving on the tenure and promotions committee (AAUP, ACE, and United Educators, 2000).

References

Adams, M. L. (2006). The quest for tenure: Job security and academic freedom. *The Catholic University Law Review, 56*(67), 189–190.

American Association of University Professors. (1999). On collegiality as a criterion for faculty evaluation. Retrieved July 7, 2010, from http://www.aaup.org/AAUP/pubsres/policydocs/contents/collegiality.htm

American Association of University Professors, American Council of Education, & United Educators Insurance Risk Retention Group. (2000). *Good practice in tenure evaluation: Advice for tenured faculty, department chairs, and academic administrators.* Retrieved July 7, 2010, from http://www.acenet.edu/bookstore/pdf/tenure-evaluation.pdf

Connell, M. A., & Savage, F. G. (2001). The role of collegiality in higher education tenure, promotion, and termination decisions. *Journal of College and University Law, 27*(2), 833–843.

Pertnoy, L. (2004). The "C" word: Collegiality real or imaginary, and should it matter in a tenure process. *St. Thomas Law Review, 17,* 201–224.

Tacha, D. R. (1995). The "C" word: On collegiality. *Ohio State Law Journal, 56,* 585–587.

University of Baltimore v. Iz, 716 A.2d 1107 (Md. Ct. Spec. App. 1998).

CHAPTER 28

Conflict of Interest Issues in the Faculty Role

CASE STUDY

Conflict of Interest Issues in the Faculty Role

Your role: You are the associate dean for the nursing programs.

You are newly appointed as the associate dean. One of your faculty members, Dr. Rhea Walton, age 66, is a tenured faculty member and chair of the graduate nursing department. She has served in the position for 10 years. She is what you would call a minimalist. She allows the graduate faculty to have free rein and rarely calls them on their behavior. She has not published in years and is basically coasting until she can retire. Previous administrations have not addressed Dr. Walton's lack of productivity because her husband is the vice provost for research at the university. In reviewing the merit increases, you learn that the previous associate dean awarded Dr. Walton 6% merit increases in the past few years, whereas other, more productive faculty have received 2% to 4% merit increases. Further, those lower raises had also been approved by the dean. Many of the productive academic administrators are quite unhappy, as they feel that Dr. Walton receives special treatment because of her husband's position. It is difficult for you to encourage a culture of productivity and meritocracy with Dr. Walton in her current role.

Questions

- How would you proceed in addressing the perceived disparity?
- What are the political implications if you remove Dr. Walton? Would the dean allow you to do so?
- How should you best manage this situation from a legal perspective?

Conflict of Interest: Legal Principles and Review of the Literature

In general, a conflict of interest occurs when there is a divergence between a faculty member's private interests and his or her professional obligations to the university, such that an independent observer might reasonably question whether the faculty member's professional actions or decisions are determined by any considerations other than the best interests of the university ("Faculty Conflict," 2007).

In academia, conflicts of interest typically arise in research when scientists or others involved in research have a financial stake in companies sponsoring the research or in companies that may stand to profit from it. The likelihood of such conflicts has increased in recent years, as the percentage of research funding that comes from industry has grown, especially in medicine, biology, chemistry, and engineering. To date, institutional policies on conflicts of interest have been inconsistent; many focus on disclosure of conflicts rather than on prohibition of them (American Association of University Professors [AAUP], 2001). Strong policies surrounding such conflicts are needed in the academy.

Another common area ripe for potential conflict of interest is the academic couple, who seem to be pervasive in universities. The term *academic couple* refers to two people who are partners or spouses and work at the same college or university. A potential conflict of interest exists when one or both members of the academic couple hold administrative positions and/or one faculty member in the couple or dyad is not held to the same standard as other faculty because of the position his or her spouse or partner holds in the university community. The spouse or partner may serve as a senior administrator or generate substantial research dollars or beneficial publicity for the university. To prohibit universities from hiring academic couples would seriously hurt their recruitment of talented faculty, administrators, and researchers (Sugarman, 2005). But allowing discrimination to occur on bases other than merit will contaminate the community, whether the preference (or perceived preference) is given on the basis of sex, race, national origin, or family relationship.

This concern has been expressed at the institutional governance level as well. Nonprofit institutions must file a report each year with the Internal Revenue Service that confirms compliance with their charitable tax exemptions. In 2008, the IRS issued a new Form 990 that digs far more deeply into their activities. Among other things, it now asks for disclosures about members of the governing board and about other interested persons—persons or organizations having some kind of close relationship with the nonprofit that might use that relationship to their own benefit, whether through jobs, salary, or contracts, at the risk or disadvantage to the nonprofit. The form seeks disclosures about members of the family, organizations in which the person has a significant financial ownership interest, and members of the family who are employed in those organizations. These disclosures have to be made by every officer and member of the board of directors. They seek not just actual conflicts of interest, but relationships that might be perceived as causing one; and the disclosures are intended to make those relationships transparent, with the objective of forcing the nonprofit to face them and deal with them.

Faculty and administrators should disclose any and all potential conflicts of interest—including familial relationships—and these relationships should be periodically reviewed for any conflict. Members of the same family should not be employed in a situation in which one member of the family works under the administrative supervision of another. Managing interpersonal conflicts and perceptions of favoritism also need to be addressed by administration, as these issues can affect morale and productivity.

Discussion of Case

The associate dean was new to the university, but quickly realized that Dr. Walton was not as productive as the other department chairs. After noting the measurable difference in productivity between Dr. Walton and her colleagues, the associate dean discussed the situation with the dean and her inability to hold all department chairs to a high level of productivity with Dr. Walton in her current position. More concerning was that the MSN department outcomes were not as high caliber as they were in other departments. To move the organization forward, it was decided that Dr. Walton needed to increase her level of productivity or a change of leadership would be required. The dean agreed with the data provided by the associate dean regarding Dr. Walton and the MSN department's lack of productivity and stated that she would inform the provost in the event that the vice provost for research discussed the issue with him.

WHEN TO CONSULT THE UNIVERSITY COUNSEL
Consult the university counsel for advice with a potential or real conflict of interest.

Findings and Disposition

The associate dean discussed Dr. Walton with legal counsel, who was quick to note the complexity of the situation. On one hand, department chairs serve at the discretion of the dean: there is no "right" to them. On the other hand, academic titles and the additional benefits that come with them (increased salary, reputation, and status) are property and liberty interests that cannot be summarily taken away. (See Chapter 8 for a discussion of due process.) In this situation, Dr. Walton had received good performance reviews and very healthy salary increases for several years: whether deserved or not, they existed in the file and would raise the inference that any demotion would be based on something other than merit, which could easily appear to be her age—a factor prohibited by federal law. Legal counsel stressed the critical importance of documenting the performance deficiencies in terms that were as objective as possible, and making sure the record was adequate to withstand review by independent third parties (judicial or otherwise). Counsel also noted that it might take longer than a year to achieve the objective unless Dr. Walton agreed to the change.

The associate dean also met with the dean, and asked about the dean's role in the annual evaluations and salary increases. The dean was not able to explain why Dr. Walton had earned merit increases so far above the norm, and admitted that she just signed off on the recommendations made by the prior associate dean as long as the total stayed within budget.

The associate dean met with Dr. Walton to address her individual productivity as well as her unit's productivity. She also explained to Dr. Walton her intention to seriously enhance the unit's performance, and the additional level of oversight and involvement and commitment of time that this would require of the department chair. Although Dr. Walton was able to demonstrate the extent and quality of her scholarly activity over the past years—bringing new information to the associate dean and persuading her that there had been good reason to award her significant salary increases—she also indicated that she did not want to take on the additional duties that the associate dean had in mind to revamp the department. Accordingly, Dr. Walton agreed to step down as the chair and to return to her position as a member of the tenured faculty.

Relevant Legal Case

Lewis v. St. Cloud University, 467 F.3d 1133 (Minn. 2005)

Dr. Richard Lewis filed suit against St. Cloud State University, claiming age discrimination in violation of the Age Discrimination in Employment Act (ADEA) and Title VII of the Civil Rights Act. He also made parallel claims under the Minnesota Human Rights Act (MHRA).

Dr. Lewis has been a history professor at the university for 30 years. He was named interim dean of the College of Social Sciences (COSS) in 1997 and was promoted to dean of COSS in 1999 at the age of 62. When Dr. Lewis returned to work in the spring of 2002 after suffering a mild heart attack, his supervisor told him that "the president had told her that there were rumors that he wanted to retire and that a plan had been developed, a plan in which a search could be completed and he would be replaced as of the following January." Dr. Lewis denied this rumor in a formal written response to the university President Saigo, stating, "I found this news of my rumored retirement and the search for a new Dean, profoundly disturbing. Clearly this action by the president is trying to force me to resign. This rumor creates a hostile work environment for me and constitutes blatant age discrimination." The university took no further action to remove Dr. Lewis as dean at that time.

Around the time that Dr. Lewis had returned to work, the university reorganized its administration and, beginning in June 2002, Dr. Lewis began reporting to Dr. Spitzer, the newly hired provost and vice president for academic affairs. In April of 2003, 11 months after Dr. Spitzer became provost, he recommended to President Saigo that the university replace Dr. Lewis as dean, and President Saigo assented.

In May, Dr. Spitzer met with Dr. Lewis, told him that he needed "to plan his retirement from the Deanship," and asked Dr. Lewis to propose an exit strategy by the following week. Throughout the ensuing months, Dr. Lewis and his lawyer worked with Dr. Spitzer on an exit strategy, but no agreement was reached.

To state a claim for illegal discrimination on account of age, Dr. Lewis had to show that he was at least 40 years old, suffered an adverse employment action, was meeting his employer's reasonable expectations at the time of the adverse employment action, and was replaced by someone substantially younger. In large measure, the university did not contest those facts. The burden then shifted to the university to prove that age was not the motivating factor for his removal as dean.

The university produced three legitimate, nondiscriminatory reasons for demoting Dr. Lewis: (1) he created a divisive environment between the faculty and the administration, (2) he was ineffective in handling interpersonal conflicts among faculty, and (3) he engaged in favoritism and bias in some of his personnel evaluations. The provost was able to provide specific incidents and supporting details that supported his bases, and in large measure Dr. Lewis did not dispute them; rather, he claimed that they were not the real reason, but pretext and a subterfuge. In rebuttal, Dr. Lewis pointed to his series of annual performance reviews, all of which had been positive, as evidence that the university's stated reasons for demoting him were not accurate or credible. The last of those reviews was prepared by Dr. Lewis's previous supervisor shortly before Dr. Spitzer became provost and just a year before the demotion, "an inference of age discrimination." Because the material facts were not disputed, both Dr. Lewis and the university moved for summary judgment, which the district court granted to the university on all claims. In doing so, the court stated, "While favorable performance reviews sometimes provide evidence of pretext, the receipt of positive reviews in the past, in and of itself, does not necessarily raise an inference of age discrimination." This decision was affirmed on appeal.

Summary

The responsibility of proving illegal discrimination rests with the party alleging the violation. The plaintiff must establish that he or she is a member of a protected category and that an unfavorable employment decision was rendered as a result of being a member of a protected category. A personnel file that contains consistently positive evaluations is sufficient evidence to carry that burden, as it raises the inference that the adverse employment action resulted from some cause other than merit. If the university is not able to prove (to the fact-finder's satisfaction) that there was some good cause, that absence of proof will actually be enough to support a finding of illegal discrimination.

Faculty members (like all university employees) are counseled to report incidents of age, gender, or race inequity to their office of equality officer prior to any negative employment decisions. This is not just a matter of personal interest, but communal: universities are pledged to preserving and maintaining a community that acts on merit. The American Association of University Professors (AAUP) advocates that universities take allegations of discrimination seriously and allow for an adequate review of such assertions (AAUP, 1995). At the same time, administrators are counseled to make sure that evaluations are accurate and personnel records are complete. Being "kind" to someone actually breaches the same obligations of objectivity and merit; it just does not violate the law.

It must be noted that legal proceedings cannot always capture the interpersonal conflicts, motives, and nuances that exist in the work environment. Legal cases are decided on facts provable by admissible evidence, and the legal casebooks are filled with decisions that were wrongly decided because the real evidence never got to the judge or jury. Administrators must be careful to keep focused on objective data when making adverse employee actions, and must figure out ways to deal with the subjective, personal, and political, issues that can also greatly affect the performance of individuals and units.

PREVENTION TIPS

Faculty and administrators should disclose any and all potential conflicts of interest—including familial relationships—and these relationships should be periodically reviewed for any conflict by an objective body.

CRITICAL ELEMENTS TO CONSIDER

- Refer to the university's conflict of interest policy.
- Report any potential conflicts to your supervisor and those noted in the conflict of interest policy.
- If you are an administrator, treat all direct reports equitably, regardless of "special" relationships.
- Refrain from participating in any employment, salary, or other important decision regarding an immediate family member or person with whom you are in a personal relationship.

CRITICAL ELEMENTS TO CONSIDER—cont'd

- To avoid a perception of conflict of interest, members of the same family may not be employed in a situation where one member of the family works under the administrative supervision of another.
- Document performance issues in a formal and timely fashion—do not wait until there are numerous performance concerns that result in negative employment decisions.

References

American Association of University Professors. (1995). On discrimination. Retrieved July 18, 2010, from http://www.aaup.org/AAUP/pubsres/policydocs/contents/ondiscrimination.htm

American Association of University Professors. (2001). Conflict of interest guidelines proposed. Retrieved July 18, 2010, from http://www.aaup.org/AAUP/pubsres/academe/2001/MJ/NB/conflict.htm

Faculty conflict of commitment and conflict of interest, 2007–2009. (2007). *Northwestern University faculty handbook*. Retrieved June 16, 2009, from http://www.research.northwestern.edu/policies/faculty-conflict-of-interest.html#iii

Lewis v. St. Cloud University, 467 F.3d 1133 (Minn. 2005).

Sugarman, S. D. (2005). Conflict of interest in the role of the university professor. *Theoretical Inquiries in Law, 6,* 255–275.

CHAPTER 29

A Discussion of Professional Liability: When a Student Is Sued

CASE STUDY

Discussion of *Benedict v. Bondi:* Medical Error by a Student Nurse

Your role: You are an undergraduate faculty member.

A 3-year-old child became seriously ill one evening and was rushed to McKeesport Hospital where an emergency operation was performed by Dr. Frank R. Bondi. Several nurses and an assistant to the surgeon were also present in and around the operating room. Your student, Jean Streigel Waddell, was then a student nurse at the hospital working in and about the operating rooms. Someone asked her to get two hot water bottles and, when she brought them back, she was told to fill them with hot water, which she did from the hot water faucet in the instrument scrubbing room off the operating room. Knowing that the bottles needed to be covered, she did so with pillowcases. Dr. Bondi instructed Ms. Waddell to give the bottles to Irma Bieda. He then told Mrs. Bieda to apply them to the child's feet. Mrs. Bieda, who was a nurse intern, placed the hot water bottles still in the pillowcases on the outer sides of the child's feet.

The operation took appropriately 2 hours. At the end, the hot water bottles were removed from the child's feet. Ms. Waddell then saw that the feet were bright red and blistered. She also saw Dr. Bondi quickly cover the feet, as if to hide them.

Ms. Waddell comes to you in your office and tells you what happened, expressing her concern and worry for the child.

Questions

- What if anything should you do?
- Is your student exposed to legal liability? Are you?

Legal Principles and Review of the Literature

Professional liability (medical malpractice) claims are a fact of life for those in the healing arts. Television shows that always show successful diagnoses and remarkable recoveries, all brought about by wonderful, empathetic, emotive physicians, establish a false sense of the possible and set a very high bar for physicians and their assistants. The American justice system, which allows attorneys to represent plaintiffs on a contingency fee basis (they are paid only if they win, by settlement or verdict), also makes it relatively easy for patients and their families to sue.

Judges and juries must decide in cases of alleged medical error whether the conduct (act or omission) fell below the standard of care that is applicable to the situation. What that standard is can be defined by the individual professions, by the hospital, by the physicians' or nurses' organization, by the medical school that provides the physicians and nurses, or by experts who testify in court and speak (from experience or education, from practice, or from the published literature) to what the standard is. Someone who performs below that level of care is called negligent and is responsible for the harm that the negligence caused, even if other people came in afterward and added to it (or failed to rectify the situation).

A person is qualified to testify as an expert if, on the basis of experience or education, he or she has a reasonable pretense to expertise in the field; if the parties to the lawsuit do not agree about that, the judge is required to make a ruling. If an expert is allowed to testify, the jury is not obligated to accept his or her testimony, but can give it the weight it deserves, crediting all, part, or none of it. A jury is never asked whether they found an expert (or any specific witness) to be credible.

Lawsuits must be filed within a certain amount of time after the event occurs; after that time passes, no claim can be filed. The statutes of limitation, as the barriers are called, force attorneys often to file lawsuits before they know exactly who did what, or who was responsible for what. It is often not typically the case that people who are sued at the beginning are dismissed from the lawsuit before it goes to trial, because either the parties agree that they did nothing wrong or the judge grants them summary judgment.

Lawyers will sue not only the persons who performed the allegedly negligent act but also those who were responsible for them. This will often mean that supervisors are sued for negligent supervision, and employers are sued for having allowed the negligence to occur. In academic hospitals, the universities have been sued as well for having negligently trained the student or resident, or for policies and procedures that allowed its faculty to perform in a negligent way, or for simply being the employer of those allegedly at fault.

A hospital nurse is primarily responsible for administrative and ministerial acts (those not involving the exercise of discretion). These include such things as placing clean sheets on the operating table, preparing gowns and gloves, sterilizing the instruments to be used in the operation and seeing that they are available for use, making ready the sterile drapes, placing the patient on the operating table, and so on. In performing these duties, he or she would be regarded as an employee of (and an agent of) the hospital. When a nurse gets involved in the actual care being provided, the nurse can be viewed as the agent of the physician, even if there is no employment relationship: it is the ability to instruct the nurse that provides the legal theory of liability. In providing service to a particular patient, the nurse can both be subject to personal liability and provide a reason to hold a physician negligent.

Within the operating room, the law calls the physician in charge "the captain of the ship":

> And indeed it can readily be understood that in the course of an operation in the operating room of a hospital, and until the surgeon leaves that room at the conclusion of the operation, . . . he is in the same complete charge of those who are present and assisting him as is the captain of a ship over all on board, and that such supreme control is indeed essential in view of the high degree of protection to which anaesthetized, unconscious patient is entitled. (McConnell v. Williams, 361 Pa. 355, 362, 65 A.2d 243, 246)

The law imposes this authority, and liability, on the physician out of concern for the patient: How can the patient know who did what when anaesthetized or unconscious? The doctor is awake, giving instructions; and if she or he feels that someone else was really responsible for the error, then he or she can join that person as a defendant in the litigation.

Employees are often protected by their employers from claims of negligence. They may have provisions in their contracts or in their faculty handbooks by which the university agrees to indemnify, defend and hold harmless from such claims as long as the actions (or omissions) occurred in the course of employment and within the scope of duties. This means that the university will provide the attorney, defend the employee, reimburse the employee for all costs or judgments against the employee, and otherwise make sure the employee does not suffer any harm as a result of the action. This employee benefit can often be provided by way of the promise of insurance, but the insurance is subject to its own rules. There may be deductibles that the insured might have to pay, or limits on the amount of money it will pay to a patient/plaintiff, or it may refuse to defend the employee at all if the employee has done something to disqualify him- or herself from coverage (e.g., for failure to follow the employer's policies and procedures). Universities can also impose their own requirements on the right to indemnification: many, for example, have protocols that require the prompt reporting of events that might lead to claims, or requirements that the employee take a certain minimum number of hours of continuing medical education, or the requirement that the employee has acted in accordance with the university's own standards of care. It should be noted that the fact of indemnification or insurance coverage does not change the fact that the employee is personally responsible (liable) for the malpractice: indemnity is only a promise to reimburse the employee for what the employee has already paid.

Discussion of Case

After listening to the student, you tell her that it was exactly the right thing to do to report the problem, and you refer her to the university's policies and procedures applicable to the reporting of unexpected adverse events. You ask that she formally make the report, so that she can learn how it is done and what happens when a report is filed. You also tell her that you will contact the head of nursing for the hospital to make sure they know about the problem.

With respect to what happened, the student tells you that the bottles were very hot to the touch after she filled them, and that she covered them with muslin pillowcases that she found in the hallway. Hospital policy, as well as the standard of care, requires that hot water bottles be covered with flannel. The student admits that she feels bad about this and responsible for it, but thinks that it should have been corrected by the graduate student nurse who actually applied the bottles to the child's feet. You tell her that although that may be true, that does not absolve her from the fact that she did not do what she should have, and counsel her to be much more careful in the future, including asking questions or giving people warnings if she feels something is amiss.

You learn that after the operation was over, the child was taken to his room in the hospital, whereupon the floor nurse discovered that his feet were badly burned. A later examination disclosed that he had suffered third-degree burns with destruction of the subcutaneous tissue down to the bone.

When the student came back into the operating room, she covered the bottles, not with flannel covers as was the proper practice, but with muslin pillowcases. Experts later determined that to have caused the injury it produced, the water must have been at the 212°F boiling point; the right temperature for hot water bottles should not be hotter than 115° or 120°F.

Findings and Disposition

To recover for the child's injuries, his father as guardian and also in his own right brought suit against Dr. Bondi, Dr. Fred Battaglia (another doctor in the room), Ms. Waddell, Mrs. Bieda, the university, and the hospital. The university agreed to identify and defend Ms. Waddell and Mrs. Bieda because they were there as part of their academic program, and a lawyer was appointed for them (and the university). Mrs. Bieda was reprimanded for not having made a report of the incident as required by university policies and was required to write a paper on the importance of complying with university clinical policies.

The trial judge granted summary judgment to all of the defendants. On appeal, the court agreed that neither the university nor the hospital could be held liable for this accident, but held that claims could be asserted against the doctor and the nurse and student nurse, and ordered that a trial be held. All three were held responsible. The judge rejected the argument that the student should be held to a reduced standard of care—that of student nurses—because they had knowingly been involved in the care of a patient and therefore assumed the duties owed to a patient by professionals.

Dr. Bondi had the complete authority and control in the operating room as to which Dr. Corsello testified, and he was therefore legally responsible as "the captain of the ship," even though he had no idea that the water bottles were too hot. In fact, it was he who actually gave orders to the one nurse, the student nurse, not to apply the hot water bottles to the child, and orders to the other nurse, the graduate nurse, to do so. As a result, his legal responsibility did not begin merely at the moment when he started to make an incision in the child's body (which is typically the time that liability attaches), but when he started issuing orders about the child's care. This included the application of the hot water bottles to the child's feet, because they were intended to assist in the rehabilitation and restoration of the patient's strength, health, and well-being.

Relevant Legal Cases

Aubert v. Charity Hospital of Louisiana, 363 So.2d 1223 (La. App. 1978)

Central Anesthesia Associates, P.C. v. Worthy, 333 S.E.2d 829 (Ga. 1985)

Champagne v. Mid-Maine Medical Center, 711 A.2d 842 (Me. 1998)

Brown v. Southwest Mississippi Regional Medical Center, 989 So.2d 933, 934 (Ms. App. 2008)

Luettke v. St. Vincent Mercy Medical Center, 2006 WL 2105049 (Ohio App. 6 Dist. 2006)

Gavigan v. Zerlin, 269 A.D.2d 563, 703 N.Y.S.2d 273 (2000)

There do not appear to be many published cases wherein student nurses are named individually in a medical malpractice action; rather, generally their employers and supervisors are named for the student nurses' alleged negligent actions or inactions, or for allegations of failing to supervise and/or negligent selection. *Benedict v. Bondi* is one of the few cases that directly addresses the issues.

Aubert v. Charity Hospital of Louisiana involved two separate appeals from a judgment rendered in a medical malpractice action. The action involved the death of Aubert during childbirth by cesarean section at Charity Hospital. Her widower, individually and as the parent of the surviving child, filed suit against Charity and other defendants, including Elvyn Lee, a student nurse anesthetist. The claim against Charity was tried by the judge who found Charity vicariously liable for plaintiffs' damages. The claim against the individual defendants were tried by a jury who found that none of the individual defendants were liable. Plaintiffs and Charity filed separate appeals. The Louisiana Court of Appeals reversed the judgment of the trial court to include student nurse Lee, and Dr. Chung, and found that Lee, along with defendants Dr. Chung and Charity Hospital, were liable for plaintiffs' damages for improper intubation.

Central Anesthesia Associates, P.C. v. Worthy was a medical malpractice action brought against several defendants including Castro, a student nurse anesthetist, for negligently administering anesthesia resulting in cardiac arrest and brain damage. The trial court granted plaintiffs' motion for partial summary judgment against all defendants except Dr. Moorehead, finding that they had violated a state law, O.C.G.A. §43-26-9(b). Defendants appealed and the court of appeals affirmed as to Central Anesthesia Associates, Castro, the physician's assistant, and three named anesthesiologists, holding that "all of these defendants had breached their statutory duty in allowing an uncertified student nurse anesthetist to administer anesthesia while not 'under the direction and responsibility' of an anesthesiologist as required by O.C.G.A §43-26-9(b), supra." Partial summary judgment was reversed as to Dr. Moorehead.

The Supreme Court of Georgia affirmed the holding that partial summary judgment against Central Anesthesia Associates, the student nurse, the physician's assistant, and three named anesthesiologists was proper. The Supreme Court of Georgia rejected the student nurse's contention that "she should not be held to the standard of care and skill of a certified registered nurse anesthetist, but only to the standard of care and skill of a second year student nurse anesthetist."

In *Champagne v. Mid-Maine Medical Center* (1998), the student nurse, Priscilla Hutchins, mistakenly brought a newborn baby to another patient in the maternity ward of defendant hospital. The patient breast-fed the baby for 3 to 5 minutes before discovering that the baby was not hers. The baby was then returned to the nursery and suffered no injuries. Plaintiff-mother filed a lawsuit against the student nurse and the hospital for invasion of privacy, battery, intentional infliction of emotional distress, and negligent infliction of emotional distress. The Superior Court of Kennebec County granted summary judgment for defendants. The Supreme Judicial Court of Main affirmed the judgment.

In *Brown v. Southwest Mississippi Regional Medical Center* (2008), plaintiff brought a medical malpractice action against a hospital and its employees (including a student nurse) for allegations of negligently administering an intramuscular injection into plaintiff's right hip and buttocks by the student nurse. The plaintiff alleged that his sciatic nerve was pierced, and consequently he was permanently injured as a result of the student nurse's alleged negligence in administering the injection. Ultimately summary judgment was entered for the hospital and student nurse for a procedural reason, because the plaintiff had not given notice of the claim as required by the Mississippi Tort Claims Act.

Luettke v. St. Vincent Mercy Medical Center (2006) was an appeal to the Court of Appeals of Ohio brought after a jury found in favor of defendants. The action involved a perforation of plaintiff's esophagus during a procedure that involved a student in training. A registered nurse, Lynn was enrolled as a student in the certified registered nurse anesthetist-training program at Wayne State University. Prior to the procedure, Lynn did not identify herself as a student in training, and no one disclosed that she would be performing all anesthesia aspects of the surgery. Lynn followed the instructions that she was given by her supervisors, who were in the operating room during the procedure, although she was left alone at certain aspects of the procedure. A perforation ultimately occurred, and plaintiff suffered complications postoperatively. Suit was brought against the student nurse's supervisors, as well as the professional practice group, and St. Vincent. At the trial court level, the plaintiff withdrew the claims against Lynn because she had no malpractice insurance.

In *Gavigan v. Zerlin* (2000), a nursing student from Adelphi University was participating in a clinical internship established by education affiliation agreements with Long Island Jewish Medical Center (LIJMC). Alleging negligence in the care he received from the student, the patient sued the nursing student, LIJMC, and one of its employees for negligent supervision. LIJMC and the employee sought contractual indemnification for Adelphi for the expenses arising out of the action. The court held that indemnification clauses in the education affiliation agreements required the university to indemnify the hospital.

Summary

Student nurses can be held liable for their actions and can be sued. A student nurse is held to the same standard of care as a registered nurse when performing RN duties. If a student nurse cannot safely function in the performance of these duties while unsupervised, the student should not be carrying out the duties. In another set of circumstances in which a nursing instructor is present, the instructor might have been found liable on the basis of inadequate supervision had the nursing instructor given the task to the student knowing the student was not capable or competent to perform the task.

CRITICAL ELEMENTS TO CONSIDER

- Make sure that nursing students know where to find, and understand, university and hospital procedures regarding reporting incidents of adverse outcome and their obligations to report in accordance with those procedures.

Continued

CRITICAL ELEMENTS TO CONSIDER—cont'd

- Be brief, accurate, and objective in reporting events. Do not give opinions or provide more information than is requested. It is important not to volunteer information on the forms; information other than what is required should be shared with the faculty member supervising the student and then, as directed, risk manager and/or university attorney.
- Do not speak to the hospital's attorney or risk manager until you have first consulted with the university attorney.

References

Aubert v. Charity Hospital of Louisiana, 363 So.2d 1223 (La. App. 1978).

Benedict v. Bondi, 384 Pa. 574, Pa: Supreme Court 1956

Brown v. Southwest Mississippi Regional Medical Center, 989 So.2d 933, 934 (Ms. App. 2008).

Central Anesthesia Associates, P.C. v. Worthy, 333 S.E.2d 829 (Ga. 1985).

Champagne v. Mid-Maine Medical Center, 711 A.2d 842 (Me. 1998).

Gavigan v. Zerlin, 269 A.D.2d 563, 703 N.Y.S.2d 273 (2000).

Luettke v. St. Vincent Mercy Medical Center, 2006 WL 2105049 (Ohio App. 6 Dist. 2006).

McConnell v. Williams, 361 Pa. 355, 362, 65 A.2d 243, 246.

Paterson, C., & Lane, L. (2000). An analysis of legal issues concerning university based nursing education programs. *Journal of Nursing Law, 7*(2), 7–18.

Best Practices in the Nursing Education Legal Environment

CHAPTER 30

Management of Students at Risk for Clinical Failure: Best Practices

CASE STUDY

Remediation of a Nursing Student Failing to Meet Clinical Objectives

Your role: As the clinical instructor in a pediatric nursing rotation, you are responsible for teaching, supervising, coaching, and evaluating eight nursing students who are in their third clinical rotation.

One of your students, R.J., is not progressing as expected. In particular, R.J. is not meeting clinical objectives related to comprehensive patient assessment and to the safe performance of previously learned technical skills. You feel that R.J. is highly likely to fail the clinical rotation unless she shows immediate improvement.

The students have been through a fundamentals and an adult health (medical-surgical) rotation at other hospitals. Their current clinical placement, with you, is on an acute care general pediatric unit. It is the fourth week of an 8-week clinical rotation. During week one, students had an orientation to the rotation, clinical objectives, expectations, and clinical unit, and then obtained a health history and provided basic nursing care to a pediatric patient and family. The following 3 weeks involved progressively more complex daily clinical objectives, including, but not limited to, comprehensive assessment; maintaining safety; providing comprehensive care; and administering medications, treatments, fluids and other prescribed or independent interventions for an infant or child and family members, consistent with pediatric nursing standards.

Identifying Best Practices in Nursing Education

Clinical Evaluation Plan

The foundation for management of a student who is struggling to meet clinical objectives is established through the overall clinical evaluation plan. Evaluation of clinical performance may be compared to the tracking of a moving target, subject to multiple variables and changes in the patient care situation.

> Evaluation of student learning and mastery of clinical learning objectives or clinical performance criteria can be very challenging in the patient care setting. Students need to demonstrate understanding of information, develop particular competencies, and demonstrate the development of critical thinking, decision-making, clinical judgment, and technical skills in an unstable, rapidly evolving patient care environment. They need to learn skills to distinguish what works from what does not work in a rapid-fire setting where the context of patient care is not static and where patient care needs and expectations can change in an instant.

Clinical evaluation, and thus management of failure to meet clinical objectives, begins with a full understanding, by the clinical instructor, of the end objectives (clinical objectives) for the clinical experience, along with a clear understanding of the benchmarks, daily objectives, or progression objectives that gauge students' progress toward these objectives. In addition, the instructor should keep in mind the need for students to learn and practice before being evaluated. Providing adequate time for development of skills and judgment is important. Evaluation also involves the clinical instructor's assessment, which involves subjectivity. However, this challenge can be addressed by attention to the connection between performance behaviors and explicit clinical objectives or competency standards.

A clinical evaluation plan includes both formative and summative evaluation; students (and faculty) benefit from concrete daily performance objectives that are clearly related to the overall clinical objectives for the rotation and unbiased, iterative feedback, including daily feedback, to each student about clinical performance along with opportunities for improvement. Instructors should keep documentation of each student's progress via weekly summaries and incident-specific anecdotal notes. Figure 30.1 illustrates the components of a clinical evaluation plan that supports management of student difficulties achieving clinical objectives.

Communicating Clinical Performance Issues

Evaluation of performance is a high-stakes process that can have financial, academic, legal, and personal consequences for the student, and can have similar consequences for the faculty member. Discovering that he or she is at risk for or has failed objectives in the clinical setting can be devastating for students; it is often also personally difficult for faculty to communicate failure to students and will

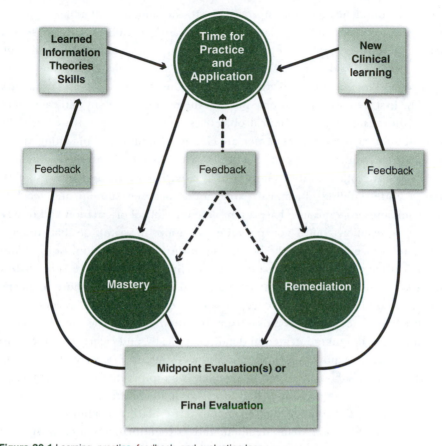

Figure 30.1 Learning, practice, feedback, and evaluation loop.

From Gardner, M., & Suplee, P. (2010). Handbook of clinical teaching in nursing and health sciences. Jones and Bartlett Learning, Sudbury MA. www.jblearning.com. Reprinted with permission.

require that faculty fully justify and document objective data to support the decision. It is therefore important to ensure that clinical evaluation is free from bias, based on behaviors linked to clear clinical objectives, and that communication of both expectations for clinical performance and the results of evaluation are explicit and in writing so that both student and faculty have a shared understanding of the issues and the process for correction if needed. Rapport with the student, coupled with effective communication of clinical performance, is also crucial for both student progression and preservation of the student's sense of efficacy and self-worth.

Faculty should be familiar with and adhere to the academic and clinical policies in their academic institution. They should consult with experienced colleagues such as the respective course or program director or dean to assist in accurately assessing clinical performance problems, documenting and communicating clearly and objectively, ensuring explicit and timely notice of problems, making recommendations for improvement to the student, and adhering to the established policies and regulations as well as law. Information presented here represents general concepts related to clinical evaluation of nursing students. Faculty should consult with their program's academic administrators and legal counsel for guidance and advice related to any student issues and problems.

The first step, which must take place at the beginning of any clinical experience, is to ensure that the clinical objectives, both summative as well as daily objectives for each clinical encounter, are clearly communicated in writing as well as orally to all students. The clinical instructor should also discuss the meaning of each objective and provide examples of related behaviors, and thus establish shared understanding of clinical expectations between student and teacher. Some nursing programs may have a template for clinical orientation and discussion of expectations, but if not, put all expectations in writing so that students have a reference point from the beginning of the clinical rotation. At the point of clinical concern, assess the nature of the clinical performance issue. Safety issues may require immediate intervention and/or immediate failure. Expectations related to safe clinical practice, as well as consequences for breaching safe practice guidelines, such as removal from the clinical setting and/or clinical failure, must also be communicated in detail, specifically, and clearly to students in writing, prior to beginning a clinical rotation. A student who is grossly unsafe in the clinical area, who needs continual supervision to provide safe nursing care, or who does not recognize his or her deficits or limitations may be one who cannot continue in the rotation because patients are placed at significant risk for injury. In this case, immediate, detailed, and written documentation of student behaviors related to clinical objectives; immediate communication with the academic administrator; and careful, frank communication, both orally and in writing, with the student will need to take place. Other issues related to clinical objectives, such as preparation, skills performance, care planning, or organization among others, may allow for a more prolonged remediation and opportunity to demonstrate improvement. In any case, attention to students' rights to academic due process along with a perspective focused on student learning, performance improvement, and the likelihood of success are needed. Students' clinical performance issues should be discussed directly and immediately with them, and documented in writing, so that opportunities for improvement can be provided and students are fully aware of their problems and the resources available to help them improve. Be sure to obtain a student signature and date for all communication related to clinical performance. All of these actions must take place within a context of respect for the student, confidentiality and privacy, timely notification with adequate time allowed for remediation, and adherence to regulatory guidelines including academic policies as well as the Family Educational Rights and Privacy Act (FERPA), the Health Insurance Portability and Accountability Act (HIPAA), the Americans With Disabilities Act (ADA), and other regulations.

Clinical Probation and Remediation

Once an assessment has been completed, place the performance in the context of clinical learning objectives by tying it tightly to one or more clinical objectives. It is essential to document in writing any serious concerns that need follow-up or improvement and explicitly communicate these to the student. If the clinical issue is one that can be improved with practice, review, further study, or clarification, a remediation plan is appropriate. Most nursing programs will have a template or form for documentation of clinical issues, but any of these should include a description of the behaviors of concern linked to clinical objectives from the formal clinical evaluation tool, a clear outline of the steps the student must take to improve clinical performance, behavioral criteria for evaluation of improvement, a time line for improvement, the date by which improvement must be shown, and consequences, should remediation not take place or should improvement in clinical performance not occur. Although the focus of the remediation plan should be support of student learning and mastery of competencies, it is important that students are informed fully of their rights, including due process rights outlined in program or university policies, as well as requirements, expectations and responsibilities, and the risk for clinical failure or other consequences. The written documentation may take the form of a clinical memo, warning, or learning contract, depending on the severity of the problem and the policies of the program.

Schedule an immediate meeting with the student in private, and sensitively, but explicitly, outline the concerns, clinical objectives, and remediation requirements. Although privacy and confidentiality are essential, so is safety of both faculty and student. Students receiving this type of feedback about their performance may become upset, defensive, disruptive, or angry, or may dispute the instructor's feedback or threaten legal or other actions. (A private session should not continue if the instructor feels unsafe in any way; the instructor should tell the student that the meeting has ended and will be rescheduled, seek assistance and consultation from the academic administrator, and involve the health system or academic unit's security department if indicated.) When students are informed in writing of expectations; are treated equally and fairly with respect to expectations, assignments, evaluation, and grading (absence of arbitrary or capricious action by the instructor); have written feedback and opportunities for improvement; are informed about progress or lack of progress; and the instructor has followed established program and university policies (including attention to due process rights) and documented such, students' legal challenges to poor grades, including those related to clinical evaluation, have not been upheld.

In giving feedback about clinical performance standards or the need for improvement, be timely and specific, and clearly outline the specific area of concern and the steps to be taken to improve. Provide an opportunity for the student to voice his or her perspective, explanations, and questions. Ask the student to describe the problem and requirements for improvement in his or her own words. Further document all of these, along with date and time. The student and instructor should both sign the form or memo. Copies of the signed documentation should be provided to the student and remediation faculty, learning laboratory staff, or other individual who would be legitimately involved with the student's performance and improvement plan in accordance with program policies and FERPA regulation. The remediation plan should be clearly outlined so that the student has a full understanding of the steps to take and the time line involved. Figure 30.2 provides a schematic of the process of clinical remediation.

Outcomes of Remediation

Follow-up to the remediation plan should include close communication among the clinical instructor, laboratory or instructional faculty involved with the student (if any), and the student him- or herself. Once the student has completed the prescribed remediation, he or she should provide documentation to the clinical instructor. The student should be provided opportunities to demonstrate mastery of the specific objectives, along with formative and then summative evaluation. If the student fails to complete the required remediation within the prescribed time line, or does not meet the respective clinical objectives, the consequences may include a clinical failure. This consequence should be clearly outlined in writing to all students prior to the beginning of any clinical rotation or experience. Daily formative feedback to each student during each clinical experience across the clinical rotation will ensure that all students are aware of their progress toward achievement of the clinical objectives. Both formative and summative feedback should be provided, including at the minimum a written midpoint or midrotation formative evaluation and a final written summative evaluation at the conclusion of the clinical rotation. Feedback for unsatisfactory clinical performance should be provided in writing and discussed with the student. Clear and full documentation of the instructor's communication of the clinical performance problem, the process of evaluation, the opportunities for remediation, and behavioral data supporting the judgment of the instructor that the student did not meet objectives after remediation are essential. A discussion and review of the documentation with the course leader and/or academic program director, depending on program policies, should occur as soon as possible, respecting program and academic policies as well as FERPA regulations related to communication of student information.

Once the decision to issue a failing clinical grade to a student has been made, the instructor should schedule a conference with the student to discuss the

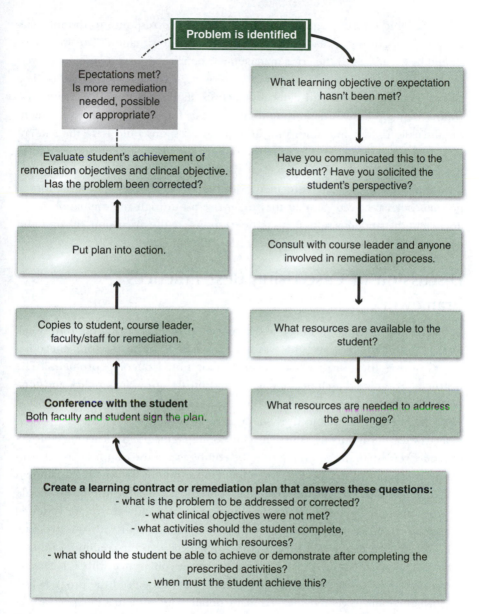

Problem is identified

Epectations met?
Is more remediation
needed, possible
or appropriate?

What learning objective or expectation
hasn't been met?

Evaluate student's achievement of
remediation objectives and clincal objective.
Has the problem been corrected?

Have you communicated this to the
student? Have you solicited the
student's perspective?

Put plan into action.

Consult with course leader and anyone
involved in remediation process.

Copies to student, course leader,
faculty/staff for remediation.

What resources are available to the
student?

Conference with the student
Both faculty and student sign the plan.

What resources are needed to address
the challenge?

Create a learning contract or remediation plan that answers these questions:
- what is the problem to be addressed or corrected?
- what clinical objectives were not met?
- what activities should the student complete,
using which resources?
- what should the student be able to achieve or demonstrate after completing the
prescribed activities?
- when must the student achieve this?

Figure 30.2 Remediation.

*From Gardner, M., & Suplee, P.(2010). Handbook of clinical teaching in nursing and health sciences. Jones and
Bartlett Learning, Sudbury MA. www.jblearning.com. Reprinted with permission.*

failure. A clear, explicit, but empathetic and sensitive approach is needed. To
acknowledge emotional difficulties that students may have when confronting a
clinical failure, it may be helpful to remember common strategies for breaking
bad news: providing privacy; speaking objectively and using data, not labels;

acknowledging effort; gauging comprehension of and response to the information; and supporting a realistic perspective about the situation. The instructor should be familiar with the crisis management policies of the program or university, as well as academic and counseling resources available for students. The clinical evaluation form and clinical objectives, along with observed behavioral (rather than subjective) data, should be the basis for the discussion. Document the discussion, date and time, and the student's response and have the student sign the written evaluation. Provide the opportunity for a student to respond to the evaluation in writing. The student should be informed that the signatures do not necessarily indicate agreement with the feedback, only that the information has been received. Should the student refuse to sign the evaluation form, document the student's refusal, his or her response to the discussion, the date and time, and seek consultation from the academic administrator.

Discussion of Case Using Best Practices Framework

Verbal feedback was given to R.J. about specific problems during the third week of the clinical rotation and this was documented in the instructor's anecdotal notes. During the fourth week, the instructor noted ongoing problems. The instructor completed a clinical memo (based on the program's policy and template) that summarized data about the student's performance, and related the data directly to clinical objectives about assessment skills and about safe performance of technical nursing skills. The clinical memo included a learning contract outlining remediation requirements to be completed in the campus clinical skills learning laboratory, a time line for remediation, criteria by which the student would be reevaluated, and the potential consequence—clinical failure—should improvement not been seen. After developing the memo, the instructor reviewed the memo, remediation plan, and approach to the student with the program director in accordance with FERPA guidelines specific to the communication of educational information, and scheduled a private conference with R.J. During the conference, instructor and student reviewed and discussed the progress and performance and reviewed the memo in detail. The student's perspective was elicited. R.J. initially emphatically denied that there were clinical performance problems. After listening to R.J.'s perspective, the instructor brought the student's attention to the behaviors documented on the clinical memo, emphasizing remediation as an opportunity to improve performance but realistically identifying risks for clinical failure. R.J. reluctantly agreed that remediation and additional practice were needed. R.J. was asked to sign the clinical memo and copies of the signed clinical memo were sent to the learning laboratory faculty.

R.J. completed the prescribed remediation within the prescribed time frame and was provided additional opportunities to demonstrate competency in the clinical skills. Despite additional practice and remediation, the student was unable to meet the clinical objectives for the rotation. Ongoing feedback was provided to the student. A detailed evaluation of student performance, tethered to clinical objectives, was written and all of the documentation was reviewed with the nursing program administrator. The clinical instructor then scheduled a conference with the student and reviewed the clinical evaluation point by point. R.J. signed the evaluation form and was offered the opportunity to respond in writing to the evaluation. The student was directed to the university handbook outlining due process procedures (e.g., student academic grievance procedure) and was encouraged to consult with her faculty adviser and with the program director. The clinical instructor offered support, and a reminder that no-cost student counseling services were available. R.J. successfully repeated the course and clinical rotation the following semester.

Summary

A proactive approach, including a clearly defined plan for student evaluation, is the starting point for effective evaluation and remediation. Clear and explicit communication of student progress toward clinical objectives, along with documentation based on observed behaviors, will support realistic, unbiased appraisals of clinical achievement. When adequate progress toward achievement of clinical objectives is not apparent, a clear, explicit, written plan for improvement, tied to the clinical objectives of the rotation, should be designed, discussed with the student, and implemented. Once adequate opportunities for improvement, if appropriate, are provided, further appraisal of student achievement of objectives should occur before a failing grade is levied.

 CRITICAL ELEMENTS TO CONSIDER
Critical elements of the process include the following:
- Clearly defined performance objectives.
- Clearly outlined expectations and possible consequences for not meeting expectations.
- Discussion and written communication to ensure shared understanding of clinical objectives and expectations.
- Formative feedback after each clinical experience, tied to daily and overall clinical objectives.
- Documentation of student progress using weekly as well as incident-specific instructor notes.
- Opportunity for improvement with a clearly outlined plan, time line, and criteria for remediation.

Continued

CRITICAL ELEMENTS TO CONSIDER—cont'd

- Feedback on outcomes of remediation.
- Clear, objective, detailed documentation of facts and behaviors.
- Empathetic but clear communication.
- Attention to program and university policies and procedures, in line with higher education regulations and laws.

References

Benor, D. E., & Leviyof, I. (1997). The development of students' perceptions of effective teaching: The ideal, best, and poorest clinical teacher in nursing. *Journal of Nursing Education, 36*(5), 206–211.

Boley, P., & Whitney, K. (2003). Grade disputes: Considerations for nursing faculty. *Journal of Nursing Education, 42*(5), 198–203.

Brown, Y., Neudorf, K., Poitras, C., et al. (2007). Unsafe clinical performance calls for a systematic approach. *Canadian Nurse, 103*(3), 29–32.

Diekelmann, N., & McGregor, A. (2003). Students who fail clinical courses: Keeping open a future of new possibilities. *Journal of Nursing Education, 42*(10), 433–436.

Electronic code of federal regulations. (n.d.). Title 34, part 99. Washington, DC: U.S. Government Printing Office. Retrieved August 3, 2011 from http://ecfr.gpoaccess.gov/cgi/t/text/text-idx?c=ecfr&rgn=div5&view=text&node=34:1.1.1.1.34&idno=34#PartTop

Gaberson, K., & Oermann, M. (2010). *Clinical teaching strategies in nursing* (3rd ed.). New York: Springer.

Gallant, M., McDonald, J., & Higuchi, K. S. (2006). A remediation process for nursing students at risk. *Nurse Educator, 31*(5), 223–227.

Gardner, M. R., & Suplee, P. D. (2010). *Handbook of clinical teaching in nursing and health sciences.* Sudbury, MA: Jones & Bartlett.

McGregor, A. (2007). Academic success, clinical failure: Struggling practices of a failing student. *Journal of Nursing Education, 46*(11), 504–511.

Westrick, S. J. (2007). Legal challenges to academic decisions. *Journal of Nursing Law, 11*(2), 104–107.

CHAPTER 31

Best Practices and Procedures to Avoid Post-Graduation Low NCLEX Scores

CASE STUDY

Best Practices in NCLEX Preparation

Your role: You are the chair of the undergraduate nursing program.

You receive a phone call from an irate parent, Mr. Strazzoli. His daughter, Alyssa, is a senior in the undergraduate nursing program. Mr. Strazzoli asks to meet with you and the dean to discuss his daughter's academic performance. Alyssa has failed the comprehensive examination and states that she is unable to graduate in 2 weeks if she does not pass the exam on her second attempt. Mr. Strazzoli is quite angry and tells you that he just spent over a $100,000 on his daughter's education and that this policy is complete nonsense. He threatens to retain an attorney. You inform Mr. Strazzoli that Alyssa must complete the Student Authorization to Discuss and Disclose an Education Record form, in accordance with the Family Educational Rights and Privacy Act (FERPA). You explain that FERPA is a federal law that protects the privacy of student education records. Under this law, the university cannot generally disclose educational records about a student to a person or entity outside the university without the student's prior authorization. You are not permitted to allow him to see his daughter's records until Alyssa signs the Student Authorization to Discuss and Disclose an Education Record form.

Background

Students and faculty are equally concerned about student performance on the NCLEX-RN because the cost of failing can result in student embarrassment and additional test anxiety, potential job loss, and an increased chance of failing the NCLEX-RN on the second attempt without the appropriate academic support. Nursing programs also risk damage to their reputation and a possible loss of new students (Frith, Sewell, and Clark, 2008). Although schools make every effort to select the best applicants for their respective programs, some students struggle because of academic or personal issues during their academic experience. Identifying trends in poor NCLEX performance is critical. Such factors may include previous course failures, significant absenteeism, borderline science and clinical nursing grades, and decreased study time because of personal commitments.

Identifying Best Practices in Nursing Education

When developing academic admission and progression policies for undergraduate nursing programs, it is critical for the faculty to determine factors that promote success in their respective academic program and NCLEX-RN. By analyzing the data, faculty can determine the following:

1. Trigger courses necessary for NCLEX preparation
2. The number of maximum nursing failures allowed before dismissal
3. Science grade-point average on admission
4. Other unique factors required for student success, such as proficiency with the English language and number of course withdrawals

One finding unreported in the literature is the difficulty that part-time students experience when acclimating to full-time nursing study. (For example, students may have taken one or two prerequisites on a part-time basis, which means that they took only one or two courses at a time.) With full-time nursing study, the student is faced with taking 12 to 20 credit hours on a full-time basis including the requisite clinical hours, which could result in the student feeling completely overwhelmed. Providing an immersion experience or "boot camp" has proved successful with respect to NCLEX preparation (Nagorski Johnson, 2009) and may have similar success in student retention. Nagorski Johnson (2009) also reports the need to attend to the students' spiritual and emotional health during a boot camp experience. Strategies such as aerobic exercise, meditation, and journaling may prove helpful.

 WHEN TO CONSULT THE UNIVERSITY COUNSEL

- Consult the university counsel to approve the FERPA Authorization Policy and Student Authorization to Discuss and Disclose an Education Record form.
- Consult the university attorney when a parent or student threatens suit.

Discussion of Case Using Best Practice Framework

In reviewing Alyssa's transcript, you note that she barely passed the adult health/medical-surgical courses in the curriculum. The passing grade was a 77, and Alyssa consistently received a grade of 77 and 78 in adult health exams and has average Health Education Systems Inc. (Hesi) scores in clinical courses. (Note: Hesi exams are standardized exams that evaluate students' knowledge of a clinical specialty or course or entire nursing curriculum.) Alyssa has done well in nonclinical courses and has satisfactory clinical evaluations. Alyssa is also a cheerleader and has missed quite a number of classes because of the basketball team's schedule. You ask Alyssa to complete a FERPA authorization form so that you and the dean may speak to her father. You and the dean meet with Mr. Strazzoli and Alyssa to discuss her academic record and to explain the rationale for the comprehensive examination and its relation to students' NCLEX-RN pass rates at your school, which is greater than 97%. You also explain that Alyssa can walk in graduation despite not passing the comprehensive exam. After the meeting, you agree that Alyssa will take a NCLEX-RN review course and meet with the remediation coordinator to review test taking strategies.

Speaking to Parents About Standardized Testing

- A standardized test is a test that is administered and scored in a consistent, or standard, manner so that nursing programs can easily compare results from students across the entire country.
- A comprehensive standardized testing program (within clinical courses, midprogram, and final comprehensive exam) has been used to identify specific areas of content weakness. The trends in scores on standardized computerized tests, in addition to grades in science courses and grades in medical-surgical courses, are used to identify students who are at risk for failure in the nursing program and/or on the NCLEX-RN.
- With available standardized test results data, faculty can advise at-risk students and assist them in developing individual plans of study as well as provide additional study and testing resources so that results may improve.
- Generally, standardized tests are perceived as being fairer than nonstandardized tests. The consistency also permits more reliable comparison of outcomes across all test takers.

  Source: Jacobs, P., & Koehn, M. L. (2006). Implementing a standardized testing program: Preparing students for the NCLEX-RN. *Journal of Professional Nursing, 22*(6), 373–379.

Nurse Advocacy

Nurses need to advocate for sick and vulnerable patients; therefore, nursing majors need to learn to advocate for themselves so they can later advocate for patients. Parents who understand this issue are far less inclined to intervene unless the issue is very significant. It is important that parents are educated during new student orientation. The dean or department chair should also ask parents directly for their cooperation in facilitating their child's independence. Although this approach will go a long way in addressing the issue, some parents will inevitably call. For those, some suggestions include the following:

1. Try to defuse the situation. If a parent comes to the dean or faculty member with an issue, the first thing one should do is to encourage the parent to allow the child to solve his or her own problems and insist that the student speak to you or the respective faculty member directly. Tell the parent, for example, "Alyssa needs to approach the faculty on her own and discuss study alternatives, but it needs to be *her* voice. You can coach Alyssa from the sidelines."

2. If the parent still insists on speaking with you, tell the parent that you will not speak with him or her unless you have the student's written permission to do so. Taking the time to do so perhaps allows the parent to reflect on his or her request to meet with the dean or department chair.

3. If the student chooses to grant permission for you to speak with his or her parents, make it clear that this action gives you authorization to speak with the parent about the student's academic record in detail, such as clinical or class absences.

4. Remind the parent about the use of standardized testing in the curriculum as mentioned in orientation and the student notification letter.

5. Discuss with the parent that you both have the same goal—his/her child's academic and professional success.

Findings

Alyssa passes the comprehensive exam on her third attempt. She walks in graduation and ultimately passes NCLEX-RN on her first attempt. In the event that a speedy resolution was not possible, Alyssa would have been referred to the remediation coordinator, who would work with her on an individual basis to correct her deficiencies. She would continue to enroll in senior seminar with varied teaching strategies to assist Alyssa in passing the comprehensive Hesi exam.

Summary

It is in the students' best interest for faculty to emphasize the importance of standardized exams early in the curriculum and assist students in mastering content and improving scores rather than waiting to bolster weaknesses in the last term. This approach will reduce anxiety for students and also decrease associated stress on the faculty (Frith, Sewell, and Clark, 2008). A comprehensive approach to NCLEX-RN success that includes content-specific computerized assessment exams, test-taking seminars, learner style inventory, incorporation of NCLEX-RN practice test items, and NCLEX-RN advisement system is warranted (Davenport, 2007).

Last, nursing faculty must establish clear policies that promote students' success. Rather than offer a stand-alone, comprehensive exam at the end of a program, faculty members need to design a comprehensive integrated approach to NCLEX-RN preparation. Such a system includes the use of clinical specialty assessment exams as well as the use of a review course with a comprehensive exam and remediation throughout the program of study.

PREVENTION TIPS

- Discuss the use of required diagnostic and standardized testing in the curriculum in open houses and new student orientation. Example: Each student is required to take the following comprehensive exam (Hesi Exit) and standardized exams (Hesi Specialty Exams) throughout the curriculum. The Hesi Specialty Exams will gradually increase in percentage of the total course grade throughout the curriculum to assist the student with mastery of content and proficiency in standardized testing. Students will be required to take a Hesi in all clinical nursing courses.
- Send a letter to new nursing students addressing the use of standardized testing in the curriculum and the use of a comprehensive exam. Require students to sign the notification letter, indicating that they have read and understood it.

CRITICAL ELEMENTS TO CONSIDER

- Have students complete the FERPA authorization form if you need to discuss their academic records with their parents.
- Review the student's transcripts for science and nursing grades below a B.
- Review student data related to pass rates on both the comprehensive exam and NCLEX-RN.
- Provide remediation support to the student, someone who is well versed in testing and the NCLEX-RN.

Continued

CRITICAL ELEMENTS TO CONSIDER—cont'd

- Designate a faculty expert on the NCLEX test plan. Send the faculty member to the annual National Council of State Boards of Nursing meeting for current updates on the NCLEX test plan.
- Allow student to engage in a personal preparation plan (Herrman and Nagorski Johnson, 2009).
- Offer a NCLEX-RN review course to student.
- Allow students the opportunity to take NCLEX practice tests.
- Offer the comprehensive exam within an academic course such as senior seminar. Consider a diversified approach to the course, such as testing of core competency skills review, simulation and clinical evaluation, and content/test review to ensure competent practitioners.
- Offer counseling services to student to decrease anxiety.
- Do a comparative analysis to find out who has not passed NCLEX-RN using students' admission criteria, science grades, and clinical course grades.
- Discuss NCLEX-RN in new-student orientation.
- Identify high-risk students and offer appropriate support early; supports include English language support, tutoring, test-taking strategies, and other academic support assessments.
- Strengthen policies on admission and progression based on data.
- Institute a cumulative midpoint comprehensive exam.
- Provide faculty development on test construction, test analysis, and NCLEX-RN test plan.
- Provide faculty development on test-item writing.
- Review curriculum in conjunction with NCLEX-RN test plan and pass rate on an annual basis.
- Use standardized testing in your curriculum (ATI, Kaplan, ERI, Hesi, etc.) with remedial supports.
- Ensure test security by using test proctoring protocol (see Chapter 17).
- Offer test-taking strategy workshops to students.
- Offer refresher courses and skill remediation as students wait to sit for NCLEX-RN.

References

Davenport, N. C. (2007). A comprehensive approach to NCLEX-RN success. *Nursing Education Perspective, 28*(1), 30–33.

Frith, K. H., Sewell, J., & Clark, D. J. (2008). Best practices in NCLEX-RN readiness preparation for baccalaureate student success. *CIN: Computers, Informatics, Nursing, 23*(6), 322–329.

Herrman, J. W., & Nagorski Johnson, A. (2009). From beta-blockers to boot camp: Preparing students for the NCLEX-RN. *Nursing Education Perspective, 30*(6), 384–388.

Nagorski Johnson, A. (2009). NCLEX-RN success with boot camp. *Nursing Education Perspective, 30*(5), 328–329.

CHAPTER 32

Best Practices in Evaluating Student Performance

CASE STUDY

A Senior BSN Student in Her Last Semester Fails Clinical and Does Not Graduate on Time

Your role: You are Professor Han, a clinical assistant professor teaching a clinical section of NURS 400: Adult Health II and Critical Care.

You have a student, Belinda Dastrovsky, who repeatedly demonstrates unsafe nursing practice, and despite the fact that she is only weeks away from graduation, you give her a failing grade in clinical.

At week seven of the final semester for the current BSN class, you determine that you can no longer assign Ms. Dastrovsky to even just one patient on the critical care unit to whom you can be certain she can provide nursing care safely without continual and direct supervision. You update your clinical coordinator for the course, Dr. Yellow, and by phone indicate that you have thoroughly documented a clinical failure that has not responded to two attempts at remediation. Before the next clinical day Ms. Dastrovsky meets with you, and you inform her that she has failed clinical and will therefore not graduate on time. Ms. Dastrovsky stiffens up with a look of anger on her face, but she says nothing. She walks out of the room and immediately e-mails the dean of the college that she is appealing her grade. A few hours later you receive an e-mail from the dean about the student.

Background

Professor Han was assigned to teach a clinical section of NURS 400: Adult Health II and Critical Care. However, when the clinical rotation commenced, Ms. Dastrovsky immediately did not seem able to answer even basic questions during the first weeks of preconference. She was assigned to two patients on the progressive coronary care unit each week, and she was barely able to complete her nursing activities within the allotted 6-hour clinical day. After receiving a verbal warning in week two about her lack of preparation for preconference, Ms. Dastrovsky was written up in week three for her poor time management and her failure to properly document her nursing care. With her written warning she was given a prescription for learning to return to the nursing tutorial laboratory (NTL) where she was directed to work on time management and documentation. Professor Harry runs the NTL and had decided to use a simulation case for the student to demonstrate competency in prioritizing care and time management. The simulation case would also integrate documentation skills. Ms. Dastrovsky was required to complete and pass the remediation before her next clinical day in week four.

Ms. Dastrovsky returned to clinical with a written evaluation of her successful remediation but again had major problems in clinical in her fourth week. She was required to do a sterile dressing change and after two unsuccessful attempts in which she had contaminated the sterile field, she was given a second clinical warning. This resulted in a conference at which she was informed she was at risk for clinical failure. In this nursing program, a second clinical warning always results in a conference at which the risk of clinical failure is discussed and documented. A second prescription for learning was given, and Ms. Dastrovsky undertook the remediation and received feedback on her performance from Professor Harry in the NTL. Professor Harry then e-mailed Professor Han and informed her that, although Ms. Dastrovsky completed the second Prescription for Learning successfully, his assessment was that the student was exceptionally slow and weak and unlikely to be able to handle the complexity of successfully taking care of two moderately ill patients. Professor Han therefore decided to make a point to spend even more time observing Ms. Dastrovsky's student nursing practice as she had to ensure that the student was practicing safely. However, she was worried that so much focus on Ms. Dastrovsky was resulting in her having significantly less time to observe her other students, including the ones who were excelling.[1]

Identifying Best Practices in Nursing Education

In a clinical or practice discipline it is essential that there be sound evaluation procedures that ensure the production of safe practitioners. It has also been recognized that developing effective interpersonal communication and a having a high bar for

---

[1] This topic is rarely written about in clinical nursing education—how having to focus on unsafe or marginally unsafe students causes a deteriorated learning environment for others in the clinical group, especially those who are excelling and who could also benefit from a clinical instructor who has time to challenge them and push them to exceptional heights. Those who really excel in clinical are the ones most likely to seek higher education and become the next generation of nursing leaders. Leaving them to their own devices, even in a clinical environment, seems like a lost opportunity to really nurture, encourage, and truly mentor young nursing talent.

ethical standards and conduct are requisite features in any practice discipline such as nursing (Dreher, 2011). Although tuition revenue–dependent nursing programs may sometimes have deans and other academic nursing administrators who may waive a policy or override a failing grade in favor of an individual student, these administrative practices ultimately can destroy the morale of a faculty work unit, not to mention the perpetuation of unsafe nursing student performance.

Van Eerden wrote in 2001, "Despite intense laboratory instruction, however, [some] students inconsistently demonstrate skill mastery in the context of actual client interactions" (p. 231). Some 10 years later this is still true. This is largely because of the gap between what kind of graduate nurse nursing educa-tion programs can practically produce within their allotted degree time frames *and* the largely unrealistic expectation of the nurse executive of what that new graduate nurse should be able to do in the health-care agency (usually the hos-pital) on day one. In other words, nursing schools cannot produce anything but a novice, and nursing practice environments should not expect anything more (Benner, 2000). The focus, however, to ensure best practices for clinical evalua-tion purposes should be the production of a more highly competent, critically thinking graduate (on the nursing education side) and the improvement (on the nurse executive and practice side) of more highly developed nurse residency programs for new graduates that have a long history of improving new graduate retention (Gillespie and Patterson, 2009; Institute of Medicine, 2011).

Bourbonnais, Langford, and Giannantonio (2008) described a new clinical evaluation tool for senior BSN students that was developed because they observed the following:

1. Inconsistency in clinical evaluation tools used from one year to the next, including new clinical faculty annually using any given tool for the first time.
2. Limited ability of evaluation tools to discriminate and evaluate progressive depth and scope of nursing students' practice from years one to four.
3. Inconsistency with faculty use of a clinical evaluation tool within the same year.
4. Difficulties expressed by faculty that it is challenging to properly evaluate attributes of professionalism.

These findings are likely very widespread, and therefore solid tools are necessary to document student performance while not becoming overly burdensome to the clinical nursing faculty (who often may be adjunct faculty and not full- or part-time faculty).

Oermann and Gaberson (2009) indicate that the evaluation process is basi-cally a faculty member's responsibility to make a judgment about an individual nursing student's performance and answers the questions "how *well* did the student perform and is the student *competent* in clinical practice" (p. 10). The process of determining safe, competent nursing practice and then documenting and evaluating it is not simple, and it is incumbent that new nursing professors and new clinical faculty be mentored to conduct this important activity with seriousness and precision.

There are two types of evaluation: formative and summative, and each is conducted very differently (Seldomridge and Walsh, 2006). Formative evaluation is designed not to be graded, but to give feedback. A quiz found at the conclusion of a nursing text (with answers provided) is an example of a type of formative evaluation. Most clinical nursing evaluation tools fall into this category whether they are done weekly (in some programs) or more typically at midterm and at the end of the quarter or semester. Summative evaluation generally takes place at the end of a course, and the student is compared to some previously established standard. A final examination in which a standard of 76 must be achieved to pass is an example of this type of evaluation.

In a recent survey ($N = 1,573$) of National for the National League for Nursing accredited pre-licensure programs (including associate, diploma, and baccalaureate programs) by Gillepsie and Patterson (2009), 70% of programs indicated they modify a single type of evaluation for use in different clinical nursing courses and 83% use a pass/fail grading system rather than a letter grade for clinical (Oerman, Yarbrough, Saewart et al., 2009). From our experience, clinical nursing evaluation tools are developed more at the undergraduate level than they are at the graduate level, although many graduate nursing programs, particularly nurse anesthesia and nurse practitioner programs, have moved to more Web- and competency-based evaluation tools that can be completed electronically, sometimes on handheld devices, by the preceptor or evaluator in the clinical agency (Cullen, Stiffler, Settles et al., 2010). Carlson-Sabelli and Delaney (2006) have also introduced informatics-based evaluation procedures that can be used when evaluating nurse-practitioner (NP) students at a distance. This is a new problem in nursing education—evaluating students (often from a distance) who are taking clinical nursing courses online (true more for RN/BSN than for generic AD, diploma, or BSN programs) and particularly when online graduate NP programs, for instance, no longer have a faculty member onsite to make routine evaluation visits (Falkenstein et al., 2007). These new types of programs require new evaluation testing strategies and include new technologies such as secured testing using Remote Proctor (Software Secure, 2010).

Some of the best-practice evaluation procedures at Drexel University in its 5-year BSN co-operative degree (BSN-Co-op) and 11-month second-degree accelerated BSN degree (BSN-ACE) undergraduate programs include using the standardized patient in the last two quarters of Co-op and last quarter of ACE to evaluate comprehensive health assessment skills (Wilson et al., 2007). Students in both programs must demonstrate competency in 10 specified critical clinical skills in the nursing skills laboratory in their last quarter prior to graduation. Critical skills vary year to year, but include such things as properly setting up an IV pump with 100% accuracy calculations and sterile dressing changes. These final check-offs prior to graduation ensure two goals: (1) the students have demonstrated mastery of the critical clinical nursing skill, particularly if their performance during real clinical time was perhaps not held to the high bar the program normally requires (e.g., due to variability in grading among faculty and variability in enforcing rigor); and (2) they have refreshed their learning so that the skill demonstration is recent and may enhance actual real-life recall in their first nursing position postgraduation (they may not have even performed the skill live in the clinical agency before). These are not simple exercises that every student can pass, and a number of students over the years have failed either skill (standardized patient comprehensive assessment or critical skills checkoff), failed again in their one chance to remediate, and did not graduate on time. Finally, in undergraduate nursing education there are trends in which simulation learning is becoming the preferred pedagogy for remediation and clinical makeup (Gaberson and Oermann, 2010), but there may be other trends in which simulation might be replacing actual clinical time because of the scarcity of clinical agency access to patients (Katz, Peifer, and Armstrong, 2010).

In the graduate nursing programs, particularly programs that prepare advanced practice nurses at the master's or post-master's doctoral level (doctoral advanced practice nursing), the standardized patient has become a very integral part of our pedagogy—mostly in the NP and nurse anesthesia programs. Human simulation is used frequently, including prior to entering the NP clinical sequence (to demonstrate competencies gained from the physical health assessment course) and at the end of the program as a comprehensive practical exam. All students who take the master's-level physical health assessment course use live models (trained professional surrogates) for both gynecological and breast examinations in females and rectal, prostate, and testicular examinations in males. Progressive nursing programs will view these skills as essential to learn with real patients instead of opting to use mannequins. The cost for this kind of testing is added to the advanced practice nurse's technology fee that the college charges clinical students in their respective MSN programs. NP programs are also moving to add even more human simulation to the online programs, requiring students to come back more frequently for competency checkoffs and on an as-needed basis for remediation. Further, for 3 years Drexel has used electronic evaluations of students by preceptors using a Web-based or handheld device, and this is becoming standard practice in many master's nursing programs. Many advanced practice programs have also implemented some type of electronic clinical log so that students may track and document their clinical time (Squires, 2009).

Discussion of Case Using Best Practices Framework

Professor Han was certainly shaken by the dean's e-mail. She was aware that the nursing program's student handbook had a clear written policy and procedure for resolving student appeals of grades and clinical evaluations. The published appeal policy required the student to first ask the professor to reconsider the grade or evaluation and, if not satisfied with this reconsideration, the student could then appeal to the department chair, then to the dean and with a final appeal to the provost. Therefore, the professor was surprised the dean had not instructed the student to follow the appeal process or had forwarded the complaint to at least the department chair, which would have been the normal chain of command in these instances. Professor Han nonetheless prepared a very detailed e-mail that outlined her documentation of the student's clinical experience; when she sent it to the dean, she copied both her department chair and her course coordinator, Dr. Yellow. Hearing nothing for several days, Professor Han e-mailed her department chair, Dr. Cotez, who subsequently informed Professor Han that the dean has scheduled a meeting with the student to discuss the case. Dr. Cotez agreed with Professor Han that she would have preferred to have handled the appeal first herself, because that is the normal appeal procedure, but because Ms. Dastrovsky went directly to the dean, the dean had obviously decided to handle the case herself.

Upon examination, the clinical evaluation process in this program is very tight. The student handbook lists how student performance in the clinical agency will be handled and the student was given several well-documented remediation attempts before the clinical failure was determined. One of Professor Han's colleagues asked whether it was fair of her to fail Ms. Dastrovsky so close to graduation. Professor Han remarked that she was very frustrated that a student with such poor organizational and basic skills got through to her final semester without having received a clinical warning (which she had checked for). Professor Han further replied that clinical evaluation begins the day that students walk in, and it continues until the day they walk out.

Ideally, the proper procedure for handling the student's appeal would have been for the dean to refer the student back to Professor Han for a reconsideration of the grade, especially because she would perhaps have to make an independent ruling on the student's appeal if it moved through the system and wound up with her.

Viewing this case study from a legal perspective, it will be extremely difficult for the student to legally challenge the academic evaluations and grades given her faculty members. Chapter 2 of this book described two important U.S. Supreme

Court decisions that establish the general principle that judges should show great respect for the faculty's professional judgment when courts review the substance of a genuinely academic decision. The U.S. Supreme Court stated in its 1978 decision in *Board of Curators of the University of Missouri v. Horowitz*, "university faculties must have the widest range of discretion in making judgments as to the academic performance of students and their entitlement to promotion or graduation."

In due process[2] cases involving students and faculty evaluations, it is always prudent to adhere as closely as possible to published policies and procedures, particularly as this is the function of various levels of academic administrators—to use their judgment in the exercise of the roles and responsibilities they have been charged to perform. This case, or any other like it, may often be resolved in steps and by others prior to the dean's intervention, leaving a dean to focus more on the best use of his or her role to promote the college. Nevertheless, in this case, the dean did not advise the student to follow the normal grade appeal process, but asked Professor Han to respond. The dean then requested to see the documentation herself, and when she met with Professor Han she questioned whether Professor Han had evaluated her too harshly. Professor Han stated that she had not and requested the dean look at the totality of her comments in which she emphasized in her midterm evaluation that she had actually praised the student for behaviors that were positive, while being ethically bound to pay a greater emphasis on the student's safety and competency behaviors. The dean ultimately ruled against the student, who then appealed to the provost. The provost upheld the dean's ruling.

The nursing program has a responsibility to uphold safe clinical practice and, in the course of doing so, routinely fail students who do not meet the standard. This author once recalls interviewing a prospective faculty member who for some 25 years admitted she had never failed a student in clinical. To the search committee, this was likely a sign of lack of rigor on her part because the committee found it unimaginable that every student she had supervised in clinical was proficient and met the standard for passing. The search committee was looking for faculty who could keep the bar high because our NCLEX passing rates had exceeded 95% per year for very large and diverse classes for some 10 years, data largely documented by MacFadyen in 2008 in *Nursing Education Perspectives*.

---

[2] Remember – a student can raise a constitutional due process claim only in public institutions. At both state and private institutions, students challenging a grade will also try to raise a breach of contract claim relying on a material failure to follow the appeal and grievance policies and procedures that are established by the institution. Because many appeal and grievance policies at state institutions provide more "due process" than courts require to meet minimum constitutional due process requirements, faculty and administrators at state institutions still need to be careful to follow applicable institutional policies and procedures as closely as possible.

Using a best practices framework, it is absolutely the responsibility of the profession to admit and graduate safe nursing students even if there are faculty, institutions, or administrators who want to bend rules or regulations to pass students. Admittedly, there are many reasons why a faculty member might not provide a candid and complete evaluation of a student's performance. There may also be enormous pressures from students, parents, and administrators to change a grade. However, nursing faculty are not properly adjudicating their responsibilities in the faculty role if they do not uphold and enforce reasonable standards. It is hoped that there are willing nursing academic administrators who will support them when their actions are based on the reasonable academic and clinical judgment of the faculty member.

Summary

In 2006 a report by the prestigious National Academies indicated that medication errors are among the most common medical errors and harm at least 1.5 million people every year. The report further indicates that the extra medical costs of treating drug-related injuries occurring in hospitals alone amounts to at least $3.5 billion a year, not including lost wages and productivity or additional health care costs. Moreover, a 2009 study by the Hearst Corporation indicates an estimated 200,000 Americans a year will die needlessly from preventable medical mistakes and iatrogenic hospital-acquired infections. Finally, a recent study that followed approximately 100 nurses in Australia for two years and was published in the *Archives of Internal Medicine* (Westbrook et al., 2010) indicated that 80% of medication errors made by nurses were caused by not following proper procedures for medication administration. Interruptions occurred during more than half (53.1%) of all administrations, contributing to both procedural and clinical errors. Whereas 70.2% of the errors were minor and caused the patient no harm, 2.7% were serious (Westbrook et al., 2010).

It is critical that nursing schools graduate only competent and safe professional, advanced, and now doctoral advanced practice nurses in particular (Dreher and Montgomery, 2009). The public has a right to be protected from unsafe nursing practitioners (used generally to describe nursing practice at any level), and it is incumbent on nursing schools to maintain rigor, uphold reasonable evaluation standards, and have nursing academic nursing administrators act with moral courage to support clinical and teaching faculty who fail students for cause. This view is not designed to be punitive, but to embrace the importance of safe and competent nursing practice. Nursing educators have a responsibility to society and themselves to be fully accountable in their teaching role to enforce standards and recognize that not all students are competent and some just cannot be remediated.

CRITICAL ELEMENTS TO CONSIDER

- Evaluation is a serious endeavor, and faculty must adhere to all proper procedures for the responsible evaluation of their nursing students at all levels.
- Comments such as "Mary is a pleasure to work within the clinical area," "Linda is an affable student who enjoys taking care of others," or "Tony has minimally met the objectives for NURS 200" are simply unacceptable and are of no value to the student. Faculty need to clearly communicate to the student that they are not meeting academic, clinical, or professional standards and expectations. Contemporaneous documentation of performance issues helps demonstrate that the grade or evaluation ultimately received was based on the faculty member's reasonable academic and professional judgment.
- For accreditation purposes, most nursing schools keep all clinical evaluations until the individual student passes NCLEX. Your institution may also have a policy that governs how long student educational records must be kept.
- New faculty, particularly new clinical adjunct faculty, must be properly oriented to the evaluation systems used both in clinical and the classroom.
- If at all possible, procedures for grade appeals and monitoring and adjudicating unsafe clinical performance should be outlined in the student handbook, which should be updated yearly.
- At the beginning of each new nursing class, students should sign a statement indicating they have read the student handbook and will abide by its guidelines; these written attestations should be kept on file.
- Clinical and teaching faculty should always at minimum keep their course clinical coordinator up to date with the progress of students in their clinical rotation, particularly students who are experiencing problems. Normally, the course coordinator should then make sound decisions about how and when to inform the respective department chair of relevant student issues.

References

Benner, P. (2000). *From novice to expert: Excellence and power in clinical nursing practice.* Upper Saddle River, NJ: Prentice-Hall.

Bourbonnais, F. F., Langford, S., & Giannantonio, L. (2008). Development of a clinical evaluation tool for baccalaureate nursing students. *Nurse Education in Practice, 8,* 62–71.

Carlson-Sabelli, L., & Delaney, K. R. (2006). Evaluating clinical competence of distant nurse practitioner students. In H.-A. Park et al. (Eds.), *Consumer-centered computer-supported care for healthy people* (p. 1006). Amsterdam, Netherlands: IOS Press.

Case study: Drexel University College of Nursing. (2010). www.softwaresecure.com. Retrieved February 11, 2011, from http://www.softwaresecure.com/US/Case%20Study% 20PDFs/Case% 20Study_Drexel(1).pdf

Cullen, D., Stiffler, D., Settles, J. S., & Pesut, D. (2010). A database for nurse practitioner clinical education. *CIN: Computers, Informatics, Nursing, 28*(1), 20–29.

Dreher, H. M. (2011). Nursing as a practice discipline. In M. D. Dahnke & H. M. Dreher, *Philosophy of science for nursing practice: Concepts and application* (pp. 23–54). New York: Springer.

Dreher, H. M., & Montgomery, K. E. (2009). Let's call it "doctoral" advanced practice nursing. *Journal of Continuing Nursing Education, 40*(12), 530–531.

Falkenstein, K., Pearlman, F., Davis, S., Kennedy, M., Poyss, A., Portwood, C., et al. (2007, February). *Evaluation of distance nurse practitioner students using secured online testing and a standardized patient lab: Is this the best of both worlds?* Poster session presented at the American Association of Critical-Care Nurses master's education conference, Masters Nursing Education: Variations on a Theme, Albuquerque, NM..

Gaberson, K. B., & Oermann, M. H. (2010). *Clinical teaching strategies in nursing* (3rd ed.). New York: Springer.

Gillespie, M, & Patterson, B. L. (2009). Helping novice nurses make effective clinical decisions: The situated clinical decision-making framework. *Nursing Education Perspectives, 30*(3), 164–170.

Hearst Corporation. (2009, August 9). Hearst national investigation finds Americans are continuing to die in staggering numbers from preventable medical injuries. hearst.com. Retrieved February 12, 2011, from http://www.hearst.com/press-room/pr-20090809b.php

Institute of Medicine. (2011). *The future of nursing: Leading change, advancing health.* Washington, DC: The National Academies Press.

Katz, G. B., Peifer, K. L., & Armstrong, G. (2010). Assessment of patient simulation use in selected baccalaureate nursing programs in the United States. *Simulation in Healthcare: The Journal of the Society for Simulation in Healthcare, 5*(1), 46–51.

MacFadyen, J. (2008). Drexel University's five-year work/study undergraduate program. *Nursing Education Perspectives, 29*(2), 66–67.

National Academies. (2006, February). *Preventing medication errors.* Committee on Identifying and Preventing Medication Errors, Board on Health Care Services, Institute of Medicine of the National Academies. Washington, DC: National Academies Press. Retrieved February 11, 2011, from http://www.nap.edu/openbook.php?record_id=11623&page=R1

Oermann, M. H., & Gaberson, K. (2009). *Evaluation and testing in nursing education* (3rd ed.). New York: Springer.

Oermann, M. H., Yarbrough, S. S., Saewert, K. J, Ard, N., & Charasika, M. E. (2009). Clinical evaluation and grading practices in schools of nursing: national survey findings: Part II. *Nursing Education Perspectives, 30*(6), 352–357.

Seldomridge, L. A., & Walsh, C. M. (2006). Evaluating student performance in undergraduate preceptorships. *Journal of Nursing Education, 45*(5), 169–176.

Squires, E. D. (2009). Electronic clinical logs. *Topics in Advanced Practice Nursing eJournal. 9*(3). Retrieved February 11, 2011, from http://www.medscape.com/viewarticle/708590

Van Eerden, K. (2001). Using critical thinking vignettes to evaluate student learning. *Nursing and Health Care Perspectives, 22*(5), 231–234.

Westbrook, J. I., Woods, A., Rob, M. I., Dunsmuir, W. T. M., & Day, R. O. (2010). Association of interruptions with an increased risk and severity of medication administration errors. *Archives of Internal Medicine, 170*(8), 683–690.

Wilson, L., Gallagher Gordon, M., Falkenstein, K., Smith Glasgow, M. E., Dreher, H. M., Rockstraw, L., et al. (2007, May/June). *Human simulation: Preparing nurses for the unexpected.* Paper presented at the International Council of Nurses (ICN) International conference: Nurses at the Forefront—Dealing With the Unexpected, Yokohama, Japan.

CHAPTER 33

Best Practices in Evaluating Faculty Performance

CASE STUDY

A Department Chair's Faculty Evaluations Become Highly Politicized

Your role: You are Dr. Flack, the department chair for the biobehavioral nursing division.

As the department chair, you have 17 full-time faculty (including both tenured and tenure-track faculty) in your department. You report directly to the assistant dean, Dr. Veebray, who oversees the biobehavioral, women's health, and child and adolescent health nursing divisions in the college and includes both undergraduate and graduate faculty.

Just prior to leaving for a 6-month Fulbright fellowship, you gave 17 faculty members their written evaluations after having met with each one personally to go over their accomplishments, areas to focus on more (or improve), and future goals (both short and long term). As has been your practice for many years, you instructed any faculty member who disagreed with your evaluation to contact you. You would then review the contested comments, meet to discuss them, and make a determination whether to change, not change, or modify the original comments. Four of the faculty evaluations in particular were very challenging for you (consequently, Dr. Veebray had helped you with three of them), but you were comfortable that the evaluations included both praise for accomplishments as well as some difficult feedback in other areas. You knew the four faculty would not be happy with their evaluations, and you expected to hear from them. But, strangely, no one contacted you to appeal their evaluation.

Background

Dr. Flack had been awarded a prestigious 6-month Fulbright fellowship. She was stepping down as chair temporarily while she traveled to Toronto to serve as visiting nursing professor at the highly regarded University of Toronto. After seeing an ad posted specifically for a short-term Fulbright in nearby Canada, Dr. Flack had applied for it, although, based on an earlier conversation with Dr. Veebray, she worried that he might not support her application. To her s urprise, Dr. Veebray immediately endorsed the idea saying, "This will be a good opportunity for you!" and he quickly wrote a support letter. A little astonished, Dr. Flack submitted her application that fall. In the spring, Dr. Flack was notified that indeed she had won the fellowship that would take place the following fall for a total of 6 months. Dr. Flack began her preparation to hand over the reins of the department to an interim chair. She considered who might be best qualified to serve as chair in her absence, but when she nominated a seasoned faculty member for the interim appointment, she was informed by Dr. Veebray that he, in consultation with the associate dean, had decided that another faculty member would be selected. Dr. Flack protested that this individual was much too inexperienced and thought her short time in the department was not sufficient to acclimate properly to the role. Nevertheless, Dr. Flack was informed this was not her decision and that the choice was final. Dr. Limb, a relatively new tenured professor who had just arrived from a university on the west coast (who was granted transfer of tenure upon hire), was announced as the interim chair.

As part of Dr. Flack's preparation for her leave, she wrote all the faculty evaluations. For 2 years, Dr. Veebray and her supervisor, Associate Dean Carraway, had been complaining about the low productivity of the faculty in the biobehavioral division. Dr. Flack suspected that a second year of strong complaints from her superiors about the lack of productivity in her department warranted even more substantive feedback in these evaluations. Dr. Flack indeed discussed this issue with Dr. Veebray, and he volunteered to look at the evaluations that had been difficult or challenging for her to write. Dr. Flack therefore sent three particularly prickly evaluations to Dr. Veebray, for feedback. Dr. Veebray returned them with blistering comments, which Dr. Flack decided she would temper before completing a final version to be delivered.

Identifying Best Practices in Nursing Education

The issue of faculty evaluation should not be so extraordinary; employees are evaluated in practically every organization. Furthermore, satisfactory performance is often associated with retaining one's job, advancing or being promoted, and merit raises or salary increases. But the evaluation of faculty is fraught by several considerations that are different from those in the corporate world. First, many faculty are evaluated by supervisors who are also their colleagues (e.g., both may have a PhD and both may be reputable scholars in their own right) (Hecht, Higgerson, Gmelch et al., 1999). This creates tension when the department chair, for instance, in some deliberations may be speaking simply as another tenured member of the faculty and on other issues may speak as the supervisor of the faculty who report to her or him.

Second, some faculty may be tenured and therefore even with poor evaluations are not eligible to be fired except for cause, which is usually further defined in the tenure policy (U.S. Department of Labor, 2009). The common assumption is that there is a decline in faculty performance once faculty are tenured (often these are also older faculty) because tenured faculty have a "job for life" unless they are fired for illegal acts or fiduciary reasons (e.g., the classics major is eliminated and there is now room for only three of five tenured faculty to teach non-major courses and there are no alternative academic positions appropriate for the other two tenured faculty) (Goodwin and Sauer, 1995; Kemper, 2010; Mangan, 2011). Although Tighe (2003) disputes the evidence of a decline in faculty productivity post-tenure proclaimed by Goodwin and Sauer and others, we have indeed seen this phenomenon on an anecdotal basis. The normal progression in academia is that an assistant professor who is tenured and promoted to associate professor will want to maintain productivity to achieve full professorship. However, tenured faculty have been heard to say, "I have no goal to become a full professor" or "I haven't decided if I want to become a full professor or not." For this reason, many colleges and universities have instituted a *post-tenure review* system in which tenured faculty are formally evaluated on a scheduled basis—often every 5 years (Morreale, 1999).[1]

One of the most prominent leaders in the contemporary faculty evaluation movement is Peter Seldin, Distinguished Professor Emeritus of Management in the Lubin School of Business at Pace University. Dr. Seldin has conducted hundreds of faculty performance workshops at colleges and universities across the country. Dr. Seldin, in his 2006 book *Evaluating Faculty Performance: A Practical Guide to Assessing Teaching, Research, and Service*, indicates that there are seven essential components of well-constructed faculty evaluation:

1. Practicality
2. Relevance

---

[1] Morreale (1999) outlines three common but different kinds of post-tenure review: (1) annual review (which often unfortunately focuses on short-term goals and is often and unfortunately a perfunctory exercise; (2) comprehensive review (periodic/consequential) in which the review is not written by one person (e.g., the tenured faculty member's supervisor) but instead by a committee of tenured faculty; and (3) triggered review (episodic/consequential), which is usually initiated by some prior indication of unsatisfactory performance.

3. Comprehensive evaluation
4. Sensitivity
5. Freedom from contamination
6. Reliability
7. Acceptability (2006, pp. 2–3)

Although most of these are fairly easy to interpret, "Freedom from Contamination" refers to not penalizing a professor, for example, for not having certain equipment if the university cannot provide it. Finally, "Acceptability," according to Seldin, is the most important criterion of them all, as the evaluation format itself must be acceptable (and agreed on) by all parties using it (supervisors and faculty themselves). In other words, all parties must agree that the evaluation process is fair, reliable, and valid—especially when it is used in merit pay decisions, for example.

At the heart of faculty evaluation is the measure of faculty productivity. In Middaugh's (2000) book *Understanding Faculty Productivity: Standards and Benchmarks for Colleges and Universities*, the real complexities of defining faculty productivity (mostly quantitatively) are discussed and he writes:

> Any methodology that hopes to measure faculty productivity must first take cognizance of what faculty do. Clearly, they do more than teach. But is this the case at only research universities, where the institutional mission is a complex combination of teaching, research, and service? (p. 10)

Middaugh, however, indicates that triumvirate mission of teaching, research,[2] and service may hold true at many more colleges and universities than just the research extensive/intensive ones. In the past decade we have seen many more midlevel universities pushing faculty more heavily to secure funded research and program grant monies. Even liberal arts colleges, at which teaching is the central mission, have moved to requiring more scholarly productivity of their faculty (the old publish or perish adage) as the bar for tenure continues to rise higher and higher. The recent high-profile case of Brown University (although it is an Ivy League school, it has traditionally been more of a teaching university than a research university) at which the tenure rate is 70% (some 20% higher than its peer institutions), the administration's highly controversial call for reform (hoping to rein in the high tenure rates) include proposals geared toward more research activities, not improved teaching (Jaschik, 2010).

Most universities and colleges will devise their own metric to determine faculty productivity. By tradition, at research-oriented or intensive universities, faculty productivity may be measured primarily by the following:

1. Grantsmanship (number of grants written and received)
2. Publications (peer reviewed, non–peer reviewed, or invited—including both journals and books and book chapters)
3. Presentations (both peer reviewed and invited)

---

[2] We would be more expansive of the word *research* and write *research/scholarship*.

4. Service to the discipline (e.g., being editor or on the editorial board of a journal; chairing or serving on the organizing committee for a national conference; participating in blind-review editing for peer-reviewed journals; serving as an officer of a national//international organization, etc.)

The Faculty Scholarly Productivity Index is now used by many universities for ranking purposes and includes the following:

- Number of faculty
- Percentage of faculty with a book
- Books per faculty
- Percentage of faculty with a journal publication
- Journal publications per faculty
- Percentage of faculty with journal publications cited in another work
- Citations per faculty (*chronicle.com*, 2011)

Interestingly, teaching may or may not be a major factor in evaluating productivity. Although measures of quality teaching are prevalent, mere satisfactory teaching may not harm a tenure case, but unsatisfactory teaching often will. Alternatively, even excellent teaching may not save a candidate who has weak or even satisfactory scholarship (American Council on Education, 2000). It is important for any faculty member to gauge the academic culture within his or her respective college or university and ascertain what a new faculty member needs to accomplish to receive a good evaluation and, separately, what is required to present a strong tenure case. If a faculty member is nontenure track, teaching is almost always emphasized much more, but the presence of some scholarship and service (e.g., serving on program, departmental, college, or university-wide committees; student advisement; undergraduate and graduate new student recruitment) is usually required if the faculty member wants to achieve a merit raise, to be promoted, or to retain the year-to-year contract for employment, which is standard in academia for non–tenure track faculty positions.

From a legal perspective, courts may consider standards and criteria established by an institution for appointment, nonreappointment, promotion, or granting of tenure to be legally binding on the institution, as part of the faculty member's contract with the institution. For reasons discussed in earlier chapters, courts will be very deferential when reviewing the substance of standards and criteria established by the institution in the evaluation and promotion decision; even so, they will not be as deferential when they are reviewing the process and procedure followed by the institution in reaching those decisions (Kaplin and Lee, 2007). Therefore, administrators must be cognizant of applicable standards and criteria when preparing their evaluations.

Performance evaluations are critical documents when it comes to defending an employment decision made by the organization. For example, if a department chair decides not to reappoint a faculty member because of long-standing performance and behavior issues that were not documented in the annual evaluation (or through some other disciplinary warning), the chair will have a difficult time explaining the decision to a jury when the faculty member disputes the reasons for termination and claims he was not aware of any issues the chair had with his performance or conduct. For juries (as for judges, as for people), if it is not written down and "in the record," it probably did not happen.

In summary, faculty evaluation is an important enterprise, especially as universities seek to improve their ranking, better serve their stakeholders, and advance higher education in the United States. And with higher education budgets throughout the United States and around the world being scrutinized and reduced because of the recent global recession, any one individual faculty member's job security may rely more heavily in the future on his or her own individual faculty productivity (Douglas, 2010).

Discussion of Case Using Best Practices Framework

As Dr. Flack subsequently prepared for her fellowship, word got back to her that all four faculty were highly upset with their evaluations and had complained to the new interim chair, Dr. Limb. Dr. Limb shared the evaluations with Dr. Veebray who was sympathetic to the faculty involved, However, Dr. Veebray never shared with Dr. Limb or the four faculty that he had been personally involved in writing three of the evaluations. Both giving and receiving feedback can be challenging to any supervisor administering a difficult evaluation, and likewise the employee on the receiving end of such an evaluation may be very defensive. A best practices framework would necessitate that supervisors (e.g., department chairs and especially new chairs) undergo some formal human resources training on how to deliver difficult or negative comments in the evaluation process. Similarly, and we suspect this is rarely done in organizations, employees (including faculty) need to be oriented to the supervisor's role to include all aspects of faculty performance (both good and bad) in the evaluation process.

Anticipating that these four faculty members might challenge the negative parts of the evaluation, Dr. Flack had been particularly careful in wording the negative feedback and had cited numerous indisputable examples of low productivity to support her evaluation. Nevertheless, in this case Dr. Flack wondered why these four faculty members never contacted her, as had usually happened in the past. However, from experience Dr. Flack also knew that passive-aggressive faculty would rather complain to others than constructively sit down to have a discussion about what was written.

During the 6 months that Dr. Flack was away, the four faculty members could not let go of their anger, and they acted accordingly. Unfortunately, Dr. Limb herself was new both to the college and to the leadership role, and she did very little to bring a sense of civility back to the department. In academic medicine it has been recognized by Grigsby, Aber, and Quillen (2009) that "it is clear that high attrition rates of academic department chairs have created the need for skilled interim leaders of academic departments. However, it is unclear whether persons serving as interim department chairs are prepared for the job" (p. 1329).

In Dr. Flack's absence, Dr. Limb and Dr. Veebray began to make substantive changes to the department. One of Dr. Flack's colleagues, the chair of the social work department, called her and told her that changes in the biobehavioral nursing division were consistently being announced. She said that she had never heard of changes being made in a department when the department chair was away for a fellowship or a sabbatical, and she prayed it didn't happen to her when she took her first sabbatical. Using a best practices framework, it is standard practice (including in academia) that interim administrators (no matter their position) be given very direct guidelines concerning the scope of their interim authority, or as Novielli (2009) states, to be given strategic plans/considerations on "what *not* to do." However, as institutions are different, this scope may vary.

Dr. Flack called a dean with whom she was very friendly and informed her what was happening back in her department. The dean said that this would never have happened in her college. She said whenever one of her department chairs or associate deans went away for any kind of temporary leave, she was very clear with any interim administrator what his or her responsibilities were: "Simply to maintain the ship. Certainly not sink it, but also not sail in unchartered waters." She further indicated she was very sensitive that major changes in any program warranted the presence of a permanent chair and that interim administrators needed to be given very firm boundaries on what they could and could not do. Dr. Flack certainly knew this had not happened in her own institution. She reflected on this and decided to ignore as much as possible the events happening back in her department while away on her fellowship. The distraction was substantial, but she aimed to focus on her scholarship and the exciting appointment at the University of Toronto.

As Dr. Flack's fellowship progressed, she also heard about significant complaints from the division's students about Dr. Limb's performance; however, she was powerless to do anything while she was away. Just prior to the end of the 6-month fellowship, Dr. Flack assessed what she heard had taken place in her absence, and thought things were worse than ever in her department. She elected to step down from her department chair position at the end of her fellowship and return to her previous faculty role. She met with the dean to inform her of this decision and was later very happy with it.

In concluding this discussion of best practices with regard to Dr. Flack's case, many institutions use the terms *interim* and *acting* synonymously. However, Grigsby, Aber, and Quillen (2009) indicate it is important to differentiate between the two.

They make the following distinction: "An *interim chair* serves as the leader while a search is conducted to find a new department chair and is expected to occupy that role indefinitely or for a specific term of service" (p. 1328). However, "a person filling the leadership role while the permanent leader experiences a temporary absence, but who anticipates returning, is referred to as an *acting chair*" (p. 1328). We thus conclude that in this case, Dr. Flack should have therefore been replaced by an acting chair, not an interim, and this may possibly have moderated the amount of change in the department that Dr. Limb and Dr. Veebray actively initiated in the absence of the chair.

❗ CRITICAL ELEMENTS TO CONSIDER

- New faculty should be oriented to the evaluation process at the beginning of their appointment.
- New tenure-track faculty should be clearly informed what the procedures and requirements for tenure are. These are usually outlined in detail by the university and often on the university's Web site or in a faculty handbook.
- The faculty evaluation process within a college should be consistent, and evaluation procedures should be directed by human resources or in some faculty cases by the office of the provost.
- Evaluators should be oriented and apprenticed in how to write and deliver a faculty evaluation. They should be particularly schooled in how to deliver a difficult or bad evaluation and how to write them in ways that focus on facts and merit, avoiding generalizations and characterizations that will generate disputes (or, worse, legal claims).
- Evaluations should not be filled with surprises. For seriously negative evaluative statements, it is generally accepted that the faculty member has been counseled or at least notified of her or his previous behaviors before the situation winds up in an annual evaluation. In other words, evaluators should be giving feedback throughout the year and not just at the end of the year.
- Midyear informal evaluation check-ins with faculty (e.g., they can be asked to write a one-paragraph summary of what they have accomplished midyear and what they are working on the duration of the year) are often helpful. Any problems detected at the time can be quickly addressed and possibly resolved before the final evaluation.
- Giving negative feedback is very challenging, and some supervisors who shy away from confrontation may need extra managerial professional development in how to handle difficult employees and give bad news.

CRITICAL ELEMENTS TO CONSIDER—cont'd

- Always consult superiors for advice when addressing difficult items in an evaluation. Having the wise counsel of another experienced, level-headed administrator should be taken advantage of. Be familiar with any grievance or appeal process at your institution that individual faculty members might utilize to contest an evaluation. If faculty members are part of a union or collective bargaining unit, then grievance or appeal rights (which may include mediation or binding arbitration options) may be set forth in the contract or collective bargaining agreement.

- If, when giving an evaluation, a faculty member wants something changed immediately, do not be intimidated to make a decision on the spot. It is always good practice to give any such request some additional consideration, and 24 hours (at least) to weigh options and best possible courses of action.

References

American Council on Education. (2000). *Good practice in tenure evaluation: Advice for tenured faculty, department chairs, and academic administrators.* A joint project of the American Council on Education, the American Association of University Professors, and United Educators Insurance Risk Retention Group. Retrieved February 14, 2011, from http://www.acenet.edu/bookstore/pdf/tenure-evaluation.pdf

Bland, C. J., Wersal, L., VanLoy, W., et al. (2002). Evaluating faculty performance: A systematically designed and assessed approach. *Academic Medicine, 77*, 15–30.

Douglas, J. A. (2010). *Higher education budgets and the global recession: Tracking varied national responses and their consequences.* Center for Studies in Higher Education, University of California, Berkeley Research & Occasional Paper Series: CSHE.4.10. Retrieved February 14, 2011, from http://cshe.berkeley.edu/publications/docs/ROPS.4Douglass.HEGlobalRecession.3.8.10.pdf

Gimbel, R. W., Cruess, D. F., Schor, K., et al. (2008). Faculty performance evaluation in accredited U.S. public health graduate schools and programs: A national study. *Academic Medicine, 83*(10), 962–968.

Goodwin, T. H., & Sauer, R. D. (1995). Life cycle productivity in academic research: Evidence from cumulative publication histories of academic economists. *Southern Economic Journal, 61*, 728–743.

Grigsby, R. K., Aber, R. C., & Quillen, D. A. (2009). Commentary: Interim leadership of academic departments at U.S. medical schools. *Academic Medicine, 84*(10), 1328–1329.

Hecht, I. W. D., Higgerson, M. L., Gmelch, W. H., et al. (1999). *The department chair as academic leader.* Phoenix, AZ: American Council of Higher Education/Oryx Press.

Jaschik, S. (2010, April 27). Brown University profs, admin face off on high tenure rate. usatoday.com. Retrieved February 14, 2011, from http://www.usatoday.com/news/education/2010-04-27-brown-tenure_N.htm

Kaplin, W. A., & Lee, B. (20071). The law of higher education: Student version, 4th ed. San Francisco: CA: Jossey-Bass.

Kemper, S. (2010, November 14). Older professors: Fewer, and better, than you think. chronicle.com. Retrieved February 14, 2011, from http://chronicle.com/article/Older-Professors-Fewer-and/125347/

Mangan, K. (2011). At 2 Texas campuses, faculty buyouts create staffing headaches. chronicle.com. Retrieved February 14, 2011, from http://chronicle.com/article/At-2-Texas-Campuses-Faculty/125796/

Middaugh, M. F. (2000). *Understanding faculty productivity: Standards and benchmarks for colleges and universities.* San Francisco, CA: Jossey-Bass.

Morrreale, J. (1999). Post-tenure review: Evaluating teaching. In P. Seldin et al. (Eds.), *Changing practices in evaluating teaching: A practical guide to improved faculty performance and promotion/tenure decisions.* Bolton, MA: Anker.

Novielli. K. (2009). *Academic department chair turnover: The critical role of interim leadership.* Paper presented by the Group on Faculty Affairs at the annual meeting of the Association of American Medical Colleges.

Roth, R. (2009). *Higher education law in America* (10th ed.). Malvern, PA: Center for Education & Employment Law.

Seldin, P., et al. (Eds.) (2006). *Evaluating faculty performance: A practical guide to assessing teaching, research, and service.* Bolton, MA: Anker.

Tighe, T. J. (2003). *Who's in charge of America's research universities? A blueprint for reform.* Albany: State University of New York Press.

U.S. Department of Labor. (2009). *Occupational outlook handbook 2009.* New York: Skyhorse.

CHAPTER 34

How to Best Enforce Student-Faculty Boundary Areas in the Academic and Clinical Environment

CASE STUDY 1

Healthy Boundaries in the Classroom

Your role: You are Dr. Noah, a colleague of Dr. Jones who is a statistics professor.

Dr. Jones has been teaching the introductory statistics course to graduate nursing students in the evening for several years. Over the years he has routinely gone with students of legal drinking age to the local pub for drinks after class. There has never been a complaint of excessive drinking or rowdy behavior, and Dr. Jones and the students who accompany him have generally developed relationships that could be perceived as being more friendly than professional. Not all the students join these after-class gatherings and one student in particular has never attended. That student, Susan Wycliffe, files an e-mail complaint with the dean, complaining that she is being marginalized and being punished in class for "not attending these drinking binges with Dr. Jones like all the other students." The dean sends the e-mail to the statistics department chair, Dr. Zuvey, and tells him "to take care of it." Dr. Zuvey immediately notifies Dr. Jones by e-mail that there has been a complaint about his going to the pub with students and to please meet with him. Dr. Jones is horrified by Dr. Zuvey's e-mail and runs across the hall to you, his colleague Dr. Noah, and asks you what he should do.

Questions

- What should you tell Dr. Jones?
- What should Dr. Zuvey tell Dr. Jones?
- Should Dr. Jones be disciplined for fraternizing with his graduate students?
- Should there be a university policy prohibiting fraternization between graduate faculty and graduate students?

CASE STUDY 2

Healthy Boundaries in Clinical

Your role: You are Professor Fine and a close friend of Dr. Doyle.

Dr. Doyle comes to you one day and complains that she doesn't think the students in her psychiatric clinical group (junior-level BSN undergraduates) are sufficiently respectful of her or her authority and professional role as their teacher. You ask her to give her some examples. Dr. Doyle explains that sometimes when calling her Sarah they speak to her as if she is their best friend. She states, "And when they say 'Hey Sarah!' I practically cringe." She goes on to say that she is having a hard time getting them to follow her instructions and confesses she sometimes feels as if they do not look upon her as their professor but as their friend. You ask Dr. Doyle why she does not require them to address her as Dr. Doyle or Professor Doyle instead of simply Sarah. Dr. Doyle replied that she always wanted to be more collegial with her undergraduate students and avoided the formal titles to promote a more egalitarian work environment. You ask, very bluntly, because you are a close friend and colleague of Dr. Doyle, "Well, do you think it's working?"

Questions

- What should you say next to Dr. Doyle?
- Do you think the casual manner of addressing faculty by their first name is problematic?
- Will the use of Dr. or Professor bring more civility to the clinical environment?
- Similarly, should faculty also address students by their first name if they are being addressed formally as Dr. or Professor?
- Should there be a departmental policy on how students should address their professors whether in the clinical or classroom setting?

How to Best Enforce Student–Faculty Boundary Areas in the Academic and Clinical Environment: Review of the Literature

Setting professional boundaries between students and professors is no different from boundary setting in other professions, including the patient-therapist or the congregant-minister relationship, for example. However, although therapists and ministers have an established code of ethical conduct, the student-teacher relationship for some reason has never been bound by a singular standard (Kitchener, 2000; Trull and Carter, 2004). Aultman, Williams-Johnson, and Schutz (2009) indicate that successful teaching and learning are integral to the student-teacher relationship, and in their study they reported that maintaining a balance between demonstrating care while maintaining a healthy, productive level of control in the classroom was the most recurring theme. Larkin and Mello (2010) highlight the medical student/physician teacher relationship in a recent issue of *Academic Medicine* and identify that the curricular content that addresses "the ethics of appropriate pedagogic and intimate relations between teaching staff and students, interns, residents, researchers, and other trainees" (p. 752) is rarely ever addressed. They further write that "attraction and revulsion are normal aspects of the human psyche, but they must, as with all passions, be kept in check, lest one threaten the integrity of the academic environment" (p. 754).

Lack of proper student-teacher boundaries can lead to a variety of negative consequences including sexual harassment, which is commonly cited as one of the most destructive outcomes of what Aultman et al. call "crossing the line." Incidents of sexual harassment between teachers and students are not limited to higher education. Dragan (2006) reported that according to the National Center for Educational Statistics: 59% of secondary schools and 54% of middle schools reported incidents of sexual harassment with 22% of them naming a teacher as responsible for the incident. For many reasons, one can assume these percentages are even higher in the college and university setting.

Henley (2009) and others also indicate that texting, e-mailing, and social networking sites are radically changing the historically traditional student-teacher relationship and placing new strains on the maintenance of healthy boundaries. Facebook, Twitter, blogs, and other cyber-based venues only add to the likelihood that student-teacher interaction will occur outside the classroom (Larkin and Mello, 2010). In the article "The Student-Teacher Relationship in a Texting World," Trotier (2008) indicates that beyond the frequency, the words used in texting, the topics shared, and the lack of discretion invite greater intimacy than in-person interactions. She recommends the following:

- Avoid engaging in inappropriate dialogue with students through the Internet.
- Avoid sending e-mails or text messages of a personal nature to students.
- Avoid being alone or in isolated situations with students, including social networking sites; this might be perceived as inappropriate in nature.
- Exercise extreme caution in connection with contact/Internet sites including chat rooms, message boards, social networking, and news groups.

Faculty members are sometimes alone with students during office meetings or, in particular, during advisement. The important point to emphasize is that if there is any anxiety or concern about being alone with the student (e.g., the student has expressed greater than usual interest in you as the professor or has made comments or innuendos with sexual, intimate, or overly personal content), then the individual faculty member ought to meet with the student more publicly, with others around, or leave the office door open at all times. O'Connor (2005) notes that the current generation of students has a proclivity to using electronic media and gaming, and recommends that educators try to find creative ways to use these educational media. She writes of her experience using instant messaging (IM) to improve writing skills. Although there is reason to be skeptical of this

approach, especially in nursing education, Twitter, for instance, has been identified as being useful as a pedagogical approach to communicate real-time, health-
related information (Dreher, 2009; Young, 2008).

There is an absence in the literature on how to properly address a college professor or teacher. The Internet is filled with anecdotal responses and advice. It is
partly the culture of the university that often dictates the practice, and other times
it really is the discipline. At Bryn Mawr College (a women's college in Pennsylvania),
undergraduate and graduate students routinely call their professors by their first
names; however, at South Carolina State University (a historically black college in
Orangeburg, South Carolina) students universally address their faculty as professor
or doctor, creating a more formal campus culture.[1] Every possible form of address
has been used in nursing schools between students and faculty, and without exception there are more faculty-student boundary issues when undergraduate students
call the nursing professor by his or her first name. Pettigrew (2009) has a very engaging article, "What Do You Call a Professor? How to Play (and Win) the University Name Game," which gives practical advice to new college freshmen who face this
issue. With master's students who are typically more mature, there are usually fewer
boundary issues when professors request that students call them by their first name,
although it is still common to see students use doctor or professor. With doctoral
students who are being mentored as future colleagues, students are often requested
to address faculty by first name, but many of them are uncomfortable doing so. The
real question, particularly for undergraduate nursing faculty, is: What do you call
your students? And the larger question remains: Do you maintain a professional
boundary between yourself and your students?

Discussion of Cases

Case Study 1

Recall the first question from case study 1: What should you tell Dr. Jones? After
hearing of the accusation, Dr. Noah is also surprised as he does not believe that
his friend and colleague Dr. Jones would ever treat any student in an arbitrary
or unfair way. However, he always worried a bit about fraternizing with graduate
students after class and was himself careful to do so only under special circumstances (e.g., after the last day or evening of class). Dr. Noah tells his friend that
he should have been more cautious, stating, "You know, these days you have to
be really careful around students. You can be accused of literally anything at
anytime." He further advises, "You know, times have changed, I would probably

---

1 Academic dress is another example of university culture. For instance, business professors (particularly in
  MBA classes) tend to dress professionally for class (in nursing administration faculty, too), but philosophy
  professors generally do not. Dress can establish boundaries, or the lack thereof, as can other forms of
  conduct.

cut out visiting pubs with these students, at least until this settles down." Dr. Jones is glad he shared these embarrassing details with his friend, but he is very weary of the process of being accused of something he clearly believes he did not do. As there is no special ombudsman for the faculty, he feels more alone. He has heard about faculty being "thrown under the bus" even over an unproved accusation.

The second question is: What should Dr. Zuvey tell Dr. Jones? Dr. Jones met with the department chair, Dr. Zuvey, 2 days later, and Dr. Zuvey said, "Tell me about this incident. I have a disturbing e-mail from a student of yours, but I certainly want to hear your side of this." Dr. Jones is clearly appreciative of this approach by his department chair as she is well known for doing diligent fact finding before acting on accusations or gossip. Dr. Jones explains that Ms. Wycliffe is perhaps the weakest student in the class and is often unprepared. He also states she does not interact well with her peers in class. To him it is obvious that she is using the "after-class activities" as an excuse for her poor performance and "getting her excuses and offense ready" if she gets a poor grade. Dr. Zuvey asks what classroom behaviors would he perceive as contributing to her alleged marginalization, and Dr. Jones says he does not know. He mentions that he perhaps calls on her less often, but that is because she does not want to embarrass her publicly by having her demonstrate she is not prepared. Dr. Zuvey informs Dr. Jones that she is not sure anything will come of this, but she does want him to "stop socializing after class." She tells him that although he may have only the best of intentions, drinking with students, even graduate students, is likely to contribute to a diminution in proper student-teacher boundaries. She further states that students who do not participate can imagine that you are secretly sharing information with those students who socialize with you that you are not providing in class. Dr. Jones agrees to cease the after-class pub activities.

Case Study 2

Recall the first question: What should you say next to Dr. Doyle? Professor Fine had been in nursing education about 5 years longer than Dr. Doyle, and having taught in both ADN and BSN programs, she had witnessed quite consistently that informality in both the classroom and clinical courses usually was an invitation to unprofessional student conduct. She told Dr. Doyle that she probably thought it is a bit late to try to have the students suddenly call her Dr. midway through the semester, as that would draw unnecessary attention to it. She did, however, believe she could speak to her clinical group in preconference and voice her displeasure with some of informality of the clinical day. She told Dr. Doyle that her recommendation would be to remind them of the seriousness of their role as students in a clinical environment full of ill individuals and that starting today she wanted to see more professional attitudes for the duration of the semester, including less laughing and joking and a more proper professional demeanor befitting of BSN students of the highest caliber. Dr. Doyle sighed and said, "I guess you're right."

Findings and Disposition

Case Study 1

The third question is: Should Dr. Jones be disciplined for fraternizing with his graduate students? In this case, he was not, as there really was no evidence of improper behavior with students off campus (e.g., intoxication or other breach of the code of conduct), and there was no institutional policy preventing (or even addressing) graduate faculty socializing or fraternizing with graduate students. The department chair could have probably forbidden Dr. Jones from socializing with graduate students after class permanently and put a faculty memo out. However, doing so might have raised a larger issue: one of precedent and establishing a "new policy" for her department that could be broadly applicable, and she wanted to avoid that. In this case, Dr. Zuvey called the student in and inquired about her allegation of marginalization. Despite asking many different ways, the student was not able to articulate any specific conduct (acts or omissions) either inside or outside the classroom. She told the student that she had not provided any evidence to support the charge, but she did indicate Dr. Jones had decided to stop going out with students after class for the rest of the term. The student seemed content with the response, and the complaint went no further. Dr. Zuvey informed the dean that she had quashed the after-class pub activities and that she found no evidence to support the student's allegations about either binging or being treated differently in class. The dean confirmed this is in a memo for the record.

The final question is: Should there be a university policy prohibiting fraternization between graduate faculty and graduate students? In this case, Dr. Zuvey informed the dean that there was no such policy at the university level except the university policy that addressed personal relationships and power differentials (e.g., when a supervisor wrongly engages in a relationship with a subordinate), but she reiterated that the university had affirmed that all individuals are entitled to freely choose their personal associations and relationships (Drexel University, 2007, p. 1). She further stated that there was already a policy in both the undergraduate and graduate student nursing handbooks that specifically prohibited romantic or personal relationships between students and faculty who are actively teaching them and included prohibitions of such behaviors between students and any kind of preceptor or evaluator.

Case Study 2

The second question is, Do you think the casual manner of addressing faculty by their first names is problematic? Professor Fine was pretty adamant that it was problematic, and Dr. Doyle, although agreeing that she (Professor Fine) was probably correct, expressed some sadness that the lines between herself and her students needed to be drawn more rigidly. Philosophically, she would prefer to model collegiality to new and impressionable nursing undergraduates rather than the traditional behaviors she had learned from her nursing education that had put the teacher on a pedestal. She also thought this traditional divide contributed to the rigidity of nursing practice in which students viewed nursing practice as black or white, with little room for higher-level critical thinking. Nevertheless, she decided that next semester she would try to use her Dr. title as an experiment to see if there really was a difference. For her, she needed more data before she would give up on her preferred teaching mode of professional address.

The third question is: Will the use of Dr. or Professor bring more civility to the clinical environment? Dr. Doyle actually followed through with her experiment, and she found she created a more professional environment when the students addressed her as Doctor. But Dr. Doyle did not simply change the way the students addressed her; she went one step further and resolved to stop addressing them by their first names also and began to address them as Mr. and Miss. For her, this satisfied her need for an egalitarian response in which each party (both student *and* professor) were more respectful of each other in their use of personal address.

In response to the fourth question: Should faculty members also address students by their first name if they are being addressed formally as doctor or professor? it is suggested that Dr. Doyle's new practice actually be adopted. It certainly is not the most common practice in the clinical environment, but when faculty use it, it becomes a very powerful and actually equitable or democratic way to bring some formality and seriousness to the clinical environment. This does not mean, however, the clinical experience must be devoid of humor, but that humor should be used when appropriate and contribute to both a learning and healing environment.

The final question is: Should there be a departmental policy on how students should address their professors whether in the clinical or classroom setting? A mandatory policy making forms of address probably should not be a requirement, but there should be a recommended policy on forms of address for faculty in the student handbook.

Relevant Legal Case

The Case of the Tenured Professor Moonlighting as a Phone-Sex Worker

In this case, reported by Schmidt in the *Chronicle of Higher Education* electronic edition (2010), a 48-year-old tenured associate professor of English, Dr. Lisa D. Chávez, was moonlighting as the phone-sex dominatrix "Mistress Jade," and posing in promotional and sexually suggestive pictures with one of her graduate students who was also working for the same phone-sex company, People Exchanging Power, in Albuquerque, New Mexico. Once it was discovered Dr. Chávez was moonlighting in this job, she immediately quit and apologized for her serious lapse of judgment.

According to the *Chronicle* profile (Schmidt, 2010), graduate students in the creative writing program began working at People Exchanging Power because it paid well and in one case helped one of the students at the center of this case, 27-year-old Liz Derrington, gain more life experience to enhance her writing. At some point, Dr. Chávez needed extra income and also obtained part-time work there, too. Subsequently, Dr. Chávez encountered Ms. Derrington at the work site. This led to their becoming friendlier and ultimately posing for the company on its Web site. During this time, some of the graduate students in the program complained to other faculty about the sexually charged conversations occurring in Dr. Chávez's class. One professor took the allegations to the department chair, Dr. Jones, but no charges were filed. Later, photos of Dr. Chávez wound up on the desk of Dr. Jones, with a note attached that read "appalled parents" (Schmidt, para. 15). Dr. Jones then asked another faculty member (and supervisor of Dr. Chávez), Dr. Warner, to investigate.

In late 2007, the provost and university administrators ruled that "Ms. Chávez had exercised bad judgment but did not find her guilty of allegations of maintaining a hostile learning environment, sexual harassment, or any other illegal activities or violations that suggested she was unfit for her job" (Schmidt, 2010, para. 24). Other tenured departmental members did not agree with the finding and continued to protest, vigorously accusing Ms. Chávez of "abuse of academic freedom and professional ethics that must govern the relationship between a professor and her student." (Schmidt, para. 26). Subsequently, one faculty resigned because she felt she could not protect her students, and three others have filed lawsuits against the university, including Dr. Chávez, who filed a lawsuit with the state claiming discrimination because she was Hispanic and bisexual. The creative writing program and English department continue to be in disarray as the new department chair, Dr. Julie Shigekuni, states, "It becomes complicated, because I think that the lawsuits, and the kind of climate of antagonism and fear that is brought by the lawsuits, creates unpredictability. Students are uncertain about how the program is functioning and about the future of the program" (para 36). Dr. Chávez continues to teach in the department and creative writing program.

WHEN TO CONTACT THE UNIVERSITY COUNSEL

These situations are not likely to present issues for university counsel; they are most likely best handled within the department. If a student refuses to be appeased by the response to his or her complaint but continues to assert it (with greater force or to higher levels), then the dean would be wise to consider seeking legal advice before any "last steps" are taken. This is particularly true if, as her response, the student refuses to participate further in class.

Summary

This chapter has explored the landscape of the boundaries between teachers and students. Gillespie (2002) has written about a transformation of the student-teacher relationship that incorporates a humanistic approach, which fosters the learning and growth of students and teachers—much like the philosophy that Dr. Doyle was struggling to implement in her own teaching pedagogy. From both cases and the very messy real-life case of Dr. Chávez at the University of New Mexico, it is clear that the new social media technology makes the student-teacher relationship in some ways much more perilous. It is only going to get worse. Faculty now struggle with whether to give students a home phone number or a cell number, and the whole process of creating a relationship between students and faculty on the Internet is problematic. There is a lot more to navigate these days to keep the student-teacher relationship focused on teaching and learning while maintaining the highest levels of professionalism. Whereas there are no hard rules about faculty and student forms of address, students (undergraduate and graduate) ought to use professor and doctor when appropriate (without obsessing over this) in academic settings and e-mail.

CRITICAL ELEMENTS TO CONSIDER

- The best way to clear up any confusion about your preference for personal address is to simply tell the students the first day of class your requirements.. That usually clears the problem up immediately, assuming you act thereafter in conformity with your declaration.
- Visit the university Web site and human resources Web site to see if there are any institutional policies regarding faculty fraternizing with students. Appreciate the fact that the question presented in these relationships is not just "fact" but "appearance." What is perceived, accurate or not, is the reality.
- Fraternization with undergraduate students, especially in the presence of alcohol (even with undergraduates of legal age) is highly discouraged. Students are predictably enamored with professors: their knowledge, experiences, and confidence. Faculty must be on guard to detect "more" than this attitude. Signs that a student is overly attracted to, attentive to, or preoccupied with you warrant exceptional faculty measures that discourage the continuation of such behaviors. If you have not experienced the situation before, seek the advice of a colleague promptly.
- Fraternization with graduate students is more acceptable, but again it can be complicated, so we caution faculty to use good judgment.

Continued

CRITICAL ELEMENTS TO CONSIDER—cont'd

- Be very wary of participating in social media interactions with any students (especially but not limited to what you are teaching) in your class via social media sites (e.g., FaceBook, Twitter). This does not mean there are no pedagogically appropriate uses of them, but these must be devised and monitored very carefully by the faculty member.

HELPFUL RESOURCES

- Academic Coach: Earnest exhortations and random tidbits for dissertating grad students, post-doctoral job hunters and tenure-track faculty. (2005, October 26). Doctor, Professor, Hey You [Web log post]. Retrieved August 1, 2011, from http://successfulacademic.typepad .com/ successful_academic_tips/2005/10/doctor_professo.html
- thegradcafe.com: Where something is always brewing. (2010, February 18). Re: How do you address a professor? [Web log comment]. Retrieved August 1, 2011, from http://forum.thegradcafe.com/topic/9610-how-do-you-address-a-professor/

References

Aultman, L. P., Williams-Johnson, M. R., & Schutz, P. A. (2009). Boundary dilemmas in teacher-student relationships: Struggling with "the line." *Teaching and Teacher Education, 25*(5), 636–646.

Brooks, D. (2011). *The social animal: The hidden sources of love, character and achievement.* New York, NY: Random House.

Dragan, E. F. (2006). Setting boundaries for sexual harassment. *School Administrator, 11*(63). Retrieved January 21, 2011, from http://www.aasa.org/SchoolAdministratorArticle.aspx?

Dreher, H. M. (2009). Twittering about anything, everything and even health. *Holistic Nursing Practice, 23*(4), 217–221.

Drexel University. (2007). Human resource policy 5: Personal relationships. Retrieved January 22, 2011, from http://www.drexel.edu/hr/resources/policies/dupolicies/hr5/

Gillespie, M. (2002). Student-teacher connection in clinical nursing education. *Journal of Advanced Nursing, 37*(6), 566–576.

Henley, J. (2009, September 23). Blurred boundaries for teachers. Guardian.co.uk. Retrieved January 21, 2011, from http://www.guardian.co.uk/education/2009/sep/23/teacher-pupil-sexual-relationship

Larkin, G. L., & Mello, M. J. (2010). Commentary. Doctors without boundaries: The ethics of teacher-student relationships in academic medicine. *Academic Medicine, 85*(5), 752–755.

Kitchener, K. S. (2000). *Foundations of ethical practice, research, and teaching in psychology.* Mahwah, NJ: Lawrence Erlbaum.

O'Connor, A. (2005). Instant messaging: Friend or foe of student writing? newhorizons.org. Retrieved January 21, 2011, from http://www.newhorizons.org/strategies/literacy/oconnor.htm

Pettigrew, T. (2009). What do you call a professor? How to play (and win) the university name game. oncapmus.mcleans.ca. Retrieved January 21, 2011, from http://oncampus .macleans.ca/education/2009/08/30/what-do-you-call-a-professor/

Schmidt, P. (2010, September 12). In professor-dominatrix scandal, U. of New Mexico feels the pain. Chronicle.com. Retrieved January 22, 2011, from http://chronicle.com/article/ In-Professor-Dominatrix/124369/

Trotier, G. (2008, December). The student-teacher relationship in a texting world. *School Law Solutions.* Retrieved January 21, 2011, from http://dkattorneys.com/news-and-events/newsletters-and-alerts/school/?id=3346

Trull, J. E., & Carter, J. E. (2004). *Ministerial ethics: Moral formation for church leaders* (2nd ed.). Grand Rapids, MI: Baker Academic.

Young, J. (2008, January 28). A professor's tips for using Twitter in the classroom. Chronicle.com. Retrieved January 21, 2011, from http://chronicle.com/blogPost/A-Professor-s-Tips-for-Using/3643

CHAPTER 35

How to Best Manage Substance Abuse Among Students

CASE STUDY

Best Practices in Managing Substance Abuse Among Students

Your role: You are the director of undergraduate nursing.

Lisa Jacobs is a sophomore nursing student who is about to begin her clinical rotations. As per your policy, she had a background check and underwent drug screening. Her drug screen is positive for cocaine. In cases in which the drug screen is positive, the medical review officer (MRO) calls the student and requests another drug screen. Lisa refuses. At your meeting, Lisa claims that she did not use drugs but her boyfriend does use cocaine. She claims that she must have become positive through sexual intercourse.

Background

Substance abuse is an issue that must be managed in nursing education for the safety of patients, students, and the profession. "Clear policies show a commitment to professional standards by academic administrators and faculty and specify what occurs when standards are violated" (Monroe, 2009, p. 276). Substance abuse policies should address the policy and procedures related to any unlawful use, manufacture, distribution, or possession of controlled or illegal substances or alcohol, as substance abuse may significantly affect the ability of students to administer safe care to patients entrusted to them in a clinical health-care setting. The development of such a policy should include nursing faculty, academic administrators, substance abuse experts, legal counsel, and consultation from clinical affiliates and the state board of nursing.

Identifying Best Practices in Nursing Education

Clinical rotations occur at independent hospitals, health-care facilities, and organizations that are affiliated with academic nursing programs. Under the law, employers are allowed to investigate the fitness of applicants for jobs and to continue doing so after they have become employed, as long as they have provided notice to the employee of their requirements and those requirements have a reasonable relationship to the job being performed. The application for employment (or even volunteering) at a clinical site may require a fairly rigorous investigation of the applicant's past, because of the sensitive nature of the services being performed, the personal disclosures made by and vulnerability of the patients, and the accessibility of drugs. The investigation can include, among other things, a criminal background check, child abuse check, FBI fingerprinting, drug test, and a check for immunizations prior to the start of the clinical practicum rotations.

Participation in clinical practicum rotations is a required part of the curriculum for most nursing students. Students need to comply with the university's drug and alcohol policies as outlined in the student handbook. Clinical affiliates generally do not permit students with a positive drug screen into their facilities. In this chapter's case study, a student may be unable to complete the nursing program, as the clinical sites may be unwilling to allow the student a clinical placement. The ramifications are even greater than just the one job: RN-BSN and graduate nursing programs (where students hold an RN license) may be required to report any positive results of background checks and drug screens to the board of nursing in the state where the student is licensed. It is also likely that university procedures require that students with a positive drug screen for illegal substances also be referred to the office of student conduct and community affairs (or similar judicial office) for review and adjudication.

University policies may prohibit employees from working while they are taking certain kinds of prescription drugs. They may also impose sanctions for conduct involving substance abuse, even if it occurs after hours and off premises. Sample substance abuse policies should include the following language:

> The possession and/or use of narcotics or drugs, other than those medically prescribed, properly used, and in the original container is prohibited. The distribution and/or sale of narcotics or drugs are prohibited. Off-campus possession, use, distribution, or sale of narcotics or drugs is inconsistent with the university's policies and goals, and is therefore prohibited. The university reserves the right to invoke the university conduct process to the extent that off-campus drug use leads to behavior that in the university's sole judgment is destructive, abusive, or detrimental to the University's interests. The university generally considers the sanctions listed below to be guidelines when adjudicating drug policy violations. Each incident is reviewed on an individual basis. Depending on the specifics of the incident, more or less severe sanctions may be imposed. A first violation may warrant the following: suspension; loss of on-campus housing; ban from residence halls; counseling evaluation; parental notification; and possibility of expulsion. (Drexel University, 2009)

Substance abuse policies and procedures should also include methods for assessing substance abuse problems, intervention, and student follow-up (Clark, 1999), in addition to specifying the range of sanctions that can be imposed. Because nursing students are trusted with caring for patients, a nursing program may impose a harsher penalty for a drug violation than would otherwise be imposed by the university.

Nursing majors are at high risk for developing substance abuse problems. Clark (1999) noted that many impaired professional nurses were addicted as students. Students who abuse drugs typically will exhibit a pattern of objective, observable behaviors that eventually compromise patient safety and clinical standards of performance. Such behaviors include irritability, excessive absenteeism, tardiness, red eyes, hand tremors, leaving clinical area frequently, unsafe clinical performance, and impaired judgment (Dunn, 2005).

It is imperative that colleges and schools of nursing develop fair, comprehensive policies and procedures regarding this important issue (refer to the *Drexel University Substance Abuse Policy* located on http://davisplus.fadavis.com for a detailed example.) Policies need to offer assistance to the student in distress while at the same time safeguarding the needs of patients. Although most nursing academic administrators recognize that substance abuse is an illness requiring early intervention, academic administrators also need to comply with state boards of nursing, university policies, and clinical affiliation requirements.

For similar reasons, policies need to be developed for students who have separated from the school or college because of substance abuse issues and who wish to return; to do so, they must comply with the requirements of these regulatory bodies and affiliates. Such polices typically specify that students may be eligible to reenter the nursing program in certain circumstances if he or she can demonstrate satisfactory evidence of successful completion of treatment and documentation of 24 months of sustained recovery. Factors that have been identified as helpful for reentry into practice include 12-step program participation, random drug screens, and sponsorship on a peer-assisted support group. The student must also provide medical clearance from the appropriate individual coordinating the therapeutic intervention and evidence of current, active nursing licensure if enrolled in a postlicensure program. A nursing student in active recovery from substance abuse will be monitored closely, particularly in clinical practice. Frequent evaluations will be mandated and stipulated in the contract delineating the contingencies of programmatic return.

Nursing faculty and academic administrators need to be humanistic in their approach to impaired students while removing them quickly from the clinical practice site. It is the goal of schools of nursing to ensure patient safety while promoting the student's well-being (Monroe, 2009).

Discussion of Case Using Best Practice Framework

The director of undergraduate nursing first confirmed that Lisa Jacobs's urine drug screen was positive for cocaine and that she had refused to allow the medical review officer to perform an additional drug screen on her urine sample. The director then scheduled a meeting with Ms. Jacobs. Because the use of cocaine is a crime, the director sought advice from university counsel and, as a result, asked a representative from legal counsel to attend the meeting as well. In accordance with counsel's advice, the director began by warning Ms. Jacobs that using cocaine was against the law and a serious violation of the university's code of conduct; that anything she said would be written down and reported; that it was all right if she chose not to answer any questions, but that her refusal to answer would be included in her file; and that the director would refer the matter to the office of student conduct following the meeting.

Ms. Jacobs denied using cocaine but admitted that her boyfriend snorted (inhales) cocaine. She said she did not know how it came to be in her system, and suggested that maybe she became positive via sexual intercourse. The director informed Ms. Jacobs that she would not be allowed to attend clinical rotation until the matter was resolved by the office of student conduct.

After the meeting, the director consulted with a toxicologist and the medical review officer to determine if a positive drug screen for cocaine could result from sexual intercourse. The toxicologist sent documentation to the director disputing the fact that one could become positive after intercourse. The director submitted this report to the office of student conduct with the rest of Ms. Jacobs's file. In accordance with the stated process, a student judicial hearing was held, in which Ms. Jacobs refused to participate. She was expelled from the university in accordance with the nursing college's zero tolerance policy for illegal drug use.

CRITICAL ELEMENTS TO CONSIDER

- Consult the university attorney and the dean of students.
- Offer education sessions on substance abuse to students during orientation and throughout the student experience.
- Offer faculty development sessions on substance abuse among students.
- Develop clear, comprehensive policies related to student substance abuse with multiple stakeholders (faculty, dean of students, substance abuse experts, legal counsel, clinical affiliates, and state board of nursing consultation).

CRITICAL ELEMENTS TO CONSIDER—cont'd

- Include substance abuse policy in student handbook (Refer to Chapter 26, Issues Surrounding Drug Testing and Monitoring of Students). Address methods for assessing substance abuse problems, intervention, and student follow-up (Clark, 1999).
- Provide a list of support groups for students if they suspect substance abuse in their peers.
- Designate a faculty member to become a peer assistance advisor or faculty advocate who is current and knowledgeable about substance abuse as well as serves as a liaison between professional assistance programs and the school (Monroe, 2009).
- Adhere to all policies and affiliation agreement requirements.
- Provide due process to students. Suspend from clinical activities until allegations of substance abuse are cleared.
- Keep all information related to the student's substance abuse confidential.
- Consult individual state board of nursing related to reporting requirements for registered nurses.
- Develop a reentry policy for those students who are separated from the university for substance abuse.

References

Clark, C. (1999). Substance abuse among nursing students: Establishing a comprehensive policy and procedure for faculty intervention. *Nurse Educator, 24*(2), 16–19.

Drexel University. (2009). Drug policy. Retrieved August 5, 2011, from http://www.drexel.edu/studentlife/SLhandbook.htm.

Dunn, D. (2005). Substance abuse among nurses–defining the issue. *AORN Journal, 82*(4), 573–602.

Monroe, T. (2009). Addressing substance abuse among nursing students: Development of a Prototype alternative-to-dismissal policy. *Journal of Nursing Education, 48*(5), 272–278.

CHAPTER 36

Best Practices in Addressing Students With Mental Health Issues or Psychiatric Disabilities

CASE STUDY

Mental Health

Your role: You are the chair of the nursing department.

Patrick Kelly is a 23-year-old student in the BSN program. Patrick is also a member of the university's rifle club. Patrick has had several outbursts in class that he has attributed to anxiety. You receive the following e-mail from Dr. Joseph Sadler, Patrick's clinical instructor:

> *I spoke to Patrick privately in an office this morning and informed him of my assessment that he was not prepared for clinical today. He began to cry and would not stop. I was afraid to leave him in the office alone for a minute, in fear that he would do something to himself or me. I asked him to leave and he continued to cry uncontrollably when I attempted to speak with him. He was unable to listen and he would not leave the clinical site. I was tempted to call security but I did not want to create a scene. He finally left the site after much coaxing and coaching. I have other students to educate. I cannot deal with this behavior on a busy medical unit. He is not psychologically well enough to be in the program and needs extensive counseling. I do not want him back in my group at this time.*
> *Joe Sadler, PhD, MSN, RN, adjunct clinical faculty*

Background

After receiving the e-mail, the chair of the nursing department contacts Mr. Kelly to determine if he is safe. She then contacts Dr. Sadler to arrange a meeting to discuss his observations and also conducts individual phone meetings with Mr. Kelly's other nursing faculty members to determine if they have witnessed any concerning behaviors. After meeting with Dr. Sadler and other faculty, the department chair learns that Mr. Kelly has sent several disturbing e-mails to several other nursing faculty stating that he has not slept in days. The following are some of Mr. Kelly's e-mails:

April 11, 2010, 11:34 p.m. E-mail from Patrick Kelly

I don't know if people in the department talk, but last week I had what I guess people call a nervous breakdown again, I had a pharmacology midterm and army stuff…which resulted in 4 straight days of no sleep.

April 12, 2010. E-mail from Patrick Kelly

I'm sick and tired of tossing and turning, slamming four cups of coffee, crying at night because I can't sleep, losing weight, and having breakdowns. I'm unraveling still, I'm not out of the dark, and I still need help.

April 12, 2010. E-mail from Patrick Kelly

I didn't sleep last night so that makes 5 days now, but hopefully this medication will help me get back on track, and this anxiety med will decrease my energy so I can calm down at night and not have freak-outs before tests.

The chair then arranges a meeting with dean of students to discuss how to best manage the situation. After discussing the matter with the dean of students, director of disability services, director of the counseling center, and legal counsel, it is determined that Mr. Kelly will be suspended from clinical rotations until he has a psychiatric evaluation. The dean of students communicates the interim suspension with the faculty advisor to the rifle club. The director of counseling services reaches out to Mr. Kelly to assist him with referring him to a psychiatrist. The director of counseling services and chair jointly meet with Mr. Kelly to discuss their concerns for his health.

Identifying Best Practices in Nursing Education

Nursing programs are seeing higher numbers of students with mental health and related disabilities as the number of college students with psychiatric disabilities in general has increased. College counseling centers across the United States are reporting increased frequency and greater severity of students' mental health concerns, such as depression, suicidal thoughts, sexual assaults, and personality disorders (Benton, Robertson, Tseng et al., 2003; Harper and Peterson, 2005) and the prevalence of anxiety and mood disorders has grown (Kaplan and Reed, 2004). Factors such as public awareness of mental health disorders, improved assessment and diagnosis, earlier intervention, improved treatments, and decreased stigma related to mental illness account for some of these changes (Kaplan and Reed, 2004; Silverman, 2004). Interventions, including medications, diminish symptoms and enable students with mental health disorders to be more productive and academically successful (Souma, Rickerson, and Burgstahler, 2009). In addition, greater numbers of students have been diagnosed and treated effectively in high school, leading to a higher likelihood that these students are able to enter college (Osberg, 2004).

Another factor contributing to the growing number of students with a mental health issue on campus involves the timing of psychiatric illness presentation. Psychiatric illnesses are often diagnosed in young adulthood and may very well be triggered by stressful situations germane to college life (Table 36.1). Some of the stressors that contribute to the development of mental health problems in college students include living in a new environment, sharing a confined place such as a dormitory room, peer pressure, greater academic demands, and less structure (Cook, 2007). New students are faced with these multiple changes during their transitions to college life, and they may be further magnified by the physical absence of parents, family members, and structural supports available through home life and high school. Current, emerging, or previously diagnosed mental health disabilities may or may not be disclosed to those in the university.

Nursing majors have additional pressures associated with clinical education during this stressful time. The nursing major is unique in the college or university setting in that program requirements overlap both academic and clinical health-care settings; students are required to adjust to both the university's academic requirements and conduct policies and the clinical agency's policies related to practice and professional conduct. This chapter explores the challenging decisions that must be made when nursing students have mental health or related disabilities. Although awareness of the needs of this group of students and sensitivity to potential biases by the various stakeholders involved in their education are required, faculty and administrators must also consider their relationships with, and responsibilities and obligations to, both the educational and health-care institutions. As Marks (2005) has stated, "Educators in nursing schools continue to ask whether people with disabilities have a place in the nursing profession, while the more salient question is, 'When will people with disabilities have a place in the nursing profession?'" (p. 70). Marks's comment reflects an evolving understanding

Table 36.1 Estimates of Prevalence of Common Psychiatric Conditions in Undergraduate College Students

Psychiatric disorder[1]	12%–18%
Anxiety/anxiety disorder[2]	4%–18.6%
Depression[3]	11%–14%
Eating disorders[4]	1%–3.5%
History of self-injurious behavior[5] (no suicidal intent)	17%
Suicidal thoughts in past 4 weeks by self-report [6]	2.5%

1. American College Health Association (2009a).
2. American College Health Association (2009b).
3. Eisenberg, D., Gollust, S. E., Golberstein, E., & Hefner, J. L. (2007).
4. Hudson, J. I., Hiripi, E., Pope, H. G., & Kessler, R. C. (2007).
5. Mowbray, C. T., Megivern, D., Mandiberg, J., Strauss, S., Stein, C. H., Collins, K., et al. (2006).
6. Whitlock, J., Eckenrode, J., & Silverman, D. (2006).

of diversity and disability in the profession, as well as the need to reconceptualize some of the assumptions and standards associated with nursing education and practice.

Developmental Psychiatric Disabilities

An emerging challenge for universities in general and for nursing programs, faculty, and administrators specifically, is the increasing number of students on campus with neurodevelopmental disabilities such as Asperger syndrome (VanBergeijk, Klin, and Volkmar, 2008). A large cohort of children diagnosed with a neurodevelopmental disability has reached college age; an increasing number of children explicitly diagnosed with Asperger syndrome and high-functioning autism are also being admitted to colleges based on their academic skills (VanBergeijk et al., 2008). These students often have received extensive support in high school via the Individuals with Disabilities Education Act, and may require a variety of accommodations for success in the university setting. Individuals with Asperger syndrome often have comorbid psychiatric conditions, particularly anxiety and depression, which add complexity to the challenges they may face in the social, academic, and clinical realms (VanBergeijk et al., 2008). There is minimal literature documenting the academic success or career choices of college students with neurodevelopmental disorders in general, and none has been found for nursing education specifically. However, based on these students' increased prevalence in the population (Rice, 2009), it is likely that nursing programs and faculty will encounter students with complex issues and needs related to these conditions and will need to make decisions regarding their academic and/or clinical progress.

Faculty Perspective

Sowers and Smith (2004) surveyed 88 nursing faculty from eight programs about their perceptions, knowledge, and concerns related to nursing students with disabilities. The authors suggest that more than 30 years after the passage of section 504 of the Rehabilitation Act and more than 10 years since the passage of the Americans With Disabilities Act (ADA), nursing faculty attitudes toward nursing students with disabilities continue to be barriers to student success (Sowers and Smith, 2004). This study demonstrated a critical need to educate nursing faculty concerning disability laws and regulations, the provision and implementation of disability accommodations, and students with disabilities who can and do complete academic nursing programs successfully. Many nursing faculty members, regardless of educational and clinical background, are not well equipped to teach or evaluate students with disabilities of any sort, and may have false assumptions about the interactions among disabilities, learning capabilities, academic or clinical performance, and patient safety (Selekman, 2002). Unlike primary and secondary teacher preparation programs, few, if any, faculty preparation programs include content on teaching college students with mental health disabilities. Faculty may have significant knowledge deficits regarding this population of students (Ashcroft et al., 2008). Increased knowledge and understanding of the legal and educational issues involved and consideration of the unique factors related to clinical nursing education can guide faculty members to be supportive of students who are managing their disabilities effectively, to recognize students at risk, and to refer them appropriately. However, faculty must also be cognizant of the fact that students at universities are not required to disclose mental health or related disabilities, unless they are seeking disability accommodations. Nursing faculty need to be able to identify students who may have issues emerging from mental health or similar disabilities to support student learning and concurrently minimize safety risks in both students and patients (Maheady, 1999). It is recommended that faculty refer a student to the office of disability services (ODS) when he or she suspects a disability and anticipates the clinical practice implications of an accommodation if granted (Ashcroft et al., 2008).

There is a distinct and critical difference between classroom accommodations and clinical accommodations. The ODS personnel and clinical faculty members must be knowledgeable about the influence of a clinical accommodation and its impact, if any, on patient care and patient safety. For example, although it may be quite reasonable for the ODS to establish an accommodation of extended time for completing a classroom examination, an accommodation of this nature would have serious safety implications in the clinical area if provided during medication administration and testing. There is a need for collaborative dialogue and planning between the ODS and the nursing program when nursing students are eligible for accommodations that extend to the clinical area. When a person with a mental health disability is experiencing illness symptoms that could endanger the safety or well-being of a patient in a clinical setting, there must be an emergent process to address this situation to ensure that patient safety remains a priority, as well as the safety of the student. Management of these types of situations involves clear communication and full understanding of clinical practice responsibilities as well as clinical and academic policies and federal regulations. Furthermore, it is essential to ensure that university administrators address both the rights of the student with a disability, as well as the obligation to ensure the safety of others, especially patients.

Major Stakeholders

The faculty member responsible for the clinical education of nursing majors is typically an employee or agent of the university who serves as a bridge between the university and clinical institutions. Whereas the relationship between a faculty member in the classroom and the student is quite delineated, the role of the clinical faculty member in undergraduate programs is more complex. Clinical faculty members are charged with teaching and evaluating students as they learn to care for sick patients (conducting health assessments, administering medications and treatments, and performing patient teaching). Clinical faculty members are also expected to balance the needs of patients, clinical staff, and students, while at the same time serving as faculty in the educational institution where there are expectations of adherence to both university and hospital/health-care policies. Although nursing academic administrators may fully understand clinical education and the necessary safety implications, students, university administrators, and legal counsel may be less informed about the technical standards required for nursing majors and the implications of accommodations for students with disabilities functioning in the clinical setting. University administrators and legal counsel are not clinicians and may not fully appreciate the specific safety implications of an accommodation respective to the clinical arena. More specifically, these university officers may be less informed about when a student should be removed from the clinical setting based on problems that are a function of symptoms of a psychiatric illness/disability. It is also important to understand that university officers, hospital administrators, students, clinical faculty, and nursing academic administrators all have competing interests and varying levels of knowledge related to clinical education and disability law. For this reason, it essential that nursing academic administrators collaborate with the various university officers, including the ODS director, dean of students, and university counsel to discuss the nuances of clinical education in the context of clinical accommodations. This group should be knowledgeable about the legal aspects of clinical education, the rights and responsibilities of students with a disability, and the management issues and decisions related to behaviors of students with disabilities in the clinical environment. An accommodation minimizes the impact of a disability and allows students to fully participate in the educational process (Gardner and Suplee, 2010). Clinical accommodations may result in modifications in a clinical practice site and/or role function of the student. Such accommodations are to be weighed against the requirements of that setting. The legal decisions related to accommodations are grounded in the legal interpretation of the ADA.

Legal Background

Since the passage of the Americans With Disabilities Act of 1990, a variety of issues and considerations have emerged (Osberg, 2004). Universities are subject to the ADA and section 504 of the Rehabilitation Act of 1973, which prohibit discrimination against individuals on the basis of a disability in employment, state and local government, public accommodations, commercial facilities, transportation, telecommunications, or in programs conducted and funded by the federal government. These laws also require that reasonable accommodations be made to provide individuals with disabilities equal opportunities.

Accommodations for people with disabilities are those situational changes that minimize or eliminate the impact of a disability, allowing the individual equal access to the university's courses, programs, and activities and providing equal employment. A reasonable accommodation is one that does not require a substantial change or alteration of an essential element of a program or position, and one that does not impose an undue burden on the university (Drexel University, 2010). Students must be able to participate in the educational program "in spite of rather than except for their disability" (Helms, Jorgensen, and Anderson, 2006, p. 192). This chapter reflects the experiences of the authors and their suggestion that decisions about disability accommodations for students who have mental health and related disabilities have presented a substantial management challenge.

Discussion of Case Using Best Practice Framework

Recall this chapter's case study. Dr. Sadler did not manage this situation based on best practices. Fortunately, Mr. Kelly was not hurt. Dr. Sadler appeared more focused on resuming his clinical day with his other students than on Mr. Kelly's immediate mental health issues. This may be because he was ill equipped to manage Mr. Kelly's mental health needs and did not recognize the serious nature of Mr. Kelly's behavior. As cited in Ashcroft et al. (2008), few, if any, faculty preparation programs include content on teaching college students with mental health disabilities. It is for this reason that faculty, particularly adjunct clinical faculty, may have significant knowledge deficits regarding this population of students. It is incumbent on academic nursing administrators to create faculty development programs and policies that attend to students with mental health disabilities as addressed in this chapter. In this case, it would be prudent for Dr. Sadler to escort Mr. Kelly to psychological counseling and notify the department chair or appropriate person immediately.

Student-Directed Accommodation Decisions

To ensure ADA compliance, most universities have established specific policies and procedures for handling requests from students and employees for reasonable accommodations. Often management of these policies and procedures is vested in a central university office, the ODS. It can be assumed that individuals with disabilities have met the criteria for admission to whatever program he or she applied or for employment at the university. In order to obtain accommodation for an academic program, students with disabilities must first disclose their disabilities to the ODS. The student must provide the ODS with the documentation it needs to confirm the existence of the specific disability condition in order to assist the student in obtaining accommodations to fulfill his or her educational requirements (Helms et al., 2006). The ODS will also seek information from the faculty or program leader to confirm the requirements of the course or program. The ODS can determine that the condition does not amount to a disability and can deny the request, at which time the best practice is for the rejection letter to request the submission of any additional information that the student believes might make the ODS change its decision. Once the ODS determines that a disability is involved and the person is eligible for an accommodation (known as a qualified individual), the ODS engages in an interactive discussion to devise a plan that is acceptable to the ODS, the university and the student. The ADA stipulates that the individual needing services is responsible for the cost associated with the diagnosis and assessment of the disability (Drexel University, 2010).

An accommodation verification letter (AVL), issued by the ODS following the interactive discussion, is used as the communication tool to inform faculty and staff of the reasonable accommodations that have been approved for the particular student. The AVL is specific and precise and assures the student nothing other than what is specifically stated in the letter, so it eliminates any guesswork or discretion by the faculty or staff (which could then readily be perceived as unfair by students not receiving those benefits) (Fig. 36.1). Once an AVL is issued to a student by the ODS, it is the student's responsibility to share that AVL with faculty or administrators if the student wants to receive the approved accommodations. If the student never shares the AVL with any of his or her professors, then neither the university nor any of the professors assigned to teach the student will be expected or required to provide any accommodations. In fact without an AVL, faculty should never provide students with disability accommodations of any kind.

It must be noted that faculty and staff who receive the AVL, which lists the approved accommodations, are not provided with information on the underlying disability. Under the Family Educational Rights and Privacy Act (FERPA), the ODS is not permitted to share the details of a student's disability with anyone at the university unless there is a legitimate education interest. Beyond FERPA, most ODS offices consider disability information confidential and often require a student's consent before the ODS will share the details of the student's disability with anyone other than the student. An academic administrator of the nursing program will also have no knowledge of the student's underlying disability.

University-Directed Accommodations Decisions

Although many students with a disability will register with the ODS, others choose not to disclose a disability; this may be the case for students with mental health disabilities, who are concerned about stigma and believe that they will not be

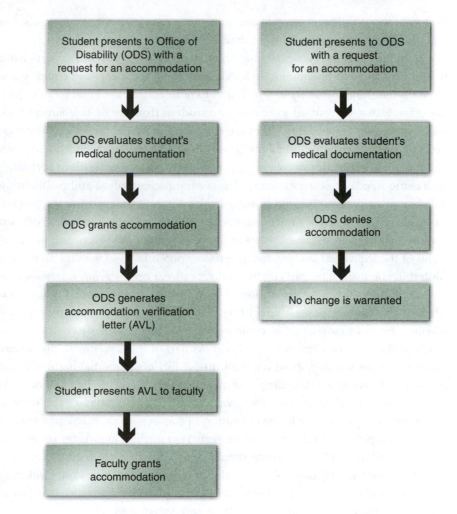

Figure 36.1 Disability accommodation process.

treated fairly. When nursing students with undisclosed conditions experience mental health symptoms and exhibit distress in the classroom and/or the clinical area, a different type of problem solving is required involving a more complex set of stakeholder considerations. For example, faculty may not be clear about how to manage an emergency situation for a student who is experiencing a psychiatric crisis. It is a best practice for a university to have an emergency student protocol in place to assist faculty in supporting the student who is an imminent danger to him- or herself. It is important that faculty members be aware of distress signals, methods of immediate intervention, and sources of help for students. Few programs appear to have such protocols (Cook, 2007), but these are necessary to protect the safety and integrity of students with emerging mental health problems.

Protocols should offer clear guidance to faculty in recognizing student distress and directing students to an appropriate intervention.

A student may not recognize that he or she is not well enough to participate in a clinical rotation providing care for sick, vulnerable patients and could refuse to take a temporary leave from the clinical experience. At the same time, university officials may be reticent to remove the student from his or her clinical rotation, as they may be fearful that they are violating the student's rights or unnecessarily harming their educational progress. Clinical faculty teaching students with emerging mental health problems have other, competing obligations including addressing needs of other students, maintaining patient safety, and maintaining collaborative relationships with nursing leadership and staff at clinical agencies. In managing such at-risk student situations, faculty, nursing administrators, and institutional officials will want to act in a manner that does not violate the legal rights of the individual student and give rise to potential legal liability. To accomplish this, the institution can conduct a direct threat review prior to initiation of any involuntary leave or suspension. The objective of this review is to assess whether the student poses a direct threat to him- or herself or to others, and whether the institution could or could not provide a reasonable accommodation that would reduce or eliminate that threat. As part of this assessment, the institution determines whether there is a high probability of substantial harm and not just a slightly increased, speculative, or remote risk. The institution will need to conduct an individualized and objective assessment about whether the student can continue to participate in the institution's programs safely, based on a reasonable medical judgment relying on the most current medical knowledge or the best objective evidence. The assessment should determine the nature, duration, and severity of the risk, the probability that the potential threatening injury will actually occur, and whether reasonable modifications of policies, practices, or procedures will sufficiently mitigate the risk (Lee and Abbey, 2008).

In the event that the student refuses to take a temporary leave from the clinical experience while having a mental health crisis, a university can convene a threat assessment task force with university officials made up of representatives of mental health counseling, public safety, student life, legal counsel, and nursing academic administration to evaluate the situation and the student's fitness for clinical educational responsibilities at this time and to consider whether an involuntary leave or temporary suspension from specific educational activities is appropriate based on an individualized assessment of the situation. Proper documentation that this assessment process was followed will help the institution defend itself in the event of legal challenge.

In an effort to manage students in crisis effectively, Drexel University has developed protocols on substance abuse and emergency student situations to guide faculty when students are in such a situation. These protocols serve as a resource in assisting faculty during interventions with students who may be in imminent danger to him- or herself or others. The need for management protocols for nursing students in crisis, particularly those with suspected mental health disabilities, cannot be underestimated. Academic nursing programs need to be cognizant of the safety of the student and the patient, as well as the student's ADA rights as they pertain to this situation, especially nursing students with mental health problems who have responsibilities in the clinical area.

Nursing Faculty Decisions

Nursing faculty members need to be comfortable addressing the technical standards or essential job competencies required for nursing students to perform patient care safely in the clinical area. Having an open, supportive dialogue about the ODS and the management of students who have a mental health disability may encourage students to seek an AVL and assist them with managing their learning process with support. In addition, nursing faculty need to learn how to have the kinds of conversations with students that employers have with employees related to essential functions of their job. Nursing students must be able to independently, with or without reasonable accommodation, meet technical standards related to (1) observation; (2) communication; (3) motor skills; (4) intellectual, conceptual, and quantitative abilities; (5) essential behavioral and social attributes; and (6) ability to manage stressful situations. For example, the student must be able to adapt to and function effectively to stressful situations in both the classroom and clinical settings, including emergency situations. Students will encounter multiple stressors while in their nursing programs. Rather than focus on the specific disabling conditions, medications, or treatment, faculty can manage a situation best by focusing on the student's behavior or function. Furthermore, when faculty encounter problems in the clinical setting when a student engages in problematic behavior or is in crisis, it is important for the faculty member to be proactive and engage the student about counseling and the ODS and its services. It is also a best practice for schools of nursing to specify these behavioral standards that they view as essential for a student to participate in a program.

Without a thorough working knowledge of disability law, nursing faculty members may devolve to their clinical nursing roles and attempt to diagnose or clinically intervene with a student. However, as noted elsewhere in this book, the legal case law clearly cautions faculty that doing so could well be held to create a special relationship that then imposes special responsibilities and liabilities. Rather than helping, faculty may be unintentionally hurting the student or at least increasing the likelihood of harm occurring to the student or others. For example, in one case, a clinical faculty member spoke to a particular student on the phone almost daily in an effort to help the student address her anxiety related to clinical performance. When the faculty member in question placed the student on clinical warning, the student felt betrayed and became depressed; the student had perceived the faculty member as a close friend and confidant. In this situation, it would have been best for the clinical faculty member to have referred the student to the student counseling center, rather than have attempted to counsel the student, as this could be considered a special relationship. It is best for faculty to refer students to the university counseling center, as would be expected from faculty members from other academic disciplines. Psychiatric/mental health nursing faculty members are especially cautioned not to establish a special relationship with students. In the academic setting, the faculty member is a teacher not a therapist (Cook, 2007).

Nursing faculty members also have an ethical duty to protect the public. The majority of clinical experiences are outside the college and in hospitals, and other clinical settings. As such, nursing programs, students, and faculty are subject to the procedures and policies of that institution. Today, distance learning adds yet another dimension to addressing anyone with mental health issues and the environment where student learning is taking place. In particular, the nursing student with mental health problems may be at a clinical site that is quite a distance from the student's respective college in today's distance learning environment. In this scenario, clinical supervision presents a new set of challenges for students with mental health issues, as well as for the faculty member attempting to supervise the student from a distance. The faculty member is not on site and is therefore unable to recognize the student who may be exhibiting mental health problems. The faculty member may make site visits only a few times a semester or may rely on a preceptor's observations. In this situation, the student is not being supervised as closely as he or she would be supervised in a usual clinical educational setting. Therefore, it would be important for the faculty member to orient the preceptor to contact him or her and document any signs that might indicate student mental health distress. Furthermore, the faculty member should be sure to share the university's emergency protocol guide and related policies with the preceptor and/or clinical faculty member, as well as other relevant policies in orientation.

In addition, faculty should understand that disability accommodations should not be provided to any student, unless a current, signed AVL has first been produced. It is also important for faculty to appreciate what is required to be kept confidential, and what is not, under both FERPA and the Health Insurance Portability and Accountability Act (HIPAA). The ability to share information is complicated if the disclosure is to be made outside of the institution (e.g., hospital to academic institution) or academic program (e.g., nursing faculty to university administrator). Many faculty incorrectly believe that FERPA and HIPAA absolutely prohibit such disclosures, and for that reason fail to make timely and critically important reports of behaviors of concern to institutional administrators. In fact, it is permissible to disclose information in connection with an emergency if knowledge of information is necessary to protect the health or safety of the student or other individuals. A failure to share such information within the university results in lost opportunities for early intervention, may complicate effective management of these situations, and may result in both harm (to student or others) and liability (to faculty or university).

Decisions to Alert Public Authorities

The shooting of U.S. Representative Gabrielle Giffords in January 2011 highlights another aspect of this situation: potential harm to the public after the university has dealt with the problem internally. The alleged shooter, Jared Lee Loughner, had exhibited behavior at Pima Community College that was so erratic that it caused his suspension and ban from campus. The college had revised its student code of conduct to better identify potentially violent students after the Virginia Tech massacre in 2007, when a student fatally shot 32 teachers and students before killing himself; however, the responses and remedies ended at the geographic borders of the campus.

College officials confirmed that Loughner attended the school from the summer of 2005 through the fall of 2010. They said he was suspended for violating the college's code of conduct after five disruptions in classrooms and libraries on two different campuses and after the discovery of a YouTube video that Loughner had posted in which he claimed that the college was illegal under the U.S. Constitution. On September 29, 2010, two college police officers delivered a letter of suspension to Loughner at the house where he lived with his parents. After meeting with administrators October 4, the college sent a second letter October 7, indicating Loughner could return to campus only if he resolved his violations and obtained "mental health clearance indicating, in the opinion of a mental health professional, his presence at the College does not present a danger to himself or others," according to a statement issued by the college.

Under Arizona law, anyone can call the county or regional health authorities with concerns about a person's mental health, and authorities are required to send out mobile units to assess the person's condition. The person who files a request for commitment must list the names of two witnesses who can attest to the subject's behavior, although they do not have to sign the document themselves. Unlike the laws in other states that allow involuntary commitment only if people pose a danger to themselves or others, or if they are profoundly disabled by their mental illness to the point of being unable to take care of themselves, Arizona apparently allows for involuntary commitment if someone is deteriorating from a mental illness and could benefit from treatment.

Laws such as these do not themselves impose obligations on individuals perceiving the mental health problem, but they do allow the observer to share the information officially and in a way that is privileged, protecting them from liability for having made a slanderous statement against a person or having violated their privacy. Under Arizona law, any one of Loughner's classmates or teachers at Pima Community College who were concerned about his behavior could have contacted local officials and asked that he be evaluated for mental illness and potentially committed for psychiatric treatment. However, none did. It remains to be seen whether any of the victims of the shootings will attempt to impose legal liability upon the college for having failed to notify the public authorities (Szabo and Lloyd, 2011).

Problem-Solving Strategies

Situational accommodation decisions would definitely benefit from the development of clear policies for both faculty and students. It would also be useful to develop comprehensive education about (1) the role of the administrator in facilitating the integration of students into the educational community; (2) the different types of accommodations that can address people's disabling conditions, helping them to be successful in completing educational requirements; (3) the best approaches to management of communication and emergency challenges; and (4) what types of campus resources are available to students with a disability. In addition, a comprehensive disabilities education program needs to be developed for nursing academic administrators, faculty members, and students to interpret clearly their legal obligations, rights, and remedies (Hirshfield and Woolf, 2005).

Universities can support their faculty members, more specifically their nursing faculty members, by making sure that they have clear policies and procedures to manage the types of emergency situations that involve the rights of the person with a disability, the care and safety of patients, the care and safety of the student at risk, and the safety of other students involved. For example, faculty development sessions can be offered to new faculty members to acquaint them with behaviors that warrant concern as well as the appropriate action to take in these situations, with periodic reinforcement of this information to ensure awareness and accessibility of these possibilities (Table 36.2).

The Buckley Amendment to FERPA was designed to establish the rights of students, inspect and review their education records, prevent the release of educational records to third parties without permission of the student, and provide guidelines for the correction of inaccurate or misleading data through formal and informal hearings. Students also have the right to file complaints with the FERPA office concerning alleged failures by the university to comply with FERPA. The university's interpretation of FERPA and its emergency exceptions should be emphasized in the university's polices and faculty development sessions (Baker, 2005).

Table 36.2 Faculty Recommendations on Managing a Student With Mental Health Issues

1. Recognize signs of psychological/behavioral distress and/or substance abuse.
2. Talk with the student privately about your concerns arising from the student's recent behavior or conduct. Share your observations and make an assessment of the urgency of the situation. *During this discussion the faculty member should focus on describing the behavior or conduct that is causing concern, rather than the suspected causes of that behavior or conduct (i.e., psychiatric illness). Even where strongly indicated, the faculty member should avoid diagnosis of psychological illness until the student mentions it.*
3. Determine if the situation requires immediate intervention. *The most basic criteria are whether the student is an immediate danger to himself, herself, or others. If this is the case, the faculty member needs to contact security or public safety representatives immediately. It is imperative that the student receive appropriate evaluation and subsequent treatment.*
4. Do not isolate yourself when dealing with a student with a serious mental health issue. Consult with academic nursing administrators and staff at the university's counseling center and legal department.

Adapted from Ashcroft, T., Chernomas, W., Davis, P., Dean, R., Seguire, M., Shapiro, C., et al. (2008). Nursing students with disabilities: One faculty's journey. International Journal of Nursing Education Scholarship, 5(1), 1–26.

Summary

It is imperative that nursing faculty bring attention to this very significant issue of educating nursing students who are living with a mental health or related disability. Although many of these students will manage their disabilities with no need for accommodations, there will continue to be a need to manage emergent problem situations related to mental health status of nursing students, particularly as these situations influence clinical practice. It is clear that faculty would benefit from both education opportunities and protocols related to the management of accommodations for nursing students with mental health or related disabilities to support the decisional procedures for both academic and clinical health-care settings.

CRITICAL ELEMENTS TO CONSIDER

- Consult the university attorney. (*Note:* University administrators and legal counsel are not clinicians and may not fully appreciate the specific safety implications of an accommodation respective to the clinical arena.)
- Consult the office of disability services.
- Consult with the student counseling office.
- Know university policies and procedures as well as the appropriate state laws. The university's interpretation of FERPA and its emergency exceptions should be emphasized.
- Initiate an emergency protocol for any reference to harm self or others or extreme emotional distress.

Continued

CRITICAL ELEMENTS TO CONSIDER—cont'd

- Focus on the academic performance and conduct of the student only, and do not diagnose the student.
- Contact the director or dean or department chair regarding the distressed student.
- Refer the student to the student counseling center.
- Do not provide an accommodation without official accommodation from the office of disability.
- Be familiar with the nursing program's technical standards.
- Implement preventive strategies such as e-mails related to student counseling services during times of high stress such as midterms and finals.
- Offer faculty development sessions to faculty related to best practices in addressing students with mental health issues and psychiatric disabilities; particularly warning signs that warrant attention.

Acknowledgment

The authors would like to acknowledge Laure Bachich Ergin, formerly Deputy General Counsel, Drexel University, and now Associate Vice President and Senior Counsel, University of Delaware, for her contributions in developing Drexel University's policies in this very complex area of educational law and her review of the chapter.

References

American College Health Association. (2009a). *American College Health Association—National College Health Assessment II: Reference group executive summary fall 2009.* Linthicum, MD: ACHA. Retrieved August 5, 2011, from http://www.acha-ncha.org/reports_ACHA-NCHAII.html

American College Health Association. (2009b). *American College Health Association—National College Health Assessment II: Reference group executive summary spring 2009.* Linthicum, MD: ACHA. Retrieved August 5, 2011, from http://www.acha-ncha.org/reports_ACHA-NCHAII.html

Andreon, D., & Durocher, J. S. (2007). Evaluating the college transition needs of individuals with high functioning autism spectrum disorders. *Intervention in School and Clinic, 42,* 271–279.

Arndt, M. E. (2004). Educating nursing students with disabilities: One nurse educator's journey from questions to clarity. *Journal of Nursing Education, 43*(5), 204.

Ashcroft, T., Chernomas, W., Davis, P., et al. (2008). Nursing students with disabilities: One faculty's journey. *International Journal of Nursing Education Scholarship, 5*(1), 1–26.

Baker, T. R. (2005). Notifying parents following a college student suicide attempt: A review of case law and FERPA, and recommendations for practice. *National Association of Student Personnel Administrators Journal, 42,* 513–533.

Benton, S. A., Robertson, J. M., Wen-Chih, T., et al. (2003). Changes in counseling center client problems across 13 years. *Professional Psychology: Research and Practice, 34*(1), 66–72.

Center for Education & Employment Law. (2001). *Higher education law in America* (2nd ed.). Birmingham, AL: Oakstone Legal & Business.

Cook, L. J. (2007). Striving to help college students with mental health issues. *Journal of Psychosocial Nursing, 45*(4), 40–44.

Drexel University. (2010). *Drexel University College Handbook 2010–2011.* Philadelphia: Drexel University College of Nursing and Health Professions. Retrieved from http://www.drexel.edu/cnhp/nursing/undergrad_handbooks.asp

Eisenberg, D., Gollust, S. E., Golberstein, E., et al. (2007). Prevalence and correlates of depression and suicidality among university students. *American Journal of Orthopsychiatry, 77*(4), 534–542.

Gardner, M. R., & Suplee, P. D. (2010). *Handbook of clinical teaching in nursing and health sciences.* Sudbury, MA: Jones & Bartlett.

Harper, R., & Peterson, M. (2005). Mental health issues and college students. *NACADA Clearinghouse of Academic Advising Resources.* Retrieved August 5, 2011, from http://www.nacada.ksu.edu/Clearinghouse/AdvisingIssues/Mental-Health.htm

Helms, L., Jorgensen, J., & Anderson, M. A. (2006). Disability law and nursing education: An update. *Journal of Professional Nursing, 22*(30), 190–196.

Hirshfield, S. J., & Woolf, S. R. (2005). Sex, religion, and politics: New challenges in discrimination law. *The Chronicle of Higher Education, 51*(38), B10.

Hudson, J. I., Hiripi, E., Pope, H. G., et al. (2007). The prevalence and correlates of eating disorders in the national comorbidity survey replication. *Biological Psychiatry, 61*(3), 348–358.

Kaplan, B., & Reed, M. (2004, March). College student mental health: Plan designs, utilization, trends and costs. *Student Health Spectrum,* 31–33. Retrieved from http://www.chickering.com/uploads/documents/spectrum/2004%20Spring%20-%20Mental%20Health%20On%20Campus.pdf

Lee, B. A., & Abbey, G. E. (2008). College and university students with mental disabilities: Legal and policy issues. *The Journal of College and University Law, 34*(2), 349–391.

Lindsay, C. L. (2005). *The college student's guide to the law.* Dallas, TX: Taylor Trade.

Maheady, D. (1999). Jumping through hoops, walking on egg shells: The experiences of nursing students with disabilities. *Journal of Nursing Education, 38*(4), 162–170.

Marks, B. (2007). Cultural competence revisited: Nursing students with disabilities. *Journal of Nursing Education, 46*(2), 70–74.

Mowbray, C. T., Megivern, D., Mandiberg, J., et al. (2006). Campus mental health services: Recommendations for change. *American Journal of Orthopsychiatry, 76*(2), 226–237.

Osberg, T. M. (2004). A business case for increasing college mental health services. *Behavioral Health Management, 24*(5), 33–36.

Rice, C. (2009, December 18). Prevalence of autism spectrum disorders. *Morbidity and Mortality Weekly Report.* Retrieved from http://www.cdc.gov/mmwr/preview/mmwrhtml/ss5810a1.htm

Selekman, J. (2002). Nursing students with learning disabilities. *Journal of Nursing Education, 41*(8), 334–339.

Silverman, M. M. (2004). College student suicide prevention: Background and blueprint for action. *Student Health Spectrum,* 13–20.

Souma, A., Rickerson, N., & Burgstahler, S, (2009). Academic accommodations for students with psychiatric disabilities. *Do-It, University of Washington,* 1–4.

Sowers, J., & Smith, M. R. (2004). Nursing faculty members' perceptions, knowledge, and concerns about students with disabilities. *Journal of Nursing Education, 43*(5), 213–218.

Szabo, L., & Lloyd, J. (2011, January 13). Loughner could have been committed under Arizona law. *USA Today.* Retrieved from http://www.usatoday.com/yourlife/health/2011-01-13-arizonalaws13_st_N.htm

VanBergeijk, E., Klin, A., & Volkmar, F. (2008). Supporting more able students on the autism spectrum: College and beyond. *Journal of Autism and Developmental Disorders, 38,* 1359–1370.

Van Dusen, W. R. (2004). Basic guidelines for faculty and staff: A simple step-by-step approach for compliance. Retrieved June 20, 2009, from http://www.nacada.ksu.edu/Resources/FERPA-Overview.htm

Whitlock, J., Eckenrode, J., & Silverman, D. (2006). Self-injurious behaviors in a college population. *Pediatrics, 117,* 1939–1948. Retrieved from http://www.pediatrics.org/cgi/content/full/117/6/1939

Best Practices in Creating a Safe Nursing Education Classroom and Clinical Environment

CASE STUDY

Creating a Safe Environment

Your role: You are Professor Smith, the faculty member assigned to teach principles of nursing.

Michael Babaya is a 38-year-old international nursing student in the accelerated nursing program in his first clinical course, Principles of Nursing. Mr. Babaya has been on clinical warning for lack of clinical preparation and failure to meet clinical objectives related to basic skills. You initiated a learning contract with Mr. Babaya and the laboratory faculty member has also worked extensively with Mr. Babaya, but the results have been less than what is necessary to continue in the program. On the last clinical day, Mr. Babaya confronts you and demands to know if he passed the course. You respond by saying that his clinical performance is best addressed in your office, privately, rather than on the clinical unit, and offer to meet him there in 20 minutes. Mr. Babaya raises his voice and begins to yell, "I demand to know *now*. Do you hear me!" He approaches you as he is making this statement, and for the first time, you are afraid for your safety and start backing away. As he continues to tell you how important it is for him to pass this course, concerned staff members call security, who come immediately and escort Mr. Babaya off the unit, telling him to calm down, get a grip, and go home. Security returns and records in an official incident report what had happened.

The next evening, Mr. Babaya appears at your office at 7:30 p.m., where you are alone, working on end-of-term paperwork. Standing first in the doorway and then entering and sitting in a chair, he tries to convince you to pass him in the course. You are patient with him, and sympathetic, and you gently explain why you cannot change his grade. As the discussion ensues, he becomes increasingly angry. He stands up, leans over your desk, and in a rising voice exclaims, "You have to pass me! I quit my job and gave up everything for this program!" You are alarmed by his conduct, quite frightened, and hope that someone else is in the area and will respond.

Background

As noted in other chapters, more and more students with behavioral health issues are arriving at universities. Higher education provides a totally different environment for these students than did high school: not only does the student have more autonomy and less oversight, but also the duties owed to the student by the institution are far fewer. Moreover, core tenants of higher education are tolerance and respect for individuality and differences, meaning that "acting out" can be acceptable, and even comes close to being a right. The combination of these factors has the potential to cause uncomfortable, even threatening, situations not just in the classroom, but also anywhere—on campus and off—and anytime.

A violent event requires the combination of a person with some (high or low) predisposing potential for violent behavior, a situation with elements that create some risk of violent events, and usually a triggering event (Reis & Ross, 1993). Under the law, people have the right to be free of the threat of violence, and this is protected by both the criminal law and the civil law of torts (see Chapter 2). A person commits an assault if he or she puts someone else in reasonable fear of being harmed, and the actor intended either to do the act that causes the fear or to cause the fear itself. Words alone are not enough, but they are if they are coupled with an act that suggests the ability to carry out the threat.

Virtually all student codes of conduct prohibit students from acts of violence, and the sanctions for violation are severe. But codes will never deter emotion. On Friday, February 12, 2010, University of Alabama Huntsville Professor Amy Bishop opened fire at a faculty meeting, killing three colleagues and wounding three others. Allegations emerged that a denial of tenure for Bishop played a role in the shootings (Bartlett and Wilson, 2010). The tragedies at Virginia Tech and Northern Illinois University have focused enormous attention on mental health issues and violence among college-aged students. In two separate attacks in 2007 in Blacksburg, Virginia, 32 Virginia Tech students and faculty were killed before the gunman, who was a senior English major, killed himself, resulting in what has become not just the deadliest school shooting, but the deadliest shooting rampage by a single gunman in all of U.S. history. Less than a year later, in February 2008, on the campus of Northern Illinois University, a 27-year-old former graduate sociology student shot 22 victims and killed 6 (including himself) ("6 Shot Dead," 2008). In 2002, a nursing student shot three nursing instructors to death at the University of Arizona and then killed himself ("Gunman in Arizona," 2002). As these tragic events indicate, faculty and administrators have good reason to be concerned for their safety.

The Higher Education Security Act requires universities to report the previous year's crime statistics to the entire campus community (Siegel, 1994). The university must also report whether any of the crimes were motivated by race, gender, sexual orientation, religion, ethnicity, or disability, otherwise known as hate crimes. This will tell consumers (potential and current students, faculty and staff) how safe the area is, but it is nothing more than historical fact. "What is perhaps most troubling about campus crime is that the majority of the incidents, excluding theft but including rape and other sexual assaults, are impulsive acts committed by students themselves, according to nationwide studies conducted by Towson State University's Campus Violence Prevention Center. Students are responsible for 80% of campus crime, although rarely with weapons" (Siegel, 1994). Because universities are often regarded as protected environments, incidents of violence are particularly shocking for the college campus and extended community. "There are many types of campus violence—including rape, assault, fighting, hazing, dating violence, sexual harassment, hate and bias related violence, stalking, rioting, disorderly conduct, property crime, and suicide" (Langford, 2004, p. 2). Today, students learn about campus crime statistics and ways to ensure their safety in university orientation and other programs.

In response to acts and threats of violence, "user-friendly" harassment policies and complaint procedures are now common on university campuses. To minimize events of (and potential liability for) harassment, colleges and universities should make their antiharassment policies and procedures clear; publish and disseminate them as widely as possible; make sure there are hotlines in place to which reports can safely and effectively be made; and provide training to potential complaint handlers and faculty, staff, and students (Alger, 1998).

Identifying Best Practices in Nursing Education

Campus violence is a complex problem, and there are no easy answers. It cannot be solved by a one-time program or a single department, nor is there a one size-fits-all blueprint for successful efforts. Senior administrators must exercise leadership by establishing and supporting a long-term, collaborative process to create and sustain a comprehensive, strategic, coordinated approach to preventing violence and promoting safety on campus. (Langford, 2004, p. 6)

Faculty and administration need to be cognizant of triggering events that would cause a student with a propensity for violence to become violent. "A *triggering event* is a description of the immediate circumstances surrounding an act of violence and is not intended to convey a lack of agency or responsibility by perpetrators but rather to address conditions that may lead to violence" (Reiss and Ross, 1993).

Increased vigilance and preventive measures during times of high stress—such as during midterm and final examinations—are recommended. For nursing faculty, the award of a clinical warning notice or grade of clinical failure would also constitute a triggering event. During these times, faculty are cautioned to take preventive measures, such as alerting one's supervisor that a student will be receiving a failing grade. The faculty member should meet with the student during a high-traffic time when many faculty and staff members will be outside the conference room or office. The member should notify faculty and staff that he or she will be meeting with a student to deliver bad news. If the faculty member suspects that the student may become violent, he or she should notify security to be on standby as a precautionary measure. The university should also teach faculty how to identify behaviors that are consistent with harassment or potential violence, and it should also emphasize its zero tolerance for workplace harassment and violence (Equal Employment Opportunity Commission, 2010). Faculty and students should also be educated to report concerning behavior such as severe depression, anger outbursts, and fascination with weapons to university public safety officials. Equally important, complainants should be treated with respect and compassion, provided anonymity when possible, and given protection from retaliation or further harm.

One of the most serious present-day problems related to college safety is the peer harassment of a student or group of students. The harassment may be on the grounds of race, national origin, ethnicity, gender, sexual orientation, religion, disability, or other factors such as fraternity hazing (Kaplin and Lee, 2007). As discussed in Chapter Thirteen, to hold a university liable for monetary damages for harassment or injuries, the student would have to demonstrate that university officials had actual knowledge of the student harassment and were deliberately indifferent to the reports (U.S. Department of Education, Office for Civil Rights, 1997). After a university receives notice of the harassing conduct, it has a duty under Title IX to take some action to prevent the further harassment or harm of the student or students (Kaplin and Lee, 2007). Student-to-student harassment is also the most common form of sexual harassment on campus. Eighty percent of the students who experienced sexual harassment on college campuses were harassed by a student or a former student (Silva and Hill, 2005). The American Association of University Women (AAUW) (2005) also showed that at colleges and universities "nearly one-third [of students] experience some form of physical harassment, such as being touched, grabbed, or forced to do something sexual" (p. 8).

Collegewide prevention programs, and procedures by which there can be prompt and direct intervention, are critical in addressing and minimizing student-student harassment and violence. Harassment policies need to be widely publicized, as do the universities' methods for reporting and responding to incidents of harassment.

Discussion of Case Using Best Practice Framework

In this chapter's case study, it is important that the faculty member speak in a low tone, be empathetic to the student, and call him by his name. You can discuss how difficult the program is, how many students have difficulty in the first term, and how often students suffering from the anxiety and stress can be helped by seeking assistance from student health. You can promise to review his case again with the laboratory faculty member, and speak again with him the following day.

It is always best if faculty members have their offices arranged in a manner so that their chair is close to the door. With this arrangement, the faculty member can exit the office quickly if necessary. It is best if faculty members do not stay in their offices late at night or early in the morning, when the campus is isolated. If it is absolutely necessary to work late, then the faculty member should lock the office door and alert public safety or security that he or she is alone in the office.

Faculty should be particularly vigilant after giving students bad news. If possible, faculty office buildings should be locked during the evening hours. In this case, you should have declined to speak with the student about his situation, but scheduled a meeting with him first thing in the morning; if he refused that appointment, then you should have called security right then, before he had a chance to get upset. Now that this has occurred, you need to report him to the student conduct committee and the office of public safety for uncivil and threatening behavior. It was particularly concerning that Mr. Babaya appeared at the faculty member's office in the evening, when no one else was in the building, and could not control his anger on the clinical unit. It is difficult to predict if Mr. Babaya will resort to physical violence; however, his recent behavior is of great concern and warrants further investigation and action.

An emergency student protocol guide is also warranted in guiding the nursing faculty on the proper procedures in the event of a violent or potentially violent incident involving students or other personnel, these protocols serve as a resource in assisting faculty during interventions with students who may be in imminent danger to him- or herself or others. The need for management protocols for nursing students in crisis must be underscored. Refer to Chapters Twenty-Three and Thirty-Five for more in-depth discussions.

In cases in which a student poses a significant safety risk, a university will convene a threat assessment task force with university officials made up of representatives of mental health counseling, public safety, student life, legal counsel, and possibly nursing academic administration (depending on the case) to evaluate the situation. They will consider the student's fitness for educational responsibilities at this time and whether an involuntary leave or temporary suspension from specific educational activities is appropriate based on an individualized assessment of the situation. Proper documentation that this assessment process was followed will help the institution defend itself in the event of legal challenge. In the event of a violent act, the police would be notified and take appropriate *action*. If the alleged perpetrator and victim are still on campus, as in *Kelly v. Yale University* (2003), the university is obligated to provide academic or residential accommodations to prevent possible future harassment or harm.

Case Findings

In this chapter's Case Study, the faculty member informed Mr. Babaya that she could not make any decisions regarding his grade at that time and that she needed to review his clinical preparation sheets. She calmly told Mr. Babaya that she had to complete all the paperwork she was working on that night, told him that she would meet with him tomorrow, and asked him to leave her office, and he complied with her request. The faculty member immediately closed and locked her door and called campus security. The security officer completed a report and escorted the faculty member to her car. The case was submitted to the student conduct committee and office of public safety. Based on the two incidents (clinical unit and office incidents) and clinical failure, the committee dismissed Mr. Babaya from the accelerated nursing program and included a "no readmit" notice in the file. The office of public safety sent Mr. Babaya written communication that he was no longer permitted on campus and to cease and desist all communications with Professor Smith.

Summary

Unfortunately, there are not always red flags (e.g., harassment, anger management issues) to predict violent behavior; therefore, a comprehensive university approach that combines education, sound code of conduct policies, vigilance, and clear reporting mechanisms are in the best interest of the college community. Harassment and other violent behavior compromise the sense of community to which most universities aspire (Kaplin and Lee, 2007). Faculty, students, and staff all desire a safe campus environment. Individuals want to go about their daily lives without fear of physical, emotional, or psychological harm. Personal safety is a basic human need that must be upheld; therefore, violence prevention and safety promotion should be seen as a broader mission of all universities (Bickel and Lake, 1999; Roark, 1993).

(**HELPFUL RESOURCES**
• "Primary Prevention: Stopping Campus Violence Before It Starts." The Higher Education Center for Alcohol, Drug Abuse, and Violence Prevention: http://www.higheredcenter.org/files/prevention_updates/may2010.pdf

HELPFUL RESOURCES—cont'd

- American College Health Association: http://www.acha.org/info_resources/guidelines.cfm
- Higher Education Center Resources: http://www.higheredcenter.org/pubs/violence.html
- The National Sexual Violence Resource Center (NSVRC): http://www.nsvrc.org
- Security on Campus: http://www.securityoncampus.org

CRITICAL ELEMENTS TO CONSIDER

- Address attitudes and perceptions that contribute to violence through education, curriculum integration, and other efforts (Langford, 2004).
- Offer counseling to students at times of high stress, such as during midterm and final examinations.
- Deliver bad news to students during normal office hours in a private office located in a high-traffic area.
- Do not keep concerns related to student harassment to yourself. Alert your supervisor and public safety.
- Alert security ahead of time if you suspect that a student, faculty, or staff member may be violent when you deliver bad news.
- Alert security when you are working late, then lock your office and take necessary safety precautions.
- Educate faculty, students, and staff about the need to report concerning behavior to public safety.
- Educate and promote bystander intervention (Langford, 2004).
- Convey clear expectations for conduct among students, faculty, and staff (Langford, 2004).
- Create and disseminate comprehensive policies and procedures addressing behavior—strong enforcement of violent behavior sends a clear message about intolerance for violent behavior (Langford, 2004).
- Provide a range of support services for students, including mental health services, crisis management, and comprehensive services for victims (Langford, 2004).
- Offer campus safety classes in orientation and offer campus escort service.

Continued

CRITICAL ELEMENTS TO CONSIDER—cont'd

- Establish comprehensive alcohol and other drug prevention programs.
- Do not keep your concerns related to aggressive, disturbing, or depressive behaviors to yourself. Notify your supervisor and the office of public safety with any questions/concerns.
- Determine if a situation requires immediate intervention. (Consider whether the student is a danger to him- or herself or others. If yes, then contact security or public safety immediately.)
- If you feel uncomfortable or unsafe, trust your instincts.
- Faculty, students, and staff should register for the emergency notification system via text and e-mail on cell phone.
- Publicize victim support services on campus.
- Convene a threat assessment task force.

References

Alger, J. R. (1998, September/October). Love, lust and the law: Sexual harassment in the academy. *Academe, 34*. Retrieved July 10, 2010, from http://findarticles.com/p/articles/mi_qa3860/is_199809/ai_n8814787/?tag=content;col1

Bartlett, T., & Wilson, R. (2010, June 17). Amy Bishop is indicted in 1986 shooting death of her brother. *The Chronicle of Higher Education*. Retrieved July 25, 2010, from http://chronicle.com/article/Amy-Bishop-Is-Indicted-in-1986/65970/

Bickel, R. D., & Lake, P. F. (1999). *The rights and responsibilities of the modern university: Who assumes the risks of college life*. Durham, NC: Carolina Academic Press.

Equal Employment Opportunity Commission. (2010). Harassment. Retrieved July 10, 2010, from http://www.eeoc.gov/laws/practices/harassment.cfm

Gunman in Arizona wrote of plan to kill. (October 22, 2002). *The New York Times*. Retrieved July 25, 2010, from http://query.nytimes.com/gst/fullpage.html?res=9A02EEDD103FF932A05753C1A9649C8B63

Kaplin, W. A., & Lee, B. A. (2007). *The law of higher education* (4th ed.). San Francisco: Jossey-Bass.

Kelly v. Yale University, WL 1563424, 2003 U.S. Dist. LEXIS 4543 (D. Conn 2003).

Langford, L. (2004). Preventing violence and promoting safety in higher education settings: Overview of a comprehensive approach. The Higher Education Center for Alcohol and Other Drug Abuse and Violence Prevention. Retrieved July 25, 2010, from http://www.higheredcenter.org/files/product/violence.pdf

Reiss, A. J., Jr., & Roth, J. A. (1993). *Understanding and preventing violence: Vol. 1. Panel on the understanding and control of violent behavior*. Washington, DC: National Academy Press, National Research Council.

Roark, M. L. (1993). Conceptualizing campus violence: Definitions, underlying factors, and effects. *Journal of Student Psychotherapy, 8*(1/2), 1–27.

Siegel, D. (1994). What is behind the growth of violence on college campuses? The United States of Violence. *USA Today*. Retrieved July 25, 2010, from http://findarticles.com/p/articles/mi_m1272/is_n2588_v122/ai_15282515/

Silva, C. & Hill, E. (2005). Drawing the line on sexual harassment on campus. American Association of University Women Educational Foundation: Washington, DC: Retrieved August 6, 2011, from http://www.aauw.org/learn/research/upload/DTLFinal.pdf

6 shot dead, including gunman, at Northern Illinois University. (2008, February 14). CNN.com. Retrieved from http://www.cnn.com/2008/US/02/14/university.shooting/

U.S. Department of Education. Office for Civil Rights. (1997). *Sexual harassment guidance: Harassment of students by school employees, other students, or third parties.* Washington, DC: Author. Retrieved July 25, 2010, from http://www.ed.gov/about/offices/list/ocr/docs/sexhar00.html?

Glossary of Legal Terms

Lawyering is all about words, and lawyers use them with precision. Non-lawyers need to know what lawyers are talking about so that there can be meaningful lawyer-client communication. This glossary is not intended to provide the definitions that lawyers would use in court; rather, it describes what the words mean and is a guide to how lawyers talk. Words in **bold** are included in the glossary.

Administrative hearing – Formal process, short of going to court, in which disputes can be resolved. *Most disputes are decided without a hearing. Oftentimes, **due process** requires that there be an opportunity to be heard. This is typically a "hearing," although a "paper review" could also qualify. An administrative hearing is one that is held outside the judicial system, conducted by some administrative agency. Within a university, it can range from a student conduct board to a grievance panel to a tenure appeals committee; outside academia, it can involve the state human relations commission or the federal Environmental Protection Agency or Occupational Safety and Health Administration.*

Arbitration – Dispute resolution process that is less formal than going to court but more formal than mediation, where an arbitrator (like a judge) renders a decision. *This is a process for having disputes decided that is less formal than is available under the judicial system. It is typically agreed to in a **contract** between the **parties**. The parties agree that the arbitrator will decide the dispute. They also decide if it is to be binding, final, or appealable.*

Brief – Memorandum of law written by lawyers and submitted to a judge. Despite the name, these are hardly ever short.

Civil law – All law that is not **criminal.** *Civil laws include constitutions, statutes and ordinances, judicial decisions, and administrative rules and regulations. There are many* *places in which civil law and criminal law overlap, but the processes for addressing the wrongs and the* **remedies** *provided at the end are what make them different.*

Complaint – The statement of the grievances made by a plaintiff that describes the wrong that has been suffered and the basis for the claim that is being asserted. *A single complaint can include several different claims (often called "counts"). A complaint is frequently called a "charge" or a "claim" in an administrative proceeding and a "petition" in certain judicial proceedings. The defendant responds to the allegations in the complaint in an "answer."*

Contract – An enforceable agreement between parties that can be oral or written. *A contract can be oral; it does not need to be in writing. It provides greater rights and protections than a "mere promise." The difference between the two takes up much of a whole course in law school.*

Criminal law – Laws adopted by legislatures wherein the government is the plaintiff and the punishment can be incarceration, or worse. *In ordered societies, the governments announce what conduct is so offensive that it deserves special punishment "at the hand of the state." In olden times, it involved being placed in the stocks, public whippings, prison, and death—instances where the state steps in, seizes the offender, and imposes the punishment. Criminal laws are interpreted "strictly" or narrowly, on the theory that people can only be punished by the state for violating rules that are very clear. In the* **civil law,** *there is wider latitude about the scope of the regulation.*

Discovery – The process of asking and answering questions that goes on between **parties** before a dispute goes to hearing or trial.

Due process – The procedures that are either promised (by contract) or required (by law) before a decision can be made final. *There is no one thing called "due process." Treatises have been written about these two words. They appear twice in the U.S. Constitution: in the Fifth Amendment ("No person shall...be deprived of life, liberty, or property, without due process of law....") and in the Fourteenth ("nor shall any State deprive any person of life, liberty, or property, without due process of law...."). They are also fundamental to the* **civil law.** *In general, the words are invoked when a decision is going to be made that is important to someone (tenure, discipline, termination being the easy examples); and again, in general, the more process that is "due," the greater the harm that could result. "Due process" refers either to the procedures that must be followed in order to make a determination or to the minimum procedure that must be followed to make the transaction adequate under standards imposed by the civil law. Often equated with "fairness," the terms are in fact very different. A university can specify a process that is quite one-sided, and that is "the process that is due" within the university community; but if that process deprives someone of rights* *that he or she has under the state or federal law, it must also meet "due process" tests that have been developed under the law. Several chapters in this book discuss due process.*

Fifth Amendment – The right against self-incrimination (among others). *Under the amendments to the Constitution of the United States, people cannot be forced to tell the government facts that would subject them to potential criminal liability. In the words of the Bill of Rights: "No person...shall be compelled in any criminal case to be a witness against himself." The phrase "taking the Fifth" means exercising the rights not to incriminate yourself. This privilege only applies to the criminal law and administrative proceedings under color of state or federal law. There is no Fifth Amendment privilege under* **civil law** *or inside academia, unless your university is a public/state institution. (The protection against self-incrimination is actually only one of several rights protected under the Fifth Amendment.)*

Lawyer-client privilege – The rule that makes your communications with your lawyer confidential. *This is a doctrine that is meant to keep confidential (secret) anything you talk about with your lawyer. The "privilege" means that it is supposed to be exempt from rules requiring disclosure of facts relevant to a claim or controversy. There are many exceptions and exclusions to the "rule." Some are doctrinal. For example, a lawyer who is hired to represent a university in a particular matter cannot keep secret from the university's leadership information given to the lawyer by a member of the faculty. Other exceptions are made by judges in the course of deciding specific motions and cases. A "best practice" is to ask your lawyer at the very start of the conversation (or interaction) whether what you say will be kept "strictly confidential" between the two of you.*

Malpractice – Conduct that falls below the standard or performance that applies to the situation.

Mediation – An informal dispute resolution process in which a mediator helps the parties reach a voluntary agreement on the solution. *This is a process by which people agree to try to work something out amicably. The mediator often "shuttles" between the parties, helping share information and negotiate a solution; the mediator does not make a decision. The parties can either accept or reject the resolution that the mediator proposes (compare with* **arbitration***).*

Motion – A formal request to have a decision made on some issue before the **parties** get to a hearing.

Party – A person (or entity) who is involved in a transaction or dispute *whether in a contract (as in, "the party of the first part") or in a proceeding (see* **plaintiff***). Lawyers refer collectively to all of the people (or entities) involved in a transaction, dispute, or claim as "the parties."*

Plaintiff – The person (or entity) who files a "plea" (a charge or a **complaint**). *The one who is required to respond to it is called the "defendant". In some proceedings (called petitions), the plaintiff is called the "petitioner" or the "grievant," and the defendant is called the "respondent."*

Remedy – The solution that resolves a complaint. *It can be money (which lawyers call "damages") or "equitable relief," a requirement that something be done or stopped (e.g., reinstatement to a job, or cessation of some conduct) or a declaration (e.g., determining the rights of the parties or interpreting a phrase in a **contract**).*

Sanctions – Punishments for failure to comply with an order. *In life, you approve something when you sanction it (as in sanctioning a conference or an event). In law, a sanction is the opposite: a punishment, imposed because you did something that was not approved. Sanctions can be imposed during a litigation (e.g., for violation of procedural rules or a judge's order) or at the end (as part of the remedy).*

Summary judgment – Final decision without having to go through a complete hearing or process. *Lawsuits end either by settlement (amicable) or decision (verdict by a jury or judgment by a judge). Summary judgment occurs when a judge rules that there is no possible way a party (one side or another) could win (on a claim or a defense) and ends that claim without having to go any further.*

Summons – An order to participate in legal proceedings. *Once delivered by the sheriff, it was an arrest warrant, and the sheriff would physically bring the person in. Today, the summons is a civilized seizure, but if you do not do what it says (usually, appear in court on a specific day and time, or file a written response by a certain date), the judge can order your arrest or impose punishments.*

Index

Note: "f," "n," and "t" following page numbers indicate figures, footnotes, and tables, respectively.